Nanovaccinology as Targeted Therapeutics

Scrivener Publishing
100 Cummings Center, Suite 541J
Beverly, MA 01915-6106

Publishers at Scrivener
Martin Scrivener (martin@scrivenerpublishing.com)
Phillip Carmical (pcarmical@scrivenerpublishing.com)

Nanovaccinology as Targeted Therapeutics

Edited by

Kaushik Pal

University Centre for Research and Development (UCRD), Department of Physics, Chandigarh University, Mohali, Punjab, India

Scrivener Publishing

WILEY

This edition first published 2022 by John Wiley & Sons, Inc., 111 River Street, Hoboken, NJ 07030, USA and Scrivener Publishing LLC, 100 Cummings Center, Suite 541J, Beverly, MA 01915, USA

For more information about Scrivener publications please visit www.scrivenerpublishing.com.

Wiley Global Headquarters
111 River Street, Hoboken, NJ 07030, USA

For details of our global editorial offices, customer services, and more information about Wiley products visit us at www.wiley.com.

Library of Congress Cataloging-in-Publication Data

ISBN 978-1-119-85734-1

Cover image: Pixabay.Com
Cover design by Russell Richardson

Set in size of 11pt and Minion Pro by Manila Typesetting Company, Makati, Philippines

Printed in the USA

10 9 8 7 6 5 4 3 2 1

Contents

Preface

Nanovaccinology as Targeted Therapeutics explores recent breakthroughs in the exciting new field of micro- and nanofabricated engineered nanomaterials. In addition to spectroscopic characterizations, significant topics for interdisciplinary research, especially in the fields of nanogels, which deal with polymer chemistry, nanotechnology, materials science, pharmaceuticals, and medicine are explored, where their small dimensions prove highly advantageous. Nanovaccinology could potentially revolutionize conventional therapy and diagnostic methods due to its superior effectiveness over its macro-sized counterparts in almost all biomedical areas. Strong interest in this novel class of material has driven many studies to discover biogenic production methods and new areas of potential utilization in this area. Therefore, it is important to keep abreast of the development of these biomedical research aspects highlighted in the 19 chapters of this book written in diverse fields of studies, and their emerging applications utilized in next-generation techniques.

The last few decades have witnessed progress being made in the treatment of chronic human diseases via precise site-specific drug delivery. Infectious diseases are the leading cause of deaths worldwide, having a significant impact on public health and the socioeconomic development of the human population. The serious threat to public health and safety posed by the rapid development of drug resistance by pathogens to currently available therapies, as well as the significant side effects that result from their prolonged treatment, are reviewed throughout this book. In addition, trends and future prospects of tools utilized in nanomedicine and nanovaccinology research for targeted drug delivery are explored as well.

In Chapter 1, a special emphasis is given to the investigations exploring recent achievements of polymeric nanoparticles, liposomes, emulsions, and carbon-based nanomaterials in vaccine delivery systems. The biocompatibility, toxicity, and stability of nanotechnology-based vaccine delivery systems are also discussed. Chapter 2 discusses novel biomedical therapy approaches to nanomedicine and nanovaccine drug delivery tools, which, although relatively new, are transforming biomedical research at a rapid pace. They are critical platforms for controlled delivery of therapeutic drugs to the targeted sites. Chapter 3 is a unique attempt to analyze the possibilities of producing nanovaccines against notorious superbugs that pose a serious threat to humans, as many of the currently available antibiotics are not effective in treating the diseases they cause. Nanotoxoids, liposomes, VLPs, OMVs, etc., are included in some of the approaches to get biomimetic nanovaccines. Their advantages and limitations when compared to traditional vaccines are progressively illustrated.

Chapter 4 highlights the fact that nanotechnology has accelerated the evolution of newer vaccines that are safe and highly effective in eradicating SARS-CoV2. Simultaneously, nanovaccines have recently been developed in which new drugs can be accommodated through nanoparticle carriers. The similar nanosize of the nano-scaled materials and pathogens ensures optimal trigger response of the immune system, resulting in satisfactory cellular and humoral immunity responses. Targeted delivery of nanoparticles results in enhanced antibody response, improved stability coupled with longer duration drug release and prolonged immunogenic memory. Chapter 5 looks at the usefulness of nanovaccines for treatment of the deadliest diseases, including cancer, tumors, bacterial, viral and parasitic diseases, and autoimmune diseases. Moreover, it also provides information about the importance of nanoscience in the invention of various safe, potent, stable, inert and biocompatible drug discoveries.

Chapter 6 focuses on the current preclinical and clinical trials in nanoimaging and nanovaccines that are applicable to cancer immunotherapy. The recent advances in anti-cancer nanovaccines using nanocarriers constitute a delivery breakthrough expected to play a vital role in improving the stability and immunogenicity of antigens. Chapter 7 demonstrates a novel way of using nanoscale 2C4N crystals against diabetes, fungal, and inflammatory diseases, and for drug analysis with optimization; and gives the order of the lattice with ORTEP. Chapter 8 illustrates the ways in which the presence of aniline in a compound enhances antidiabetic, antifungal, and anti-inflammatory activity, which is a novel trend in recent work for nanocrystalline specimen with an IC50 value of 43 nm.

Chapter 9 denotes the recent use of macro- and nanoscale crystals of BGLBMH mainly as a novel antidiabetic agent as well as antioxidant utility with its monoclinic, $P2_1/c$ form of system with band gap of 3.139 eV. Chapter 10 focuses on the organic, crystalline N2MNM4MBH efficacy at a macro/nano-level for drug use in alpha-amylase and alpha-glucosidase enzymes against diabetes. Chapter 11 discusses the use of ZnO nanoparticles from *Mangifera indica* as ZnO-MIZN for *E. coli*, *S. typhi* and *S. aureus* inhibition zones in mm and for novel biouse as antibiotic and antidiabetic agents. Chapter 12 discusses the novel use of 2F5NA crystals in nanotube production, and antidiabetic, antifungal, anti-inflammatory interactive lattice with HF/B3LYP.

Chapter 13 discusses the use of 2-Amino-4-methylpyridinium 4-hydroxybenzoate (AMPHB) crystalline macro- and nano-scaling for nanotube generation as well as device fabrication, and as an antidiabetic, antifungal and anti-inflammatory therapeutic. Chapter 14 describes a crystalline sample of CPDMDP with base monoclinic system used for computational interaction that acts as a novel base for antidiabetic and antioxidant vaccine, with the presence of pyrazole. Chapter 15 discusses the novel modus operandi of preparing a 4M2NA crystalline sample by evaporation for an antidiabetic–insulin response and an antifungal, anti-inflammation effect with proper optimization. Chapter 16 discusses the use of *Mangifera indica*–AgO-MIZN of 43 nm used as a vaccine/drug for cancer and bacterial and fungal infections.

Chapter 17 discusses the recently surfaced nanotechnology used to resolve vaccine failures that mainly arise as a result of weak immunogenicity of vaccines, *in-vivo* instability, the need for multiple jabs, and toxicity. Liposomes, emulsions, polymeric nanoparticles, and graphene oxide nanosheets are some examples of nanovaccines. The chapter more or less summarizes the hopes as well as the gaps that need to be filled in order to achieve the targeted proposals. Chapter 18 implies that the old vaccine strategy fundamentally involves the method of utilizing either inactivated (killed) or live attenuated antigens. Live attenuated vaccines for clinical disease arise from mutated/same genotypes, while nanoparticles with higher surface properties enable them to strengthen the immune system and immunological response. Finally, Chapter 19 comprehensively covers the evolution of nanovaccines and their morphology, carriers used, formulation as well as characterization, and the role of nanovaccines in immunotherapy, with an emphasis on recent advances.

Though development of nanovaccines is still in the infancy stage, with only a few in the early phases of clinical trials, we firmly believe this new generation of vaccines has great potential for the prevention and treatment of many diseases. The information provided in this book further highlights some of the improvements in this span of work, focusing on the factors that limit nanovaccines' efficiency in optimization. Remarkable strategies to employ assemblies of the various biogenic schemes of nanovaccines are also illustrated in this book. Thus, it may become clear to all readers that vaccinology-enabled renewable energy technologies are starting to scale up dramatically. As it matures and becomes more cost-effective in the decades to come, bio-nanotechnology could eventually replace the traditional, environmentally unfriendly biomaterials and improve the performance of the biogenic industry through utilization of nanomedicine to manufacture nontoxic, highly durable materials that are cost-effective. To aid in this discovery process, this book provides an overview of key current developments that will direct future research attempts towards utilization of such tailored nanovaccinology that will play an essential role in achieving the desired goal of cheap and efficient vaccine production.

This book also covers the hottest topics based on nanovaccinology applications in the field of therapeutics and nanodetectors as per biomedical applications. It is enhanced by the welcomed contributions of biotechnologists, nanotechnologists, biochemists, medical biologists, pharmacists, materials scientists as well as academicians and research scholars. There is every indication that with appropriate liability and regulation alongside the topics, commercial production of manufactured novel composite materials can be realized. Furthermore, the diverse brilliant innovations and explorations highlighted throughout the entire book can modulate spectroscopic performances with technical excellence in the inter- and cross-multidisciplinary research of high competence.

Lastly, I would like to express my overwhelming gratitude to all the authors and co-authors for their excellent research contributions to this book. I also wish to thank the entire team at Wiley-Scrivener for their consistent support during even the most difficult stages of its publication. I am confident that within a short period of time the eBook series will be very popular in university and institute libraries worldwide, and hopefully will be highly cited in coming years.

Dr. Kaushik Pal
May 2022

1

Nanotechnology in Vaccine Development and Constraints

Tahmina Foyez[1] and Abu Bin Imran[2]*

[1]Department of Pharmaceutical Sciences, School of Health and Life Sciences, North South University, Dhaka, Bangladesh
[2]Department of Chemistry, Bangladesh University of Engineering and Technology, Dhaka, Bangladesh

Abstract
Generally, vaccinations are the most efficient prophylactic measures against infectious diseases. Despite the obvious advantages of vaccines, optimizations are required due to poor immunogenicity, instability, toxic effect, and the necessity for multiple dose of a vaccine. Nanotechnology have currently been introduced into vaccination research to address these difficulties. The nanotechnology in vaccine development can improve immune responses. Particle size at the nanoscale is critical for this benefit. Nanoparticles (NPs) used in the formulation of vaccine can improve stability of antigen and immunogenicity while also allowing for targeted distribution. A variety of NPs vaccines have been permitted for human use, with composition, size, shape, and surface qualities. However, obstacles are present because of a lack of proper knowledge of NPs activity *in vivo*, which can be used as a delivery mechanism to improve antigen processing to boost immunity. We have discussed the recent achievements of nanotechnology in vaccine delivery systems in this chapter, emphasizing the different carriers, such as polymeric NPs, liposomes, emulsions, and carbon-based nanomaterials. The basic knowledge of *in vivo* biocompatibility, toxicity, and stability of nanotechnology-based vaccine delivery systems has also been discussed.

***Keywords*:** Nanotechnology, nanovaccinology, antigen, antibody, nanoparticles

**Corresponding author*: abimran@chem.buet.ac.bd

Kaushik Pal (ed.) Nanovaccinology as Targeted Therapeutics, (1–20) © 2022 Scrivener Publishing LLC

1.1 Introduction

Currently, infectious diseases are the primary cause of mortality. They are caused by microorganisms like viruses, bacteria, fungi, or other parasites. The human immune system fights and removes foreign invading particles [1, 2]. A vaccine is a living, dead, attenuated, inactivated form of a pathogenic microbe, such as a bacterium or virus, or a component of the pathogenic microbe's structure, which enhances antibody production in the host body but is incapable of causing severe illness [3]. It develops immunity to control and adjust our immune systems from over-reactivity or underactivity [4, 5]. Vaccines have become an everyday part of life, providing a high-impact benefit to human by preventing or managing a wide range of diseases. Vaccine development has a long and glorious history that started late in the 18th century. Louis Pasteur's laboratory's first attempts to vaccine development [6]. The development of vaccines is crucial to the successful control of many deadly diseases. However, efficient preventative and therapeutic vaccinations for totally healing lethal diseases and major microbial infections have yet to be produced. On the other hand, critical challenges that need to be addressed include the design, manufacture, and global distribution of vaccines. To design a vaccine, the antigen, adjuvant, manufacturing method, and delivery strategy should be established. Antigen is a pathogen-derived foreign substance that can elicit an immunological response within the host. A vaccine can be classified into four types based on its antigen: live-attenuated vaccine, inactivated vaccine, subunit vaccine, and peptide-based vaccine. Adjuvants are immunomodulatory agents that are used to boost immune reaction. The first adjuvant, aluminum was designed to boost the production of antibodies, making it an excellent choice for vaccine development [7, 8]. If genetic and structural information about microorganisms is known, vaccinations can be developed quickly. Nanotechnology platforms are particularly beneficial in current vaccine development and have accelerated the testing of novel prospective vaccines. Recently nanoparticles (NPs), as vaccine delivery vehicles, have received tremendous attention. Nanovaccine formulations not only improve antigen integrity and immunity, but they also provide selective distribution and sustained release. A wide range of NPs antigens with varying physicochemical properties have been authorized for clinical use [9–11]. The primary goal of using NPs delivery methods is to delay antigen presentation and uptake by dendritic cells (DCs), resulting in immediate DC activation [9, 11, 12]. Antigen and adjuvant are also protected

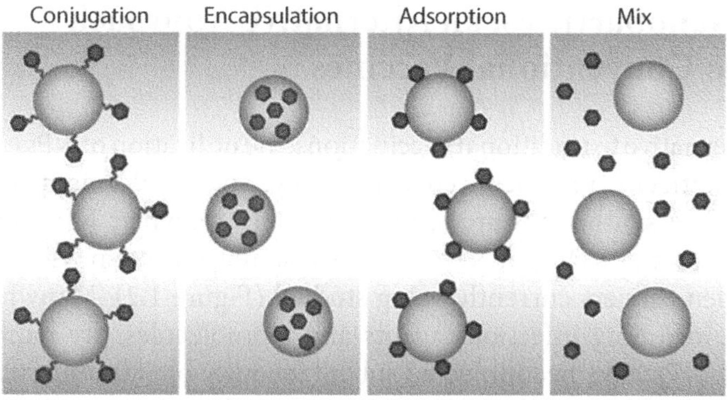

Figure 1.1 The interactions of NPs with the target antigen. Reproduced (adapted) from [19]. Copyright 2013, Elsevier.

from early enzyme and protease degradation by NPs [13]. Vaccine antigens can be administered to the target site by enclosing them in NPs or conjugated particles (Figure 1.1). NPs can be designed with peptide, protein, polymer, and other targeting ligands for vaccine formulations due to their unique physical and chemical properties, including as greater surface area, variable shape and size with various surface charges, and other targeting ligands. Although NPs have the benefits listed above, they also have drawbacks, such as a lack of mechanical stability under physiological conditions due to protein corona development and unfavorable interactions with the endothelial system [14, 15]. Biocompatible NPs have improved physical stability while avoiding unwanted interactions with immune cells and boosting blood supply [16, 17], which imitate biological membranes. The nanovaccines that use carrier biomimetic NPs allow prolonged circulation and avoid cytotoxicity when delivered to the body [18].

Nanotechnology has opened the way for developing novel vaccines based on nanomaterials, which have unique qualities and serve as antigenic delivery systems and immunomodulatory substances. Multiple research groups in the area are developing nanovaccines for a variety of diseases, and tremendous advantages from this nanotechnology are expected in the coming decades for both animal and human health.

1.2 Nanoparticles, an Alternative Approach to Conventional Vaccines

As an alternative to traditional vaccinations, the utilization of NPs exhibiting relevant antigenic moieties seems promising. These NPs might come from biological or synthetic sources. Inorganic NPs, polymer NPs, liposomes, virus-like particles (VLPs) NPs, and self-assembled protein NPs are among the antigen carriers currently being studied (Figure 1.2). Many biological systems, including infectious agents and biomolecules, are nanoscale in size [20]. NPs have been injected subcutaneously or intramuscularly, and they have the ability to pass through capillaries [21]. Recent advancements

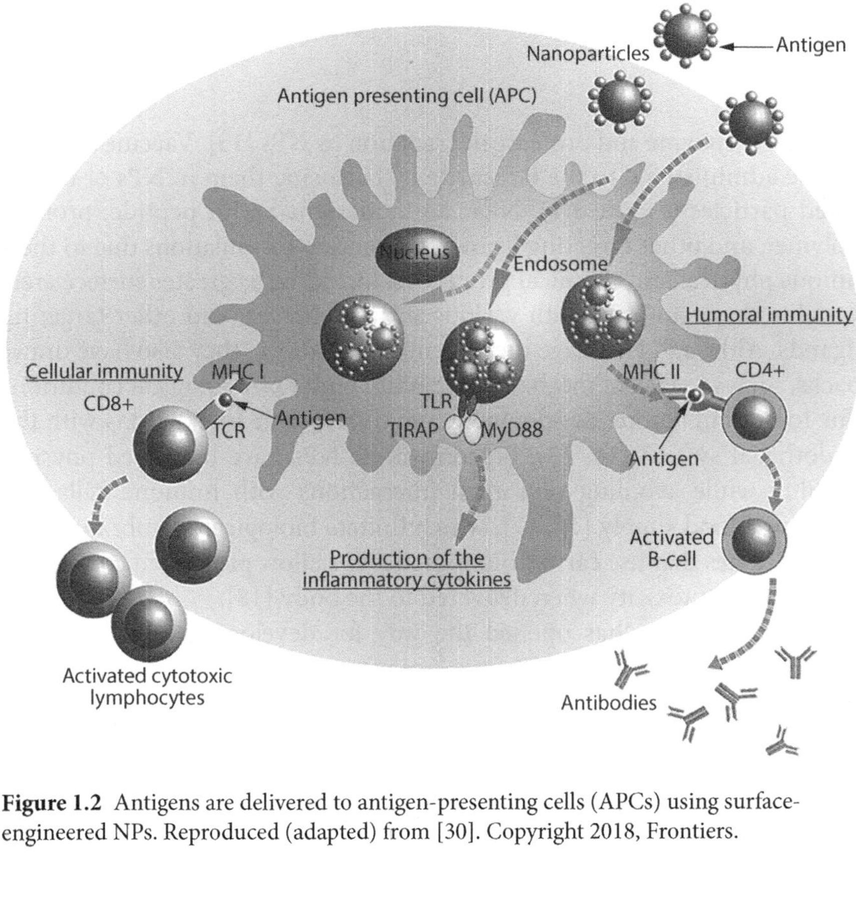

Figure 1.2 Antigens are delivered to antigen-presenting cells (APCs) using surface-engineered NPs. Reproduced (adapted) from [30]. Copyright 2018, Frontiers.

have made it possible to create NPs with distinct physical and chemical characteristics. The shape, size, solubility, surface composition, and so on can all be tuned and manipulated, allowing for the development of NPs with particular biological features. They can also be engineered to include a variety of compounds, including antigens, making them extremely valuable in vaccine development [22, 23]. Antigens can be incorporated into NPs through encapsulation or conjugation [24]. The native structure of antigens can be protected against proteolytic breakdown by NPs, and antigen transportation to antigen-presenting cells (APCs) can be improved [25]. Furthermore, NPs containing antigens have a local depot effect to ensure the presence of antigens in immune cells for a longer period of time [26]. Interestingly, carbon black (CB) NPs, carbon nanotubes (CNTs), poly lactic-co glycolic acid (PLGA) NPs, titanium dioxide (TiO_2) NPs, and silicon dioxide (SiO_2) NPs have all been shown to exhibit intrinsic immunomodulatory properties [27]. In point of fact, once ingested by APCs, these NPs transmit a signal that promote proteolytic degradation and the induction of oxidative stress, resulting in the release of lysosomal contents [28, 29]. These features indicate that NPs could be useful antigen transporters and innate immune stimulators in vaccinations.

1.3 Nanoparticles as Vaccine Delivery Vehicle

Liposomes, NPs having a phospholipid bilayer, have been used in the pharmaceutical industry since 1960 [31]. NPs have a diameter of 1 to 100 nm (Figure 1.3), whereas antigens or DNA segments have 1 to 10 nm [32]. Therefore, they are susceptible to being absorbed by biological systems, and it is the first step in eliciting immunogenicity. A nanovaccine is composed of NPs and can be composed of protein, lipid, metals, polymers, and other materials. The positive strategy of nanovaccines allows for not only antigen enhancement but also vaccine stability, immunogenicity, and effective target delivery. Due to advancements in nanovaccinology, many nanovaccines have already been licensed for clinical use, and others are in clinical trials [33–35]. Adjuvants and multiepitope antigens may be effectively co-delivered into target cells and APCs using nanovaccines, and the release of antigen in the cytoplasm and antigen cross-presentation can be precisely controlled.

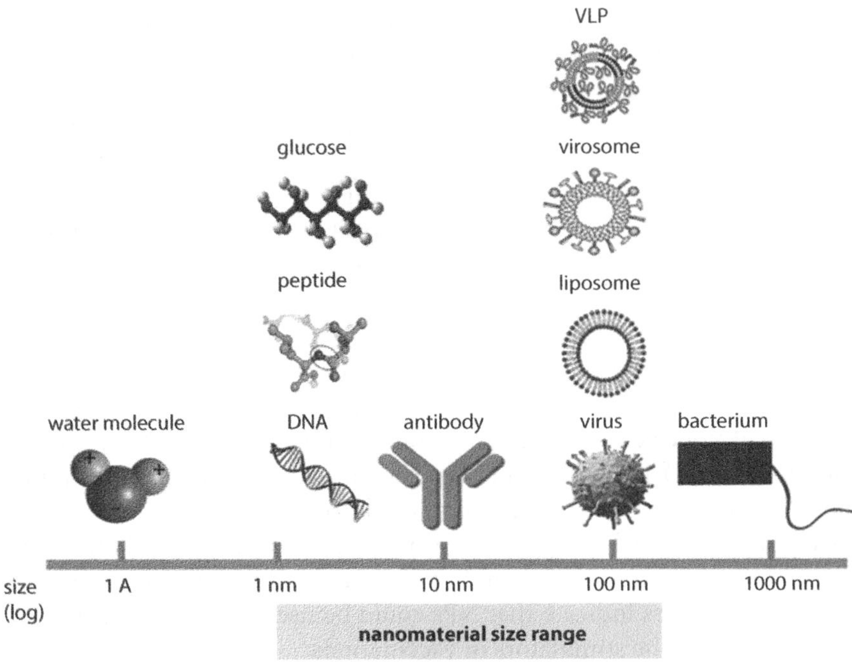

Figure 1.3 The size comparison of various biological systems used in nanovaccinology. Reproduced (adapted) from [36]. Copyright 2016, IntechOpen.

1.4 Nanotechnology to Tackle the Challenges of Vaccine Delivery

1.4.1 Polymeric Nanoparticles

Polymeric NPs can be made by polymerizing monomeric units or by using synthesized polymers. The customizable qualities, size, composition, and surface properties of these NPs make them appealing in the medical industry because they allow for regulated release and drug molecule protection [37]. Poly (lactic acid) (PLA), poly (glutamic acid) (PGA), PLGA, and chitosan are the most frequently used polymeric NPs for vaccine formulation [19]. The chemical structure of polymeric NPs is designed to behave differently in different environments to control the release rate. The function and uses of other polymeric NPs vary substantially depending on the inherent chemical and biological effects in distinct materials [38]. PLGA is a biodegradable and biocompatible polymer that can undergo *in vivo* hydrolysis [39] and encapsulate and release different biomolecules over time [40–42]. Under physiological conditions, these NPs may incorporate antigens and inhibit their destruction for one month, which is crucial for vaccination [43]. Furthermore, PLGA NPs promote antigen processing and display to susceptible cells by promoting antigen uptake by APCs [44]. Other NPs, chitosan, and *N*-(2-hydroxypropyl)methacrylamide/*N*-isopropyl acrylamide were also investigated as vaccines preparation [45–47]. Chitosan is a favorable and promising polymer for DNA vaccine formulation because of its cationic character, which allows attachment to the DNA, generating DNA–polymer interactions that protect DNA from enzyme hydrolysis. It is indeed extremely hydrophobic, inactive, and non-immunogenic, with bio-adhesive properties that facilitate mucosal vaccination techniques. Chitosan has been further discovered to have natural adjuvant properties, stimulating dendritic cell maturation to enhance T helper 1 (Th1) responses [48]. Over the years, multiple developments have resulted from chitosan-based NPs delivery technology, including a therapeutic potential anti-tumor papillomavirus (HPV) vaccine [49], treatment methods for influenza A [50], highly contagious myocarditis [51], and some livestock diseases such as Newcastle disease (ND) virus [52, 53] and Noda virus [54]. Polymeric NPs have biocompatibility, antigen encapsulation and stability, regulated release of antigens, cellular retention in APCs, microbe characteristics, and delivery feasibility [55–57]. As the research advancements of polymer science continue, vaccine technologies will develop accordingly.

1.4.2 Inorganic Nanoparticles

Inorganic NPs have sparked a lot of interest in vaccine formulation because of their simplicity in drug loading and bioactivity properties. Furthermore, their thermochemical stability makes sterilization easier [58]. Inorganic materials are relatively nontoxic and can be manufactured in a variety of sizes, forms, and dimensions. Gold (Au) NPs are a popular inorganic nanomaterial used in vaccine delivery because of decreasing toxicity, increasing immunogenic activity, and providing vaccine storage stability [59]. Another extensively investigated composition for vaccine delivery is carbon NPs [60] which has good biocompatibility [61, 62]. Protein and peptide antigens can be coupled on CNTs for delivery, which has increased IgG response levels [62–65]. Mesoporous carbon NPs have been studied for use as an adjuvant in vaccinations [62]. Silica is another promising material for nanovaccinology because of its biocompatibility and having excellent properties as nanocarriers. Silica NPs' size and form can be altered selectively to regulate their cellular interaction [66]. Many silanol groups on surface are advantageous for introducing additional functionalities, such as cell recognition, biomolecule absorption, improved cell contact, and cellular uptake [67–69]. It is revealed that DNA vaccine incorporated into SiO_2-layered double hydroxide induces antibody response as well as boosts T-cell multiplication and pushes T helper (Th1) cells toward Th1 activation [70]. Superparamagnetic iron oxide NPs (SPIONs) is another inorganic material for nanovaccinology. SPION-based vaccine delivery system is modified to improve the stability of vector and APC targeting ability to ensure prolonged exposure in the target area [71]. Other nanomaterials have been used as vaccine delivery vectors and adjuvants, including silver (Ag) NPs and calcium phosphate NPs [71, 72].

1.4.3 Biomolecular Nanoparticles

The biomolecular materials have a number of advantages that make them attractive candidates for synthetic vaccine preparation. They are biologically inspired systems that are built on the basis of biomolecules. Biomolecular materials benefit from transporting a range of carriers and displaying diverse moieties on their surfaces [19]. Although a number of biomolecular NPs have been investigated, liposomes, virus-like particles (VLPs), micelles, and immunestimulating complexes (ISCOMs) (Figure 1.4) are the four most widely used materials for vaccine applications [60].

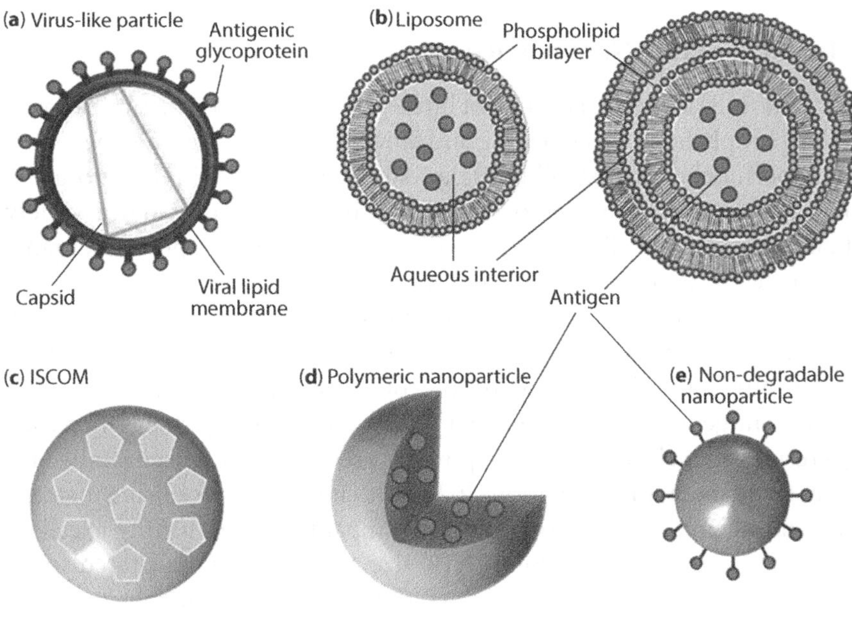

Figure 1.4 A schematic illustration of various NPs that have been used as vaccinations [60]. Reproduced (adapted) from [60]. Copyright 2013, Frontiers.

1.4.4 Liposome

Liposomes are sphere NPs comprised of lipid layers [73] which are formed when lipids with a hydrophilic part and a hydrophobic part combine in water. Liposomes can encapsulate a variety of medications and be utilized for regulated delivery for their substantial therapeutic uses [74]. There has been a lot of research done on liposomes and their vaccine potential. Liposomes have the advantage of being able to be modified to obtain desired immunostimulatory effects. A unique nanovaccine system targets inflammatory cells and increases innate immunity to T cells against a mimic antigen created by modifying liposomes to have lectin binding mannose on their surface and trapping monophosphoryl lipid A (MPLA) adjuvant [75]. While liposomes have been used to administer vaccines against various infections, one particularly intriguing application is tuberculosis prophylaxis, a fatal disease [76]. Virosomes have been used in clinical trials for a number of preventive purposes, including tetanus and hepatitis B vaccinations [77]. It is recently shown that virosomal immunizations could be programmed to selectively activate T lymphocytes, improving immunization protection against influenza infection [78].

1.4.5 Virus-Like Particles

Another biomolecular NPs known as VLP has a typical virus shape but lacks viral genome, rendering them inactive and unable of replication. They quickly and effectively produce a strong and prolong immunological response in the host [79]. Hepatitis B protection is provided first with a VLP-based human vaccination[80]. VLPs have recently been used as vehicles for several human papillomavirus (HPV) vaccines. According to a recent study, HPV vaccinations based on VLPs elicit a strong cross-protective antibody response [81]. During chronic infection, cytotoxic T cells are essential for removing damaged cells and regulating microbe load. They can really be highly effective in vaccines because they target the T-cell response.

1.4.6 Micelles

The cores of micelles, another type of biomolecular NPs, are hydrophobic in contrast to liposomes and VLPs [82]. They are widely used with weakly water-soluble drugs delivery or encapsulated amphiphilic compounds [83]. Micelles have been used in two different ways as vaccine delivery systems. First, protein vaccines may be simply covalently attached to the hydrophilic micelle. HIV vaccines have been attached to adjuvant-loaded micelles using this approach, resulting in significant APC activation *in vitro* [84]. Model peptide antigens coupled to polymer-lipid microspheres are demonstrated to attach protein albumin and travel to the lymphatic vessels, where they significantly raise T-cell numbers and act as an anti-cancer vaccination [85]. Endosome disruption can be triggered by polymer-based micelles, allowing vaccines to be transported to the cytoplasm, resulting in significant cytotoxic T-cell responses [86]. Molecules with similar or identical hydrophobic moieties can also be self-assembled and form heterogeneous micelles. This phenomenon has been utilized to create protein amphiphile microspheres capable of transporting several antigens to the same cell [87].

1.4.7 Immunostimulating Complexes

ISCOMs are biomolecular structures. They are made up of cholesterols, phospholipids, and Quil A saponins. ISCOMs have an immunostimulatory effect because they contain Quil A saponins, which are well-known adjuvants. ISCOMs have been studied for around 35 years to be highly effective as a synthetic vaccine [88]. Still, they can cause significant, unfavorable injection-site reactions [89], limiting their use to animal vaccinations [90]. ISCOMA-TRIX is identical to the traditional ISCOM except that the Quil A saponins are first filtered to give a specified group of saponins that do not induce substantial inflammation [91]. ISCOMA-TRIX has been demonstrated to produce immune responses in mice and rabbits [92].

1.4.8 Self-Assembled Proteins (SAPNs)

SAPNs are 20–30 nm icosahedrons. For the manufacture of NPs-based vaccinations, self-assembling technologies promote higher levels of protein quaternary structure. By genetic engineering technique, attaching the influenza virus with ferrintin, researchers could generate a stronger immunological response than the flu vaccine [93]. Another protein is the major vault protein (MVP). For studies of mucosal immunity, Vault NPs are utilized [94]. SAPNs have been shown to improve immunity in a various of diseases, including malaria [95], HIV [96], toxoplasma [97], and severe acute respiratory syndrome [98]. Then encapsulate two HIV protein epitopes onto SAPN surface produce epitope-specific neutralizing antibodies more efficiently. This suggests that SAPN could be used as a nanovaccine to trigger an immunological response against HIV [96].

1.4.9 Emulsions

Nano-sized emulsions are another type of NPs used as an adjuvant in vaccinations [99–101]. These NPs can be found with sizes ranging from 50 to 600 nm. It can either contain antigens in their core for optimal vaccination administration or be combined with the antigen [101]. MF59TM, an oil-in-water emulsion, which has been approved as a safe and effective vaccine adjuvant [102, 103], is one of the most regularly used emulsions. It has been undergone extensive research for application in influenza vaccines [103–105]. Another example is Montanide™ that has been used in Malaria vaccines [106, 107] and vaccines for foot-and-mouth disease [108]. Non-covalent click self-assembly has been used to produce a tailorable nano-sized emulsion platform technology for antigen and medication delivery [109].

1.5 Constraints and Challenges of Nanovaccines

A successful vaccine requires a solid understanding of the physiological and immunological characteristics of any disease. Nanovaccines are widely using for treating numerous infectious and non-infectious diseases; their efficiency in stimulating our immune response to infections may be expected to be more significant. Understanding the properties of NPs and how they interact with cells can help to develop safer nanovaccines. NPs have toxicity, which must be addressed judiciously to maximize their utilization. The toxic effects and immunological responses generated by NPs are influenced by their composition, size, charge, shape, hydrophobicity, and route of exposure. NPs cause cellular injury in a size-dependent manner because smaller nanoparticles are more active, they can do more damage. NPs can easily penetrate alveoli, where they can aggregate and cause pulmonary inflammation [110, 111]. On the other hand, repetitive exposure to NPs damages the lung cells, allowing them to penetrate blood vessels and travel from lung tissue to other organs via systemic circulation. The shape of NPs plays a role in their toxicity; for example, nanofibers are shown to be more cytotoxic than spherical NPs of the same composition [112]. NPs with a low solubility or disintegration rate accumulate in cells and tissues, where they persist for a long time, such as rat nasal exposure to Au NPs lasted 15 days. Ag NPs aggregates accumulated in the lungs for 7 days [113]. NPs that penetrate the cell can increase the reactive oxygen species (ROS). The accumulating ROS interacts with the protein machinery of cell, affecting all metabolic activities in the cell. They also exhibit mitochondrial toxicity and nuclear DNA damage. Apoptosis occurs when a cell is exposed in this way [114]. As a result, high concentrations of NPs or their accumulation cause disturbance of cellular homeostasis. It can be concluded that NPs may cause tissue damage, resulting in local and systemic pathophysiological disorders. Some of the drawbacks of nanovaccines are related to their stability [115]. Increased production of nanovaccines is also an important concern due to their activity and cost-effective manufacturing process. Several loading of various components, such as antigens and adjuvants in a single nanoplatform, is complex and becoming more complicated. These drawbacks can cause side effects and/or poor immunogenicity, making them unsuitable for clinical use. Furthermore, the understanding of the details on how NPs interact with immune cells is not adequate. In fact, their adjuvant effect and ability to activate the immune system are still unknown at the molecular level and need to be better understood [116]. As a result, a deep study of nanotoxicity, immune response, and excretion of NPs over time should be conducted for safety and reliability purposes.

1.6 Concluding Remarks

A new approach of NPs-based vaccines has revealed remarkable potential in addressing the majority of the limitations of the existing vaccines. NPs can be used as an alternative adjuvant for both humans and animals. They work as both an antigen carrier and a stimulator of innate immune responses. Modern vaccination changed to a small subunit of the pathogen instead of a traditional whole pathogen. As the purified inactivated entire pathogens and subunit or recombinant antigens are insufficiently immunogenic on their own, the use of a powerful immunostimulatory system is required to boost the immunity. This can be accomplished via NPs based methods. To successfully apply this versatile NPs-based vaccination technology, a thorough study of the effects of NPs diameter, polarity, and other physical and chemical properties is necessary. The stability of NPs under different storage circumstances, as well as their immunogenicity over time, should be prioritized in research, since these aspects will have a direct impact on the market viability of vaccines. Recent advancements in NPs-based adjuvant and vaccine delivery systems can be utilized more widely to prevent and treat infectious diseases. Nanovaccines principles offer notable benefits such as targeted delivery, prolonged transmission, minimal side effects, and activation of a powerful immune response to various biological and external stimuli by overcoming all physiological barriers. They enable antigen stability, improve antigen processing and immunogenicity with targeted administration, and inhibit antigen and adjuvant burst release. In the realm of vaccine development, inorganic, polymeric, biomolecular, and other NPs have been found to enhance weakly immunogenic antigens. Nanovaccine are now being developed for the prevention of pathogenic diseases. The therapeutic and tolerogenic vaccines are used to treat cancer and autoimmune disorders, respectively, expand the possibilities of the synthetic vaccine platform. The development of new vaccines, such as single-dose, needle-free injection, gradual release, targeting, alternate administration techniques, and delivery channels will become more demanding in the near future.

Acknowledgments

A.B. Imran gratefully acknowledges the support of the Capacity Utilization Programme under Special Allocation for Science and Technology (BS-182 and PHY'S-467) from the Ministry of Science and Technology, Peoples Republic of Bangladesh. A.B. Imran is also thankful to the Committee for Advanced Studies and Research (CASR) in BUET. T. Foyez cordially acknowledge the support from North South University.

References

1. Arias, C.A. and Murray, B.E., Antibiotic-resistant bugs in the 21st century–A clinical super-challenge. *New Engl. J. Med.*, 360, 439–443, 2009.
2. Rosenblum, M.D., Remedios, K.A., Abbas, A.K., Mechanisms of human autoimmunity. *J. Clin. Invest.*, 125, 2228–2233, 2015.
3. Whitney, C.G., Zhou, F., Singleton, J., Schuchat, A., Benefits from immunization during the vaccines for children program era - United States, 1994-2013. *MMWR. Morb. Mortal. Wkly. Rep.*, 63, 352–355, 2014.
4. Wraith, D.C., Therapeutic peptide vaccines for treatment of autoimmune diseases. *Immunol. Lett.*, 122, 134–136, 2009.
5. Anderson, R.P. and Jabri, B., Vaccine against autoimmune disease: Antigen-specific immunotherapy. *Curr. Opin. Immunol.*, 25, 410–417, 2013.
6. Plotkin, S., History of vaccination. *Proc. Natl. Acad. Sci. U.S.A.*, 111, 12283–12287, 2014.
7. Shin, M.D. *et al.*, COVID-19 vaccine development and a potential nanomaterial path forward. *Nat. Nanotechnol.*, 15, 646–655, 2020.

8. Munks, M.W. *et al.*, Aluminum adjuvants elicit fibrin-dependent extracellular traps *in vivo*. *Blood*, 116, 5191–5199, 2010.
9. Zhang, X.Q. *et al.*, Potent antigen-specific immune responses stimulated by codelivery of CpG ODN and antigens in degradable microparticles. *J. Immunother. (Hagerstown, Md.: 1997)*, 30, 469–478, 2007.
10. Hokmabad, V.R. *et al.*, A comparison of the effects of silica and hydroxyapatite nanoparticles on poly(ε-caprolactone)-poly(ethylene glycol)-poly(ε-caprolactone)/chitosan nanofibrous scaffolds for bone tissue engineering. *Tissue Eng. Regener. Med.*, 15, 735–750, 2018.
11. Krishnamachari, Y., Geary, S.M., Lemke, C.D., Salem, A.K.J.P.r., Nanoparticle delivery systems in cancer vaccines. *Pharm. Res.*, 28, 215–236, 2011.
12. Joshi, V.B., Geary, S.M., Salem, A.K., Biodegradable particles as vaccine delivery systems: Size matters. *AAPS J.*, 15, 85–94, 2013.
13. Bishop, C.J., Kozielski, K.L., Green, J.J., Exploring the role of polymer structure on intracellular nucleic acid delivery via polymeric nanoparticles. *J. Control. Release: Off. J. Controlled Release Soc.*, 219, 488–499, 2015.
14. Corbo, C., Molinaro, R., Tabatabaei, M., Farokhzad, O.C., Mahmoudi, M., Personalized protein corona on nanoparticles and its clinical implications. *Biomater. Sci.*, 5, 378–387, 2017.
15. Corbo, C. *et al.*, The impact of nanoparticle protein corona on cytotoxicity, immunotoxicity and target drug delivery. *Nanomedicine (London, England)*, 11, 81–100, 2016.
16. Fang, R.H., Kroll, A.V., Gao, W., Zhang, L., Cell membrane coating nanotechnology. *Adv. Mater. (Deerfield Beach, Fla.)*, 30, e1706759, 2018.
17. Gao, W. *et al.*, Surface functionalization of gold nanoparticles with red blood cell membranes. *Adv. Mater. (Deerfield Beach, Fla.)*, 25, 3549–3553, 2013.
18. Vijayan, V., Uthaman, S., Park, I.K., Cell Membrane-camouflaged nanoparticles: A promising biomimetic strategy for cancer theragnostics. *Polymers*, 10, 1–25, 2018.
19. Zhao, L. *et al.*, Nanoparticle vaccines. *Vaccine*, 32, 327–337, 2014.
20. Laval, J.M., Mazeran, P.E., Thomas, D., Nanobiotechnology and its role in the development of new analytical devices. *Analyst*, 125, 29–33, 2000.
21. Schneider, C.S. *et al.*, Nanoparticles that do not adhere to mucus provide uniform and long-lasting drug delivery to airways following inhalation. *Sci. Adv.*, 3, e1601556, 2017.
22. Irvine, D.J., Hanson, M.C., Rakhra, K., Tokatlian, T., Synthetic nanoparticles for vaccines and immunotherapy. *Chem. Rev.*, 115, 11109–11146, 2015.
23. Szeto, G.L. and Lavik, E.B., Materials design at the interface of nanoparticles and innate immunity. *J. Mater. Chem. B*, 4, 1610–1618, 2016.
24. Chattopadhyay, S., Chen, J.Y., Chen, H.W., Hu, C.J., Nanoparticle Vaccines adopting virus-like features for enhanced immune potentiation. *Nanotheranostics*, 1, 244–260, 2017.
25. Pachioni-Vasconcelos, J. de A., *et al.*, Nanostructures for protein drug delivery. *Biomater. Sci.*, 4, 205–218, 2016.

26. Fredriksen, B.N. and Grip, J., PLGA/PLA micro- and nanoparticle formulations serve as antigen depots and induce elevated humoral responses after immunization of Atlantic salmon (Salmo salar L.). *Vaccine*, 30, 656–667, 2012.
27. Zhu, M., Wang, R., Nie, G., Applications of nanomaterials as vaccine adjuvants. *Hum. Vaccin. Immunother.*, 10, 2761–2774, 2014.
28. Ghiringhelli, F. *et al.*, Activation of the NLRP3 inflammasome in dendritic cells induces IL-1beta-dependent adaptive immunity against tumors. *Nat. Med.*, 15, 1170–1178, 2009.
29. He, Y., Hara, H., Núñez, G., Mechanism and regulation of NLRP3 inflammasome activation. *Trends Biochem. Sci.*, 41, 1012–1021, 2016.
30. Pati, R., Shevtsov, M., Sonawane, A., Nanoparticle vaccines Against infectious diseases. *Front. Immunol.*, 9, 2224, 2018.
31. Torchilin, V.P., Recent advances with liposomes as pharmaceutical carriers. *Nat. Rev. Drug Discovery*, 4, 145–160, 2005.
32. Mamo, T. and Poland, G.A., Nanovaccinology: the next generation of vaccines meets 21st century materials science and engineering. *Vaccine*, 30, 6609–6611, 2012.
33. Kushnir, N., Streatfield, S.J., Yusibov, V., Virus-like particles as a highly efficient vaccine platform: diversity of targets and production systems and advances in clinical development. *Vaccine*, 31, 58–83, 2012.
34. Plummer, E.M. and Manchester, M., Viral nanoparticles and virus-like particles: Platforms for contemporary vaccine design. *Wiley Interdiscip. Rev. Nanomed. Nanobiotechnol.*, 3, 174–196, 2011.
35. Roldão, A., Mellado, M.C., Castilho, L.R., Carrondo, M.J., Alves, P.M., Virus-like particles in vaccine development. *Expert Rev. Vaccines*, 9, 1149–1176, 2010.
36. Chen, Y.-C., Cheng, H.-F., Yang, Y.-C., Yeh, M.-K., Nanotechnologies applied in biomedical vaccines. *IntechOpen, J. Pharm. Pharmacol.*, 5, 85–107, 2017.
37. Kamaly, N., Xiao, Z., Valencia, P.M., Radovic-Moreno, A.F., Farokhzad, O.C., Targeted polymeric therapeutic nanoparticles: Design, development and clinical translation. *Chem. Soc. Rev.*, 41, 2971–3010, 2012.
38. Shae, D., Postma, A., Wilson, J.T., Vaccine delivery: where polymer chemistry meets immunology. *Ther. Deliv.*, 7, 193–196, 2016.
39. Acharya, S. and Sahoo, S.K., PLGA nanoparticles containing various anticancer agents and tumour delivery by EPR effect. *Adv. Drug Deliv. Rev.*, 63, 170–183, 2011.
40. Mahapatro, A. and Singh, D.K., Biodegradable nanoparticles are excellent vehicle for site directed *in-vivo* delivery of drugs and vaccines. *J. Nanobiotechnol.*, 9, 55, 2011.
41. Danhier, F. *et al.*, PLGA-based nanoparticles: an overview of biomedical applications. *J. Control. Release: Official Journal of the Controlled Release Society*, 161, 505–522, 2012.

42. Silva, A.L., Soema, P.C., Slütter, B., Ossendorp, F., Jiskoot, W., PLGA particulate delivery systems for subunit vaccines: Linking particle properties to immunogenicity. *Hum. Vaccin. Immunother.*, 12, 1056–1069, 2016.
43. Getts, D.R., Shea, L.D., Miller, S.D., King, N.J., Harnessing nanoparticles for immune modulation. *Trends Immunol.*, 36, 419–427, 2015.
44. Santos, D.M. *et al.*, PLGA nanoparticles loaded with KMP-11 stimulate innate immunity and induce the killing of Leishmania. *Nanomed.: Nanotechnol. Biol. Med.*, 9, 985–995, 2013.
45. Sawaengsak, C., Mori, Y., Yamanishi, K., Mitrevej, A., Sinchaipanid, N., Chitosan nanoparticle encapsulated hemagglutinin-split influenza virus mucosal vaccine. *AAPS PharmSciTech*, 15, 317–325, 2014.
46. Dhakal, S. *et al.*, Mucosal immunity and protective efficacy of intranasal inactivated influenza vaccine is improved by chitosan nanoparticle delivery in Pigs. *Front. Immunol.*, 9, 934, 2018.
47. Lynn, G.M. *et al.*, *In vivo* characterization of the physicochemical properties of polymer-linked TLR agonists that enhance vaccine immunogenicity. *Nat. Biotechnol.*, 33, 1201–1210, 2015.
48. Carroll, E.C. *et al.*, The vaccine Adjuvant chitosan promotes cellular immunity via DNA sensor cGAS-STING-dependent induction of type I interferons. *Immunity*, 44, 597–608, 2016.
49. Tahamtan, A. *et al.*, Antitumor effect of therapeutic HPV DNA vaccines with chitosan-based nanodelivery systems. *J. Biomed. Sci.*, 21, 69, 2014.
50. Sawaengsak, C. *et al.*, Intranasal chitosan-DNA vaccines that protect across influenza virus subtypes. *Int. J. Pharm.*, 473, 113–125, 2014.
51. Ye, T. *et al.*, M cell-targeting strategy facilitates mucosal immune response and enhances protection against CVB3-induced viral myocarditis elicited by chitosan-DNA vaccine. *Vaccine*, 32, 4457–4465, 2014.
52. Zhao, K. *et al.*, Enhancing mucosal immune response of newcastle disease virus DNA vaccine using N-2-Hydroxypropyl trimethylammonium chloride chitosan and N,O-carboxymethyl chitosan nanoparticles as delivery carrier. *Mol. Pharmaceutics*, 15, 226–237, 2018.
53. Zhao, K. *et al.*, Quaternized chitosan nanoparticles loaded with the combined attenuated live vaccine against Newcastle disease and infectious bronchitis elicit immune response in chicken after intranasal administration. *Drug Delivery*, 24, 1574–1586, 2017.
54. Valero, Y. *et al.*, An oral chitosan DNA vaccine against nodavirus improves transcription of cell-mediated cytotoxicity and interferon genes in the European sea bass juveniles gut and survival upon infection. *Dev. Comp. Immunol.*, 65, 64–72, 2016.
55. Vela-Ramirez, J.E. *et al.*, Safety and biocompatibility of carbohydrate-functionalized polyanhydride nanoparticles. *AAPS J.*, 17, 256–267, 2015.
56. Ulery, B.D. *et al.*, Rational design of pathogen-mimicking amphiphilic materials as nanoadjuvants. *Sci. Rep.*, 1, 198, 2011.

57. Ross, K.A. *et al.*, Lung deposition and cellular uptake behavior of pathogen-mimicking nanovaccines in the first 48 hours. *Adv. Healthcare Mater.*, 3, 1071–1077, 2014.
58. Liu, Y. *et al.*, Functional nanomaterials can optimize the efficacy of vaccines. *Small (Weinheim an der Bergstrasse, Germany)*, 10, 4505–4520, 2014.
59. Stone, J.W. *et al.*, Gold nanorod vaccine for respiratory syncytial virus. *Nanotechnology*, 24, 295102, 2013.
60. Gregory, A.E., Titball, R., Williamson, D., Vaccine delivery using nanoparticles. *Front. Cell. Infect. Microbiol.*, 3, 13, 2013.
61. Bianco, A., Kostarelos, K., Prato, M., Applications of carbon nanotubes in drug delivery. *Curr. Opin. Chem. Biol.*, 9, 674–679, 2005.
62. Wang, T. *et al.*, Synthesis of a novel kind of carbon nanoparticle with large mesopores and macropores and its application as an oral vaccine adjuvant. *Eur. J. Pharm. Sci.: Official Journal of the European Federation for Pharmaceutical Sciences*, 44, 653–659, 2011.
63. Villa, C.H. *et al.*, Single-walled carbon nanotubes deliver peptide antigen into dendritic cells and enhance IgG responses to tumor-associated antigens. *ACS Nano*, 5, 5300–5311, 2011.
64. Parra, J., Abad-Somovilla, A., Mercader, J.V., Taton, T.A., Abad-Fuentes, A., Carbon nanotube-protein carriers enhance size-dependent self-adjuvant antibody response to haptens. *J. Control. Release: Official Journal of the Controlled Release Society*, 170, 242–251, 2013.
65. Pantarotto, D. *et al.*, Immunization with peptide-functionalized carbon nanotubes enhances virus-specific neutralizing antibody responses. *Chem. Biol.*, 10, 961–966, 2003.
66. Niut, Y. *et al.*, Recent advances in the rational design of silica-based nanoparticles for gene therapy. *Ther. Deliv.*, 3, 1217–1237, 2012.
67. Yu, M. *et al.*, Hyaluronic acid modified mesoporous silica nanoparticles for targeted drug delivery to CD44-overexpressing cancer cells. *Nanoscale*, 5, 178–183, 2013.
68. Xia, T. *et al.*, Polyethyleneimine coating enhances the cellular uptake of mesoporous silica nanoparticles and allows safe delivery of siRNA and DNA constructs. *ACS Nano*, 3, 3273–3286, 2009.
69. He, X.X. *et al.*, Bioconjugated nanoparticles for DNA protection from cleavage. *J. Am. Chem. Soc.*, 125, 7168–7169, 2003.
70. Wang, J. *et al.*, The enhanced immune response of hepatitis B virus DNA vaccine using SiO2@LDH nanoparticles as an adjuvant. *Biomaterials*, 35, 466–478, 2014.
71. Al-Deen, F.M. *et al.*, Magnetic nanovectors for the development of DNA blood-stage malaria vaccines. *Nanomaterials (Basel, Switzerland)*, 7, 1–17, 2017.
72. Joyappa, D.H., Kumar, C.A., Banumathi, N., Reddy, G.R., Suryanarayana, V.V., Calcium phosphate nanoparticle prepared with foot and mouth disease

virus P1-3CD gene construct protects mice and guinea pigs against the challenge virus. *Vet. Microbiol.*, 139, 58–66, 2009.
73. Kraft, J.C., Freeling, J.P., Wang, Z., Ho, R.J., Emerging research and clinical development trends of liposome and lipid nanoparticle drug delivery systems. *J. Pharm. Sci.*, 103, 29–52, 2014.
74. Schwendener, R.A., Liposomes as vaccine delivery systems: A review of the recent advances. *Ther. Adv. Vaccines*, 2, 159–182, 2014.
75. Wang, N. *et al.*, Mannose derivative and lipid a dually decorated cationic liposomes as an effective cold chain free oral mucosal vaccine adjuvant-delivery system. *Eur. J. Pharm. Biopharm.: Official Journal of Arbeitsgemeinschaft fur Pharmazeutische Verfahrenstechnik e.V*, 88, 194–206, 2014.
76. Orr, M.T. *et al.*, Adjuvant formulation structure and composition are critical for the development of an effective vaccine against tuberculosis. *J. Control. Release: Official Journal of the Controlled Release Society*, 172, 190–200, 2013.
77. Felnerova, D., Viret, J.F., Glück, R., Moser, C., Liposomes and virosomes as delivery systems for antigens, nucleic acids and drugs. *Curr. Opin. Biotechnol.*, 15, 518–529, 2004.
78. Monto, A.S. *et al.*, Influenza control in the 21st century: Optimizing protection of older adults. *Vaccine*, 27, 5043–5053, 2009.
79. Noad, R. and Roy, P., Virus-like particles as immunogens. *Trends Microbiol.*, 11, 438–444, 2003.
80. Grimm, S.K. and Ackerman, M.E., Vaccine design: Emerging concepts and renewed optimism. *Curr. Opin. Biotechnol.*, 24, 1078–1088, 2013.
81. Bissett, S.L. *et al.*, Pre-clinical immunogenicity of human papillomavirus alpha-7 and alpha-9 major capsid proteins. *Vaccine*, 32, 6548–6555, 2014.
82. Zhang, N., Wardwell, P.R., Bader, R.A., Polysaccharide-based micelles for drug delivery. *Pharmaceutics*, 5, 329–352, 2013.
83. Torchilin, V.P., Structure and design of polymeric surfactant-based drug delivery systems. *J. Control. Release: Official Journal of the Controlled Release Society*, 73, 137–172, 2001.
84. Jiménez-Sánchez, G. *et al.*, Preparation and *in vitro* evaluation of imiquimod loaded polylactide-based micelles as potential vaccine adjuvants. *Pharm. Res.*, 32, 311–320, 2015.
85. Liu, H. *et al.*, Structure-based programming of lymph-node targeting in molecular vaccines. *Nature*, 507, 519–522, 2014.
86. Keller, S. *et al.*, Neutral polymer micelle carriers with pH-responsive, endosome-releasing activity modulate antigen trafficking to enhance CD8(+) T cell responses. *J. Control. Release: Official Journal of the Controlled Release Society*, 191, 24–33, 2014.
87. Accardo, A. *et al.*, Self-assembled or mixed peptide amphiphile micelles from Herpes simplex virus glycoproteins as potential immunomodulatory treatment. *Int. J. Nanomed.*, 9, 2137–2148, 2014.
88. Sanders, M.T., Brown, L.E., Deliyannis, G., Pearse, M.J., ISCOM-based vaccines: The second decade. *Immunol. Cell Biol.*, 83, 119–128, 2005.

89. Waite, D.C. *et al.*, Three double-blind, randomized trials evaluating the safety and tolerance of different formulations of the saponin adjuvant QS-21. *Vaccine*, 19, 3957–3967, 2001.
90. Hägglund, S. *et al.*, Characterization of an experimental vaccine for bovine respiratory syncytial virus. *Clin. Vaccine Immunol.: CVI*, 21, 997–1004, 2014.
91. Pearse, M.J. and Drane, D., ISCOMATRIX adjuvant for antigen delivery. *Adv. Drug Delivery Rev.*, 57, 465–474, 2005.
92. Baz Morelli, A. *et al.*, ISCOMATRIX: A novel adjuvant for use in prophylactic and therapeutic vaccines against infectious diseases. *J. Med. Microbiol.*, 61, 935–943, 2012.
93. Kanekiyo, M. *et al.*, Self-assembling influenza nanoparticle vaccines elicit broadly neutralizing H1N1 antibodies. *Nature*, 499, 102–106, 2013.
94. Champion, C.I. *et al.*, A vault nanoparticle vaccine induces protective mucosal immunity. *PLoS One*, 4, e5409, 2009.
95. Kaba, S.A. *et al.*, Protective antibody and CD8+ T-cell responses to the Plasmodium falciparum circumsporozoite protein induced by a nanoparticle vaccine. *PLoS One*, 7, e48304, 2012.
96. Wahome, N. *et al.*, Conformation-specific display of 4E10 and 2F5 epitopes on self-assembling protein nanoparticles as a potential HIV vaccine. *Chem. Biol. Drug Des.*, 80, 349–357, 2012.
97. El Bissati, K. *et al.*, Protein nanovaccine confers robust immunity against Toxoplasma. *NPJ Vaccines*, 2, 24, 2017.
98. Pimentel, T.A. *et al.*, Peptide nanoparticles as novel immunogens: Design and analysis of a prototypic severe acute respiratory syndrome vaccine. *Chem. Biol. Drug Des.*, 73, 53–61, 2009.
99. Aguilar, J.C. and Rodríguez, E.G., Vaccine adjuvants revisited. *Vaccine*, 25, 3752–3762, 2007.
100. Aucouturier, J., Dupuis, L., Ganne, V., Adjuvants designed for veterinary and human vaccines. *Vaccine*, 19, 2666–2672, 2001.
101. Shah, P., Bhalodia, D., Shelat, P., Nanoemulsion: A pharmaceutical review. *Sys. Rev. Pharm.* 1, 24–32, 2010.
102. Peek, L.J., Middaugh, C.R., Berkland, C., Nanotechnology in vaccine delivery. *Adv. Drug Delivery Rev.*, 60, 915–928, 2008.
103. O'Hagan, D.T., MF59 is a safe and potent vaccine adjuvant that enhances protection against influenza virus infection. *Expert Rev. Vaccines*, 6, 699–710, 2007.
104. De Donato, S. *et al.*, Safety and immunogenicity of MF59-adjuvanted influenza vaccine in the elderly. *Vaccine*, 17, 3094–3101, 1999.
105. Nicholson, K.G. *et al.*, Safety and antigenicity of non-adjuvanted and MF59-adjuvanted influenza A/Duck/Singapore/97 (H5N3) vaccine: A randomised trial of two potential vaccines against H5N1 influenza. *Lancet (London, England)*, 357, 1937–1943, 2001.

106. Kumar, S. *et al.*, CpG oligodeoxynucleotide and Montanide ISA 51 adjuvant combination enhanced the protective efficacy of a subunit malaria vaccine. *Infect. Immun.*, 72, 949–957, 2004.
107. Oliveira, G.A. *et al.*, Safety and enhanced immunogenicity of a hepatitis B core particle Plasmodium falciparum malaria vaccine formulated in adjuvant Montanide ISA 720 in a phase I trial. *Infect. Immun.*, 73, 3587–3597, 2005.
108. Dar, P. *et al.*, Montanide ISA™ 201 adjuvanted FMD vaccine induces improved immune responses and protection in cattle. *Vaccine*, 31, 3327–3332, 2013.
109. Zeng, B.J. *et al.*, Receptor-specific delivery of protein antigen to dendritic cells by a nanoemulsion formed using top-down non-covalent click self-assembly. *Small (Weinheim an der Bergstrasse, Germany)*, 9, 3736–3742, 2013.
110. Kumar, S., Khilnani, G.C., Banga, A., Sharma, S.K., Predictors of requirement of mechanical ventilation in patients with chronic obstructive pulmonary disease with acute respiratory failure. *Lung India: Off. Organ Indian Chest Soc.*, 30, 178–182, 2013.
111. Nho, R., Pathological effects of nano-sized particles on the respiratory system. *Nanomed.: Nanotechnol. Biol. Med.*, 29, 102242, 2020.
112. Zhu, M. *et al.*, Physicochemical properties determine nanomaterial cellular uptake, transport, and fate. *Acc. Chem. Res.*, 46, 622–631, 2013.
113. Yu, L.E. *et al.*, Translocation and effects of gold nanoparticles after inhalation exposure in rats. *Nanotoxicology*, 1, 235–242, 2007.
114. Gupta, I., Duran, N., Rai, M., *Nano-antimicrobials*, pp. 525–548, Springer, Berlin, Germany, 2012.
115. Arms, L. *et al.*, Advantages and Limitations of Current Techniques for Analyzing the Biodistribution of Nanoparticles. *Front. Pharmacol.*, 9, 802, 2018.
116. Sahdev, P., Ochyl, L.J., Moon, J.J., Biomaterials for nanoparticle vaccine delivery systems. *Pharm. Res.*, 31, 2563–2582, 2014.

2

Nanomedicine and Nanovaccinology Tools in Targeted Drug Delivery

Bogala Mallikharjuna Reddy

Abinnovus Consulting Pvt. Ltd., Technology Business Incubator, University of Madras, Guindy Campus, Chennai, India

Abstract

Infectious diseases are the leading cause of death worldwide, having a significant impact on public health and socio-economic development of the human population. The rapid development of drug resistance by pathogens to currently available therapies, as well as the significant side effects that result from their prolonged treatment, pose a serious threat to public health and safety. So, novel biomedical therapy approaches must be developed. Nanomedicine and nanovaccine drug delivery tools are relatively new, yet they are transforming biomedical research at a rapid pace. They are critical platforms for the controlled delivery of therapeutic drugs to targeted sites. These tools provide several benefits in the treatment of chronic human diseases via precise drug delivery to specific target sites. The current book chapter provides an overview of advances in nanomedicine and nanovaccinology drug delivery tools for infectious disease research, diagnostics, and therapy. Nanomedicines and nanovaccines present opportunities and challenges in the development of drug delivery systems and clinical applications. In addition, trends and prospects of tools used in nanomedicine and nanovaccinology research for target-specific drug delivery are explored.

***Keywords*:** Nanomedicine, nanovaccinology, drug delivery, nanomaterials, disease diagnosis, therapeutics

2.1 Introduction

The old saying "Prevention is better than cure" is more appropriate to the current health crisis experienced by the human population across

Email: bmreddy@abinnovus.com

Kaushik Pal (ed.) Nanovaccinology as Targeted Therapeutics, (21–52) © 2022 Scrivener Publishing LLC

the world [1]. Infectious diseases, such as severe acute respiratory infections (coronaviruses: SARS CoV-2/COVID-19, SARS CoV, and MERS) and human immunodeficiency virus (HIV/AIDS) disease are caused by pathogenic agents, i.e., viruses, bacteria, parasites, and fungi [2–4]. They are the leading cause of human mortality and account for more than 15 million deaths worldwide [3]. Viral infections cause substantial global health threats because they affect millions of people around the world, wreaking havoc on public healthcare and socioeconomic growth of human societies [3, 5]. The efficient cure of viral infectious diseases is limited by the development of resistance to drugs, particularly those linked with influenza and HIV [2, 3]. This process causes a threat to public health and safety due to enhanced mortality and morbidity, extra costs from the utilization of expensive drugs, and a huge load on public healthcare systems [3, 6]. Hence, prevention of viral infections is the greatest—possibly the only—means to alleviate the public health concerns caused by viral infectious diseases [7]. At present, vaccinations are the best efficient preventive means of defense in combating deadly infectious diseases, and they symbolize the core topics of research for human public healthcare and safety in the world [8].

Historically, vaccine formulation is based on Louis Pasteur's paradigm "isolate, inactivate, inject," and most vaccines have been developed in a manner that imitates pathogens and thus, stimulates the patient's immunity to fight against the disease [9, 10]. There have been remarkable successes in the prevention of viral infections, such as polio, smallpox, papilloma, and hepatitis A using vaccines [7, 8, 11]. However, vaccine formulation is a difficult undertaking, thus much research has been started to gain a deep understanding of the immune system's reaction to antigens, which aids in the manufacture of numerous vaccines via antibody and cell-regulated mechanisms for viral infection defense [10, 12]. Generally, issues arise when attempting to formulate vaccines against viruses, like COVID-19, HIV, hepatitis C virus (HCV), which are highly variant, where the above-mentioned traditional strategy of vaccine formulation is futile [10]. For the past few decades, high throughput tools have proven to be essential in the understanding of complex physiological immune systems and in using these pioneering technologies in the development of novel vaccines [10, 13]. New antigen production, approaches for vaccination (comprising even weakly infectious vaccines), and serial efforts of community/mass immunization have enhanced the efficiency of viral vaccines, all of which are possible merely because of the emergence of highly promising nanotechnology [7, 14].

The word "nano" is obtained from the Greek word "nanos," which implies small or dwarf [15, 16]. A "nanomaterial" is a material that has one of its dimensions in the 1 to 100 nm range [16]. Nanoscience refers to the study of materials and structures on a nanoscale, and the unique and interesting properties displayed by them [16]. Nanoscience is a multidisciplinary field involving other areas like physics, chemistry, biology, medicine, computer science, materials science, and engineering. Nanotechnology (or molecular manufacturing) deals with the design, fabrication, and application of nanomaterials, nanodevices, and nanosystems [16]. In other words, nanotechnology is related to the preparation of functional/useful materials, devices, and systems via manipulation/control of matter at nanometer scale, i.e., 10^{-9} or one billionth of a meter [16]. Although ancient humans used 'nanomaterials' for many centuries in paintings (Lycurgus cup, stained glass windows, ceramic glazes, Renaissance pottery) and weapons ("Damascus" saber blades), the theoretical underpinnings of modern nanotechnology were first provided in 1959 by Richard Feynman in his provocative lecture "There's plenty of room at the bottom" [16, 17]. The term "nanotechnology" was first coined by Norio Taniguchi in 1974 upon referring to the ability of precisely engineering materials at the nanometer level [18]. Now, nanotechnology impacts many aspects of day-to-day human life, and the potential applications of nanotechnology are numerous and diverse.

Nanoscience and nanotechnology are gaining more importance in medicine due to the excellent physicochemical and biological properties exhibited by nanomaterials [3]. They include: (i) small particle size that not only affects bioavailability and circulation time but also facilitates drug delivery into anatomically privileged sites, (ii) large surface area to volume ratios that results in enhanced solubility compared to larger particles and ensures that large drug payloads can be accommodated, and (iii) tunable surface charge of the particle that facilitates cellular entry across the negatively charged cellular membrane, gives the possibility of encapsulation and accommodates large drug payloads [3, 19, 20]. Therefore, nanomaterials are very attractive tools for targeted drug delivery in the treatment of infectious viral diseases. The emerging area of "nanomedicine" deals with the application of nanoscience and nanotechnology in the field of medicine that involves the utilization of nanomaterials and nanodevices for early diagnosis, treatment, and prevention of many diseases [21]. The word "nanomedicine" was first coined by Eric Drexler and Robert Freitas in the 1990s, whereas the first multivolume textbook on nanomedicine was published by Robert Freitas with the title "Nanomedicine" in 1999 [16, 21, 22]. Nanomedicine includes an array of systems, such as nanomaterials, nanoporous matrices, nanofibers, nanopatterned surfaces, and nanoscale coatings. Among them, nanomaterial-based applications in the formulation and delivery of drugs have evolved as the most beneficial nanomedicine system. Nanomedicine uses nanomaterials as biomedical tools in diagnosis and therapeutics or treatment of diseases (like cardiology, oncology, ophthalmology, orthopedics, neurological diseases, infectious diseases, etc) that was impossible earlier with the traditional medicine approaches [21].

The application of nanotechnology in vaccinology is known as "nanovaccinology" [8]. Nanomaterials are used in nanovaccinology to enhance the development of vaccines and in the optimization of sophisticated nanovaccine systems for advanced antigen delivery and effective induction of immunity against pathogenic diseases [7–9, 23]. These are made possible by the nanomaterials small size, which allows them to easily migrate through cells via endocytosis, delivering physiologically active antigens to predetermined target areas [10, 24]. Also, nanomaterials are relatively simple to produce, undergo surface modification, have good solubility, are biodegradable, biocompatible, possess extended circulation time, can deliver necessary doses of drugs, and protect the antigen from enzymatic degradation [7]. All these properties of nanomaterials improve the bioavailability (or stay) and circulation of the antigen in the body for longer durations, achieve target-specific action on infected organs, and control the natural and stimulated immune response, including the generation of memory cells that are critical for a nanovaccine's success [7]. In addition to the dose, size, and shape of nanomaterials, the key factors affecting the efficiency and success of nanomaterial-based vaccines are: (i) a superior antigen that triggers the immunity, (ii) a resistant adjuvant that coactivated the natural immune system, and (iii) a delivery vehicle system to permit its interaction with antigen-presenting cells or APCs [8]. Therefore, the design of nanomaterials-based vaccines must take into account all the factors that control linking/binding and delivery of antigen (size, shape, composition, and surface modification), biodistribution, bioavailability, biocompatibility, and immunogenicity of the used nanomaterials [8, 25]. Before the clinical trials, the success of the formulated nanovaccine is assessed by first investigating the nanovaccine response mechanism to enhance the immunogenicity and then, evaluating the efficiency of the nanovaccine by testing against a large group of populations with different ages, sex and health conditions [10, 26]. This book chapter mainly focuses on the recent advancements in nanomedicine and nanovaccinology tools for target-specific delivery of drugs that combat infectious diseases. Brief insights on the commercialization of nanomaterial-based medicines and vaccines for clinical trials and their future perspectives have been summarized in this work.

2.2 Nanomaterial-Based Drug Delivery Tools

There are numerous types of nanomaterials studied as potential delivers of drugs and vaccine antigens. Specifically, many researchers have focused their attention on the improvement of nanomaterial-based natural and synthetic delivery tools in the size range of viruses (20-200 nm). These delivery vehicles protect the drug/antigen from biodegradation, improve its bioavailability, and facilitate its uptake by APCs [8]. As shown in Figure 2.1, the nanomaterials-based drug delivery systems are classified into self-assembled proteins, micelles, liposomes, inorganic nanoparticles,

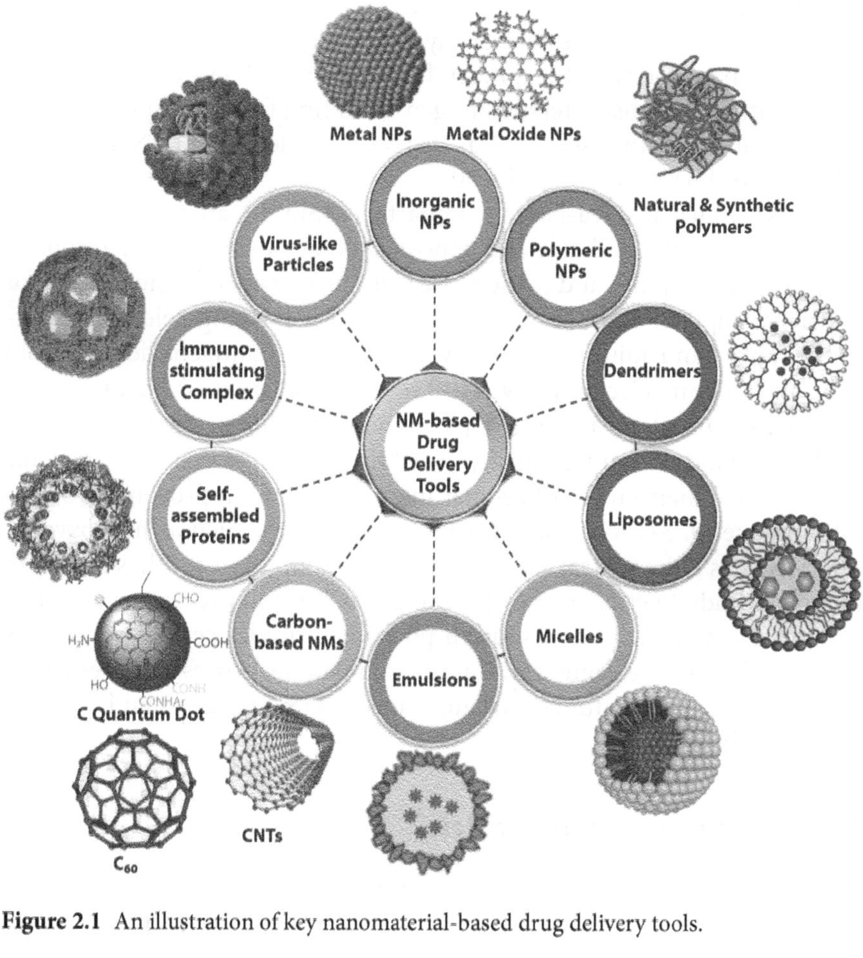

Figure 2.1 An illustration of key nanomaterial-based drug delivery tools.

polymeric nanoparticles, dendrimers, emulsions, carbon-based nanomaterials, immunostimulating complexes, and virus-like particles.

2.2.1 Inorganic Nanoparticles

Many inorganic nanoparticles (NPs) have been examined for their application in the drug delivery of nanomedicines and nanovaccines. Examples of inorganic NPs include metallic nanoparticles (MNPs) and metal oxide nanoparticles (MONPs). Though inorganic NPs are nonbiodegradable, they possess a stable structure and are synthesized in a controllable manner [8, 9, 23, 27]. MNPs, such as gold nanoparticles (AuNPs), are increasingly used in nanomedicine and nanovaccine delivery because they are simply fabricated into diverse shapes (cubic, rod, spherical, etc.), varied size (2–150 nm), and easily undergo surface-modification with carbohydrates [9, 28]. Gold nanorods have been used as a delivery vehicle for an antigen obtained from a respiratory syncytial virus via conjugating the surface of Au nanorod with the antigen [29]. Other Au NPs have been investigated either as transporters of antigens resulting from viruses (influenza and foot-and-mouth disease) or as deoxyribonucleic acid (DNA) vaccine adjuvant for HIV/AIDS virus [9, 30].

MONPs, such as silica-based nanoparticles (SiNPs), are promising inorganic NPs for nanomedicine and nanovaccinology delivery systems due to their biocompatibility and possess excellent properties of nanocarriers for a variety of applications, i.e., real-time molecular imaging, selective targeting of cancer, and adjuvants for delivery of vaccines/antigens derived from HIV and porcine circovirus [9, 31–33]. All these are possible due to the presence of abundant silanol groups on the surface of SiNPs that are modified to provide extra functionality in cell recognition, specific biomolecule absorption, enhancement of cellular interaction, and improvement of cellular uptake [9, 31]. Calcium phosphate-based NPs, such as hydroxyapatite (HAp), is either extracted from natural resources or synthesized from other methods (wet-chemical) by using the reactants (calcium chloride, sodium citrate dibasic, and sodium phosphate) under certain conditions [9, 34–36]. They are nonhazardous, biocompatible, possess different sizes (50–100 nm), and are functional adjuvant for DNA vaccines and mucosal immunity [9, 37].

2.2.2 Polymeric Nanoparticles

Natural or synthetic polymeric nanoparticles offer another way for therapeutic drug delivery because of their characteristics, such as biocompatibility, biodegradability, easy modifying ability (to desired sizes and shapes), nontoxicity, and nonimmunogenicity [9, 38]. Natural polymers based on polysaccharides are used in the preparation of adjuvant nanoparticles, such as chitosan, pullulan, alginate, and inulin [9, 8, 23, 38]. Chitosan-based nanoparticles are used in the preparation of different vaccines that include HBV vaccines, DNA vaccines, and Newcastle disease vaccines [9]. Inulin adjuvant nanoparticles (such as Advax™) have shown improvement in immune response against hepatitis B and influenza diverse viruses [9]. Many synthetic polymers are also used in the preparation of nanoparticles for drug delivery purposes, which includes poly(D, L-lactide-co-glycolide) (PLG), poly(v-lactic-coglycolic acid) (PLGA), poly(γ-glutamic acid) (γ-PGA), poly(ethylene glycol) (PEG), and polystyrene [9].

PLG and PLGA polymeric nanoparticles have been extensively studied in the entrapment of antigen and its delivery to specifically targeted cells or prolonged antigen release based on their slow rate of biodegradation [9, 39, 40]. PLGA has been used in the delivery of antigen derived from several pathogens including hepatitis B virus (HBV), plasmodium vivax (with adjuvant monophosphoryl lipid A), model antigens (tetanus toxoid and ovalbumin), and *Bacillus anthracis* [9, 39]. Poly(γ-glutamic acid) based nanoparticles contain γ-PGA units that self-assemble into nanospheres with hydrophobic inner core and hydrophilic outer shell and usually encapsulate hydrophobic antigen [9, 41]. Polystyrene nanoparticles conjugates to various antigens as their surface can be modified with diverse functional groups [9]. Both natural polymers and synthetic polymers are used in the synthesis of nanohydrogels that can form hydrophilic three-dimensional (3D) polymer networks. Nanohydrogels possess favorable characteristics that include high water content, large surface area for multivalent conjugation, high loading capacity for antigens, and flexible mesh size [9, 42]. Chitosan nanogels are commonly used in the delivery of antigen (Hc, *Clostridium botulinum* type-A neurotoxin subunit) for an adjuvant free intranasal vaccine and recombinant antigen (NcPDI) for *Neospora caninum* vaccination [42, 43].

2.2.3 Dendrimers

Dendrimers are polymeric structures with well-defined branches with widths ranging from 1 to 10 nm that form semi-globular to globular forms and have a high density of functionalities on the surface [44, 45]. Dendrimers are used for medical applications because of their confined structure, hyperbranched and low polydispersity [38]. Different polymeric-linkages, such as polyamines (polyethyleneimine, polypropyleneimine/PPI), or combination of polyamides and amines (polyamidoamine/PAMAM), and chitin can be part of dendrimer design. They are functionalized with many groups that include peptides, carbohydrates, and silanol groups [38, 44, 45]. Dendrimers are fabricated by either divergent or convergent methods, which results in the formation of cavities inside spherical dendrimer structures [38]. Drugs are delivered using dendrimers in various ways: (i) drugs are encapsulated within the interior cavities of dendrimers, (ii) formation of dendrimer-drug networks, and (iii) prodrugs are produced from cross-linking of drugs to the surface of dendrimers [45]. High efficiency of entrapment is possible with high-generation dendrimers (> 64 surface groups) in comparison to smaller dendrimers, and they are used for the delivery of therapeutic drugs. In addition, the free end groups of dendrimers are easily modified via conjugation with biocompatible molecules to decrease cytotoxicity and increase bio-permeability of the dendrimers during the delivery of therapeutic vaccines, drugs, and genes to the target-specific sites [38]. DNA has been conjugated with PAMAM dendrimers to form PAMAM-DNA dendrimer complexes (100–175 nm) and their toxicity and immunogenic potentials are studied for drug delivery applications. Also, dendrimers are used for the delivery of antisense oligonucleotides, fluorouracil, and indomethacin [45].

2.2.4 Liposomes

Liposomes are obtained from the self-assembly of biodegradable and non-toxic phospholipids into the hydrophobic bilayered outer shell and hydrophilic interior core [9, 23]. Liposomes are unilamellar or multilamellar structures of single or concentric multiple lipid shells separated by aqueous layers [23]. Liposomes are tailored to include both hydrophobic drugs (within phospholipid bilayer) and hydrophilic drugs (in aqueous core). The simplest liposome contains a lipid bilayer enclosing a hollow core of 50 to 1000 nm in diameter. The clinical drugs are incorporated into the hollow core for their delivery [38, 46]. Liposomes release drugs into the cytoplasm upon fusing with cell membranes, and therefore, they form perfect carrier tools for targeted drug delivery applications [38]. In addition, multiple types of drugs can be incorporated within two regions (lipid shell and aqueous core) of unilamellar or several hydrophilic layers (aqueous) of multilamellar liposomes [38]. Liposomes also permit the sequential release of several drugs upon gradual disintegration of lipid bilayers, i.e., from the outer shell to the inner core [38]. Surface modification/functionalization of liposomes with polymer (PEG chains) can enhance targeted delivery of drugs and prolong their circulation or bioavailability in cells [38].

Generally, liposomes are used in biomedical applications, such as encapsulation of vaccines, diagnosis, and treatment of cancer, anti-microbial activity, and targeted drug delivery to the brain [38, 46]. Currently, liposomes are under clinical trials or marketed for treating human diseases, such as Epaxal®, CAF01, Inflexal® V, RTS, S/AS01, and Stimuvax for combating hepatitis A, tuberculosis, influenza, malaria, and lung cancer, respectively [9, 47].

2.2.5 Micelles

Micelles are nanomaterials (< 100 nm) generated by self-assembly of amphiphilic (hydrophobic/hydrophilic) molecules in water, resulting in two different regions, hydrophobic inner core and hydrophilic outer surface [8]. The hydrophobic inner core of micelles can physically entrap water-insoluble or hydrophobic drugs, and it can also be covalently bonded to drugs or vaccines [38]. When amphiphile concentration exceeds the critical micelle concentration (CMC) limit, hydrophobic interactions become a major driving force for the assembly of amphiphiles in the aqueous medium [45]. Low molecular-weight hydrophobic core and amphiphilic polymers (PEG) make up the majority of nanosized micellar delivery tools [45]. Because of the hydrophilic outer surface, micelles are protected from nonspecific uptake by reticuloendothelial cells and thus, guaranteeing their great stability in biological systems. As a result, the dynamic structure of micelles makes them effective delivery tools for therapeutic drugs and therefore, allows for a slower rate of dissolution, a wide range of loading capacities, and efficient conjugation of target-specific drugs and vaccines [38, 48]. In the recent past, micelles have been studied as vaccine adjuvants and drug delivery tools, with hydrophobic drugs encapsulated in the core [8]. Micelles can deliver therapeutic vaccines/drugs in two ways: (i) antigens can be covalently attached to the hydrophilic surface; HIV antigens are attached to adjuvant-loaded polymer-based micelles, resulting in a vaccine that can trigger APCs significantly *in vitro*, and (ii) development of peptide amphiphiles (PAs), formed via linking of peptides to hydrophobic alkyl tails, which self-assemble in an aqueous medium to form micelles [8]. Spherical or cylindrical PA micelles have the correct concentration of antigen and amphiphilic adjuvants and can effectively reach lymph nodes. PAs were used as vaccine tools in mice, following subcutaneous inoculation, to induce antigen-specific IgG1 antibody response against group A streptococcus [8]. Micelles can enhance the immunostimulatory capacity of the antigen. Micelles can be exploited for endosome breakdown and subsequent release of peptide vaccines in the cell cytoplasmic matrix, antigen delivery, and greater cytotoxic T cell responses *in vivo* by selecting appropriate hydrophobic core molecules [8]. In addition, the biodistribution and pharmacokinetics of micelle delivered drugs (paclitaxel, doxorubicin, and cisplatin) are altered favorably i.e., enhanced circulation time and improved accumulation at target tumor sites, while compared to the corresponding free drugs [45, 49].

2.2.6 Emulsions

Nanoemulsions are oil-water dispersions in which the isolated phase droplets are nanosized (50–600 nm) and are stabilized by a surface-active film made up of surfactant and co-surfactant [45]. Oil-in-water (O/W) and water-in-oil (W/O) dispersions are the two types of nanoemulsions [23]. Nanoemulsions synthesis procedures include lab-scale ultrasonication, low energy emulsification (where water is added to an oil solution of the surfactant), and high energy emulsification (using homogenizers) [45]. The nanosize scale of emulsion droplets stops the occurrence of creaming or sedimentation on coalescence and storage of droplets. Nanoemulsions are clear or translucent systems. Nanoemulsions are attractive as pharmaceutical formulations because they form spontaneously (i.e., they are easy to make), are optically transparent, and are thermodynamically stable [45]. Nanoemulsion structure can affect the release rate of drugs. In O/W nanoemulsions, hydrophobic drugs are mostly dissolved in the oil droplets and they are released slowly (based on O/W partitioning) because of hindered diffusion. On the other hand, the diffusion of hydrophilic drugs is less constrained and they are quickly released from the O/W nanoemulsions. The opposite behavior is anticipated with W/O type nanoemulsions [45]. By carrying antigens inside their cores or simply mixing with the antigens, both O/W and water-in-oil (W/O) nanoemulsion types have evolved as exceptional adjuvants for efficient vaccination or medication administration [9, 45]. Nanodelivery tools, such as MF59™, Montanide™ family (ISA 50 V, 51, 201, 206 and 720), Fungizone, amphotericin, vincristine, and paclitaxel nanoemulsions are used to cure diseases, i.e., influenza, malaria, cancer, foot-and-mouth diseases [9, 23, 39, 45, 50].

2.2.7 Carbon-Based Nanomaterials

Carbon-based nanomaterials are frequently studied tools for drug and vaccine delivery because they can be easily internalized into a broad range of cell types [8, 9, 23]. Several physical and structural features of carbon-based nanomaterial tools, such as surface modifications, can influence the capability of transporting antigens and triggering immune responses [8]. Carbon-based nanomaterials are biocompatible and can be fabricated into various structures, such as nanotubes and mesoporous spheres [9, 23]. Among carbon-based nanomaterials, carbon nanotubes (CNTs) are attractive due to their excellent properties, which make them utilizable in several industries. CNTs are carbon-based tubular structures of 100-1000 nm in length and they are prepared by the wrapping of a single layer of graphite called "graphene" into a hollow cylinder, also known as single-walled CNT or SWCNT [8, 38]. Multiwalled CNT, or MWCNT, is a CNT formed from concentric multiple graphene layers (2 to 50, connected by van der Waals forces) [38]. Typically, the diameter of SWCNTs (0.4 to 2 nm), MWCNTs, (2-100 nm), and C_{60} or fullerenes (1–2 nm, internal diameters) varies from each other [8, 9, 23]. Fullerenes differ from CNTs in the 3D arrangement/network of the carbon atoms and also in several conjugated double bonds of their structure [9, 23]. Other nanomaterials based on carbon are "carbon quantum dots," which can undergo surface modification to carry different therapeutic payloads via chemical cross-linking with the surface functional groups. The appropriate size and firm shape of CNTs make them smart nonpolymeric carriers of therapeutic agents. Both SWCNTs and MWCNTs enter into cells via endocytosis or by insertion through the membrane of cells [9, 23]. The IgG response has improved after many peptide and protein antigens were linked to CNTs for delivery. The use of mesoporous carbon nanoparticles as oral vaccine adjuvants is being investigated [9, 51]. Fullerenes are used in the delivery of therapeutics such as antibiotics, antiviral and anti-cancer agents [38]. Furthermore, fullerenes shield the damaged mitochondria by supplying free radicals and thus, allowing tissue-specific targeting of mitochondria, which can be used for delivery of therapeutic agents [38].

2.2.8 Self-Assembled Proteins

Self-assembled proteins (SAPs) are an array of supramolecular protein structures formed from noncovalent interactions (van der Waals, hydrophobic, ionic interactions, and hydrogen bonding) of two or more peptide/protein subunits i.e., helical coil domains connected by a short linker region/chains [8, 52]. The obtained SAPs possess novel structures and properties that are determined by the positioning and nature of individual constituent peptides/proteins [52]. Several factors, such as protein strength, structure, orientation, protein-protein interactions, and environmental parameters (pH, temperature, and ionic strength) influence the performance of self-assembled proteins [52]. The self-assembled proteins possess various functions because of several features: (i) many proteins are functional in their natural monomeric structure, and their efficacy can be enhanced upon self-assembly (ii) SAPs have novel collective functions and properties that are not exhibited by their building block units. (iii) SAPs are capable of displaying many functions with the incorporation of new functional molecules into their core structure [52]. SAPs with higher antigen-carrying levels are studied for the fabrication of nanomaterial-based drug and vaccine delivery tools. SAPs can induce potent immune responses against vital HIV epitopes [8]. Ferritin can self-assemble into a spherical-like structure of 10 nm diameter. The recombined protein, obtained from genetically fusing influenza virus hemagglutinin (HA) to ferritin, can instantaneously assemble into an octahedral structure and transformed eight trimeric HA spikes to produce a superior immune response in comparison to trivalent inactivated influenza vaccine that is normally developed for destroying instead of building a viral structure [8, 9]. Self-assembling of 96 units of major vault protein (MVP) produces a barrel-shaped vault nanostructure of approximately 40 nm in width and 70 nm in length [8, 9]. Antigens can be packed inside vault nanostructures during the self-assembling process of MVPs. Vault nanostructures can encapsulate major outer membrane protein (MOMP) of *Chlamydia muridarum* for mucosal immunity studies [8, 9].

2.2.9 Immunostimulating Complexes

Immunostimulating complexes (ISCOMs) are open cage-like spherical structures (~ 40 nm size) that can be prepared from spontaneous mixing of adjuvant Quillaja saponins (often QuilA from *Quillaia saponaria* tree), phospholipids (phosphatidylcholine or phosphatidylethanolamine), cholesterol, and protein (antigen) under specific formulation or stoichiometric composition [9, 23, 39]. The spherical structures of ISCOMs trap antigen via apolar interactions, and they exhibit immune-stimulating properties that can be used as a vaccine adjuvant to induce longer protection and stronger immune response [9, 39]. ISCOMs are used in entrapping viral envelope proteins that are obtained from herpes simplex virus type-1, HIV, bacteria, and parasites (*Escherichia coli, Plasmodium falciparum, and Brucella aborus*), influenza, hepatitis, and Newcastle disease [9, 23, 39, 53]. Also, *Chlamydia muridarum* has been used for mucosal immunity studies [8, 9].

2.2.10 Virus-Like Particles

Virus-like particles (VLPs) are noninfectious self-assembling nanomaterials that are obtained from naturally occurring or synthesized by individual expression of viral structural proteins, and they closely resemble virus-like structures [9, 23]. VLPs of different sizes (20–800 nm) can be fabricated from various viruses (only take their good aspects) using different processing methods. Historically, the manufacturing of VLPs involves the assembly of biocompatible capsid proteins into VLPs takes place within the expression of host organisms via *in vivo* route [9]. The assembled VLPs are purified from encapsulated and adherent contaminant chemicals. VLPs are formed in multiple cell culture systems, such as bacteria, insects, mammals, yeast, and plants. Alternatively, the assembly of VLPs can be possible with an emerging approach that involves cell-free *in vitro* procedures. In this method, the conventional model of assemble-then-purify is reversed, i.e., firstly, VLP building blocks are purified from contaminants at large scales, then they are assembled *in vitro*, thus avoiding the traditional step of disassembling VLPs after their assembly inside cells structures [9]. VLPs are nonreplicating nanostructures that do not integrate into the host genome. They do not recombine with the host or defective virus. Hence, VLPs are many vaccine delivery tools. VLPs can be engineered to express multiple proteins by fusing them or by generating more antigens. VLPs can offer protection against both the virus of origin and heterologous antigens [23]. To date, VLPs have been commercialized based on the self-assembly of proteins taken from a wide range of target viral families, including retroviridae (HIV), flaviviridae (hepatitis C virus), paramyxoviridae (Nipah), parvoviridae (adeno-associated virus), and bacteriophages (Q, AP205). Though many VLP vaccines are currently in clinical or preclinical trial stages, some VLP-based vaccine formulations have already been available on market. VLP-based vaccines such as Recobivax HB, Cervarix, Gardasil, and Mosquirix have been approved against pathogenic viruses/diseases that include influenza virus, human papilloma virus (HPV), chikungunya virus, hepatitis B, and malaria [9, 23, 54].

2.3 Targeted Drug Delivery Applications

Targeted drug delivery relates to the efficient direction of therapeutic drugs and their collection at the desired target site. For effective targeted drug delivery, the nanomaterial-drug delivery tools should be available in biological systems for sufficient duration, escape the immunological system, reach the target specific cells/tissues, and deliver the therapeutic drug payloads [38, 55]. Table 2.1 lists some of the targeted delivery tools for application in nanomedicine and nanovaccinology to combat pathogens and diseases [9, 38, 56].

Table 2.1 A list of targeted delivery tools used against pathogens and diseases.

Targeted delivery tools	**Properties**	**Immunity response type**	**Target pathogen or disease**
Polystyrene NPs	40–50 nm size, conjugated antigen peptide vaccine	Cell-mediated	Cancer
Liposomes	135–158 nm diameter	Humoral	COVID-19, SARS CoV-2/ pandemic corona virus, 2019
Au NPs	40–100 nm diameter, nano-adjuvant vaccine	Specific to antigen	SARS (severe acute respiratory syndrome, CoV-1
Virus-like particles/VLPs	Self-assembly, bivalent vaccine	Humoral and cellular response	Influenza and circo viruses
Dendrimers	50–100 nm size, DNA vaccine	Humoral and cellular response	Schistosomiasis
Micelle	~171 nm diameter, bi-adjuvant neo-antigen vaccine	Antigen specific immune therapy	Cancer
Carbon nanotubes (CNTs)	SWNT, conjugated with mannosylated antigen	Cell-mediated	Rhabdovirus

(*Continued*)

Table 2.1 A list of targeted delivery tools used against pathogens and diseases. (*Continued*)

Targeted delivery tools	Properties	Immunity response type	Target pathogen or disease
Ferritin (SAP)	Self-assembled protein, dual target, therapeutic vaccine	Humoral immunity and cell-mediated	Hepatitis-B virus (HBV)
Calcium-phosphate NPs	90 nm size, cross-protective nanovaccine	Humoral and cell-mediated	*Brucella melitensis* and *Brucella abortus*
Silica-based NPs	Transferrin mesoporous silica conjugated to doxorubicin	Cell-mediated	Cancer
Ag NPs	15 nm size, vaccine scaffold	Humoral immunity	*Escherichia coli*
Liposomevesicle	150 nm size	Cell-mediated	AIDS/ HIV virus
Virus-like particles (VLPs)	22 nm size, anti-sporozoite vaccine	Humoral and cellular response	Malaria
ISCOMs	~ 40 nm size, Quil A saponin based	Cell-mediated	Newcastle disease
Emulsions	50–600 nm size, W/O emulsions	Cell-mediated	Foot-and-mouth diseases

Most of the targeted drug delivery research has been focused on passive and active targeting of nanomaterial-based therapeutic agents (drugs/vaccines) for effective treatment of infectious pathogens/diseases, such as cancer, neurodegenerative, cardiovascular, viral infections, and so on. Figure 2.2 shows a schematic of targeted nanomaterial-based delivery of drugs/vaccines to some organs of human beings for curing diseases.

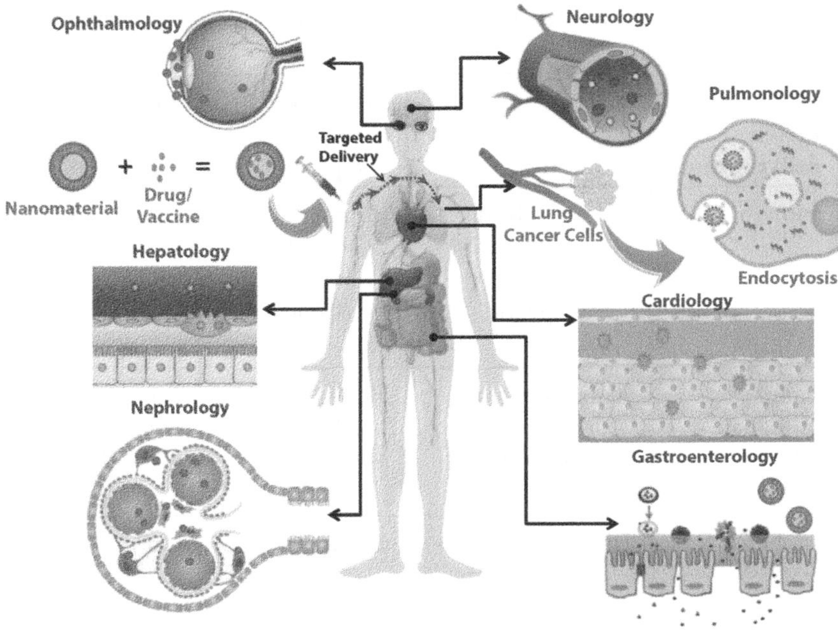

Figure 2.2 A schematic showing the nanomaterial-based targeted delivery of drug/ vaccine to some organs of human being.

2.3.1 Cancer

Cancer is one main causes of death across the world, and chemotherapy is commonly used in the treatment of different cancer types. However, chemotherapeutics involve reagents that possess poor aqueous solubility, inadequate tumor specificity, and dose-dependent toxicity [38, 57]. Multidrug resistance expels anti-cancer agents out of the cell membrane. Nanomaterial drug delivery tools prevail over the limitations by directly targeting the tumor cells and tissues, delivering therapeutic agents at controlled rates, and enhancing the therapeutic efficacy. At present, anti-cancer nanomaterials are based on reformulating the chemotherapeutic drugs by mixing with polymeric NPs. PEGylated liposomal formulation, known as doxorubicin (Doxil®) was the first nano-drug developed for the treatment of cancer. Doxil consists of cholesterol, phospholipids, and lipo-polymer (PEG) and its benefits include prolonged circulation time, extra accumulation in cancer cells, and a decrease in toxicity [38]. Another liposomal drug formulation (Marqibo®) was developed for curing acute lymphocytic leukemia disease in adult humans [38, 58]. Marqibo® is produced from cholesterol and sphingomyelin and it drastically enhances the circulation time and accelerates drug concentration in target cancer cells [38]. Cisplatin (Lipoplatin®) is prepared from cholesterol, dipalmitoyl phosphatidylglycerol, methoxy-PEG-distearoyl phosphatidylethanolamine and soy phosphatidylcholine. It is used in treatment of breast cancer, pancreatic adenocarcinoma, and gastric cancer [38]. The antibody-drug conjugate Kadcyla® is used in the treatment of breast cancer (HER2+) and it is synthesized from covalent conjugation of maytansine derivative (DM1) to trastuzumab (Herceptin®) by the antibody's lysine residues [38]. Also, the albumin-conjugated anti-cancer drug paclitaxel (Abraxane®) or reformulated rapamycin drug with micellar NPs (Rapamune®) are other nanomaterials with good therapeutic effects [38].

2.3.2 Neurology

Neurodegenerative diseases (NDs) cause a gradual loss in the function of neurons and consequently result in neuronal death. Examples of NDs include Parkinson's disease (PD), Alzheimer's disease (AD), multiple sclerosis (MS), and Amyotrophic lateral sclerosis (ALS). The patients of NDs exhibit symptoms related to movement, dementia, and memory because of progressive loss of neurons. Limited treatment of NDs exits due to restraining arrangement of the blood-brain barrier (BBB). The high selectivity of BBB permits only a few therapeutic drugs to reach the central nervous system (CNS) of the brain. Hence, more drug doses are needed, thus giving rise to unfavorable systemic effects. Once medications penetrate the BBB, nanomaterial-based therapy techniques in NDs aim for targeted drug delivery and continual local release of pharmaceuticals into the afflicted region of the brain [38, 59]. The amyloid-(A) peptide aggregates into amyloidal plaques and is a major pathological aspect of AD. Clinical drugs (donepezil, rivastigmine, galantamine, and memantine) reformulation with lipid-based NPs nonpolymeric QDs and polymeric NPs permits their transport through BBB and lowers the side effects in comparison to free drugs for AD [38].

PD is the selective deterioration of dopaminergic neurons and is characterized by the presence of protein and synuclein inclusions (Lewy bodies) in neurons [38]. Target specific delivery of dopamine and other PD drugs (bromocriptine, ropinirole, apomorphine, and mitoapocynin) via their encapsulation by liposomes or polymeric NPs is one nanomaterial-based therapeutic strategy to enhance the constant release of drugs and to lower side effects while curing of PD [38]. ALS is a progressive ND affecting motor neurons that controls voluntary muscle movements (walking, chewing, and talking) in the spinal cord and brain. Clinically, gradual muscle weakness causes death because of respiratory failure. Loading of Riluzole in solid lipid NPs improves delivery of the drug to CNS, and pH-dependent controlled drug delivery is attained with negligible biodistribution in other organs (spleen, liver, heart, lung, and kidneys) of the body [38]. MS occurs due to the destruction of the protective layer (myelin sheath) on CNS nerves, which results in faulty communication of instructions from the brain to the body. Glutamate receptor antagonist conjugated with non-polymeric fullerene (C_{60}) to form derivative NP that reduces clinical progression of chronic MS in an *in vivo* model [38]. In addition, Glatopa® was the first generic drug that is obtained from therapeutic peptide, glatiramer acetate (Copaxone®) for curing MS [60].

2.3.3 Cardiology

Cardiovascular disease (CVD) affects the cardiovascular system, brain vascular systems and peripheral, and kidney arteries. Nanomaterial drug delivery tools for the treatment of CVD mainly focus on target-specific drug delivery and in enhancing the bioavailability of drugs for vascular restenosis (VR). Liposomal sirolimus containing sirolimus drug, liposomes (cholesterol and phosphatidylcholine), and chitosan coating considerably inhibits VR. Carvedilol is an inhibitor for curing myocardial infarction (MI), hypertension, post-MI, congestive heart failure and left ventricular dysfunction (VD). However, its low aqueous solubility and predominant presystemic metabolism hinder its bioavailability. The niosome-based nanomaterial entrapping carvedilol resulted in an approximately two-fold increase in plasma concentrations in comparison to carvedilol, therefore responsible for improved bioavailability and enhanced therapeutic effect [38, 61]. Similarly, resveratrol is a cardioprotective polyphenol drug with low aqueous solubility and bioavailability. Nano-formulations of resveratrol as solid lipid NP and liposome exhibit improved bioavailability and regulated release [38]. Polymeric NPs loaded with vascular endothelial growth factor (VEGF) are potential delivery tools to enhance tissue remodeling, vasculogenesis, and in surmounting hypoxia-related side effects for myocardial ischemia angiogenic therapy [38]. Target-specific nanodelivery tools (ligand-loaded polymeric micelles or magneto-fluorescent NPs) are used in medical imaging and curing of atherosclerosis [62].

2.3.4 Ophthalmology

Currently, numerous ocular or ophthalmology therapies make use of nanomedicine delivery tools for the treatment of infection, cycloplegics miotics or mydriatics, inflammatory, diagnostic, and surgical operations. However, some barriers make the eye an impenetrable organ for several therapeutic agents, which include mucoaqueous tear layer, corneal epithelium, and blood-retina barrier [38, 63]. Target-specific nanodelivery tools possess benefits in ophthalmology disease therapy by decreasing eye irritation and improving their bioavailability, therefore facilitating an easy entry path for drugs to the eye [38]. The extensively used nanodelivery tools (liposomes and polymeric NPs) for targeted drug delivery to appropriate components of the eye by enhancing residence time on the tear film and improving corneal permeability [38]. Nanoformulation of pranoprofen with PLGA or poly(lactic-co-glycolic acid) improves ophthalmic delivery of pranoprofen and induced analgesic and anti-inflammatory effects of the drug [38]. In addition, chitosan-based polymeric NPs entrap dexamethasone or diclofenac, cefuroxime, and enhance the ophthalmic bioavailability of drugs [38]. They interact with the ophthalmic surface and shield drugs from metabolic degradation and prolong the precorneal residence time of drugs. Also, lipid-based NPs containing brimonidine are used in the treatment of glaucoma ophthalmic disease [38]. Refusal of immunologic grafts is a major concern in the corneal transplantation process. PEG- or PLGA-based polymeric formulations of curcumin and dexamethasone avoid refusal of corneal graft due to sustained delivery of corticosteroids [38, 64].

2.3.5 Pulmonology

Pulmonary lung diseases (PLD) comprise cystic fibrosis, asthma, chronic obstructive pulmonary disease (COPD), idiopathic pulmonary fibrosis (IPF), and pulmonary tuberculosis [38]. They are frequently fatal, and currently, there exists no efficient remedy for the complete restoration of lungs affected by PLDs. Traditional therapeutics are used locally or systemically to lungs as nasal drug inhalers. Inhalation of drugs, in which active therapeutic molecules are in the form of an aerosol, may result in burst discharge, and therefore higher risk of lung toxicity. Furthermore, the size of aerosol droplets restricts the efficacy of drugs, as droplets >5 μm do not pass the upper respiratory tract, particles between 1 and 5 μm mainly settle at lower respiratory tract, and drug molecules < 1 μm gets suspended in air and exhaled out of lungs. Nanomaterial-based drug delivery tools permit improved bioavailability, sustained release, reduced dosage, and decreased usage/treatment. Nanomedicine inhalation formulations consist of both natural and synthetic polymeric NPs (alginate, chitosan, PEG, PLGA, and poloxamer) [38, 64, 65]. Furthermore, pulmonary inhalation of polyamidoamine (PAMAM) dendrimers loaded with beclometasone dipropionate

(BDP) as an asthma medication was successful [66]. In addition, a variety of lipid-, polymer-, polysaccharide-, carbon-based, and metallic NP formulations are used for nanodrug or nanovaccine delivery in the therapy of pulmonary immune hemostasis (PIH) [38].

2.3.6 Tissue Engineering

Tissue engineering deals with biocompatible materials that naturally improve the repair and regeneration ability of tissues via their cellular mechanisms. Recently, the development of therapeutic nanomaterials and their direct administration to combat against diseases is gaining popularity in the effective implementation of tissue regeneration methods [67]. Nanodelivery tools used in tissue regeneration include natural polymer NPs (collagen, gelatin, albumin, and chitosan), synthetic polymer NPs (PLA and PLGA), and nonpolymeric NPs (silica-based and metallic type). Calcium phosphate-based NPs are used in the delivery of many growth factors that promote osteoblasts stimulation for the formation of bones [38]. Also, nanodelivery of polymeric NPs or nonpolymeric metallic NPs loaded with synthetic bisphosphonate drugs suppresses bone-resorbing cells, osteoclasts or promotes apoptosis of osteoclasts and thus, they are extensively used in curing osteoporosis. Nanotherapeutic material EquivaBone® (carboxymethyl cellulose, hydroxyapatite, and demineralized bone matrix) is implanted as an osteoinductive bone graft substitute to stimulate the mineralization required for dental and bone tissue regeneration [38]. Moreover, natural or synthetic polymeric NPs containing anti-inflammatory therapeutic agents are delivered to the infected bone tissue region to decrease inflammation of larger wounds, and to improve osteoblasts resorption [38, 68].

2.3.7 Viral Infections

Viral infections are related to diseases that are caused by viruses and commonly they are responsible for high human mortality and threaten public health and safety of human societies worldwide [38]. Examples of viral infections include COVID-19, SARS, MERS, HIV/AIDS, Ebola, Influenza, Yellow fever, Zika, Varicella, Viral gastroenteritis, Viral hepatitis, Human papillomavirus (HPV), and Rheumatoid arthritis (RA). For the successful treatment of viral infections, many nanomaterial-based drug delivery techniques have been created [38]. Selenium (Se) NPs conjugated with Oseltamivir drugs are used as a remedy for Influenza (H1N1). Nanoformulation Se-Oseltamivir displayed low cytotoxicity and high effectivity in the treatment of H1N1 virus-infected kidney cells and it showed higher viability in comparison to oseltamivir against Influenza. Ag NPs loaded with Amantadine exhibited low toxicity in cells infected with Influenza (H1N1 virus). Similarly, diphyllin-loaded polymeric (PLGA, PEG) NPs are very safe drug delivery vehicles with superior biocompatibility and antiviral effectiveness against influenza (H1N1) virus than diphyllin. Squalene-based NPs encapsulating α-tocopherol/adenosine showed high efficacy and good potential to regulate inflammation against COVID-19 coronavirus or SARS/CoV-2 virus. Also, an antigen lipid nanovaccine for treatment of COVID-19 has been produced using liposomes encapsulated cytosine-phosphorothioate-guanine oligodeoxynucleotide (or CpG-ODN) and monophosphoryl lipid A (or MPLA) as adjuvants. This nanovaccine effectively introduces strong humoral and CD4+ and CD8+ T-cell responses and thus shows a good *in vitro* neutralization effect. A complex of Hyaluronic acid (HA)-Au NPs and interferon α (INFα) have been used in hepatitis C virus (HCV) infection treatment and exhibited high stability in human serum medium and sustained targeted drug delivery for one week [38]. A good antiviral activity (against HIV/AIDS) was induced by dispersible and highly hydrophilic oxidized-MWCNT encapsulated benzimidazolone drugs (CHI415 and CHI360) and they further exhibited low cytotoxicityin HIV/AIDS patients. Efavirenz is entrapped into poly(propyleneimine) dendrimers (TuPPI) and is decorated using Tuftsin to obtain final TuPPI NPs that can identify mononuclear phagocytic cells via Tuftsin and significantly caused higher uptake of the drug in HIV infected macrophages in comparison to uninfected cells [69]. Targeting of inflamed tissues by non–drug-loaded or standalone C_{60} fullerenes exhibited good results in the treatment of RA by decreasing synovitis and alleviating resorption and destruction of bones [70].

2.3.8 Other Miscellaneous Types

Nanomaterials obtained by the coating of all-trans retinoic acid (atRA) with $CaCO_3$ or nanoegg-atRA has been used for stimulation of glucose-dependent insulin secretion from islets in streptozotocin-induced diabetes and they not only exhibited pancreatic duodenal homeobox1 (PDX-1) expression but also increased the number of β-cells in the Langerhans islet [71, 72]. Nanoegg-atRA may induce *in vivo* regeneration of β-cells and gives practical knowledge for future diabetes mellitus therapy. Transbuccal transmucosal system (Buccal Patch®) was developed for the delivery of remifentanil to manage cancer pain islet [71, 73]. The device's nanochannel size permits diffusion of the drug from its resource to the specific target tissue at a sustained and regulated rate, thus reducing the risk of extra dosing the patient. Intravenous introduction of ibuprofen containing lipid nanocapsules has the benefit of analgesic in comparison to normal oral formulations. Nanodelivery tools are used for extending the length of the telomeres of natural/artificial chromosomes. PLGA NPs (Telomolecular Corporation, TC) encapsulated vTRT (telomerase reverse transcriptase or nanocircles) are used in the treatment of age-related diseases. Upon mixing DNA nanocircles and oTRT for large-molecule delivery application, the TC industry aims at the development of breakthrough pharmaceutical nanodelivery tools, and it currently works on human tissue regeneration *in vivo* in age-associated disorders [71].

2.4 Commercial Nanodelivery Tools

Although pharmaceutical products of nanomedicine and nanovaccinology industries are subjected to similar testing regulations as other nonnanopharmaceuticals products, certain risks and challenges exist before their widespread commercialization. Physical and chemical factors that are critical to the performance of nanotherapeutic products must be understood in particular. Recently, studies from many clinical trials revealed the potential of nanomedicines and nanovaccines in the prevention and treatment of several infectious diseases. However, many formulations are still in the clinical/testing stages, and the number of commercial medicines is small. With encouraging results from conducted clinical trials, the innovative enhancement in the immunization field is highly anticipated for the years to come. In addition, suitable testing procedures and clinical specifications to regulate the nanomedicine and nanovaccinology products or their manufacturing methods need to be monitored regularly and new efficient strategies should be developed for rapid commercialization of nanodelivery tools. Table 2.2 lists some nanomaterial products that are approved by Food and Drug Administration (FDA) and European Medicines Agency (EMA) agencies and are marketed for targeted drug delivery applications [38].

2.4.1 Industrial Manufacturing

Many pharmaceutical companies are focusing their manufacturing on nanomedicine and nanovaccine products. Nanomaterials used in medication and vaccine delivery have been approved for a greater range of medicinal uses. Some are in premature stages of clinical trials, whereas others

Table 2.2 Some commercial nanomaterial products approved by FDA and EMA.

Nanomateral product	Nanoparticle formulation	Therapeutic agent	Disease indication(s)
Abraxane®	Albumin	Paclitaxel	Non–small lung cancer, Pancreatic cancer
EquivaBone®	Hydroxyapatite (HAp)	---	Osteoinductive bone graft substitute
Feraheme®	Superparamagnetic iron oxide nanoparticle (SPION) covered with dextran.	---	Anemia in chronic kidney disease
Glatopa®	L-glutamic acid polymer with L-alanine, L-lysine, and L-tyrosine (Glatiramer)	---	Multiple sclerosis
Kadcyla®	Maytansine derivative, DM1	Trastuzumab	HER2+ breast cancer
Krystexxa®	PEGylated uricase	Pegloticase	Gout disease
Mepact®	1-Palmitoyl-2-oleoyl-sn-glycero-3-phosphocholine and 1,2-Dioleoyl-sn-glycero- 3-phospho-l-serine liposomes	Mifamurtide	Nonmetastasizing osteosarcoma
NanoTherm®	Nanoparticles of superparamagnetic iron oxide coated with amino silane	---	Glioblastoma, prostate, pancreatic cancer
Onivyde®	Nanoliposomes	Irinotecan	Pancreatic cancer, colorectal cancer

(*Continued*)

Table 2.2 Some commercial nanomaterial products approved by FDA and EMA. (*Continued*)

Nanomateral product	Nanoparticle formulation	Therapeutic agent	Disease indication(s)
Onpattro®	Lipid nanoparticles	Transthyretin targeted siRNA	Transthyretin-mediated amyloidosis
Plegridy®	PEGylated interferon β-1a	Interferon β-1a	Multiple sclerosis
Rebinyn®	Glycopegylated coagulation factor IX	Factor IX	Hemophilia
Vyxeos®	Distearoylphosphatidyl choline, distearoyl phosphatidylglycerol, cholesterol	Daunorubicin, cytarabine	Acute myeloid leukemia

are marketed and currently used in the treatment of infectious diseases. Nanomaterial-based conjugates are promising vehicles for next-generation therapies because of their simple protocols for creation and high manufacturing yield, as well as their potential anticancer activity [71].

2.4.2 Advantages and Disadvantages

Nanomaterial delivery tools offer many advantages, beginning from their broad range in size and finishing at their improved bioavailability. Nanomaterial delivery tools are available in a variety of sizes, components, and shapes, and therefore they offer numerous and versatile applications [9, 10]. In addition, because of their special sizes quite similar to the cell components, these nanomaterials can easily enter into cells via a cellular mechanism known as 'endocytosis' [9]. Nanoemulsions vaccines can be easily accumulated in lymph nodes because of their high affinity for lymphatic systems. Similar novel nanovaccine delivery systems can be used in the treatment of cancer immunotherapy, influenza prophylaxis, and other medical applications that are under clinical research studies [10, 12]. Several types of nanosize additives, such as nanoaluminum, offer several advantages that include safety, easy preparation, and affordable prices [12]. Although many developments occurred in conventional vaccines, their toxicity and instability are major disadvantages, and therefore nanomedicines and nanovaccines present a plethora of opportunities for improving stability and safety via enhancing immune responses in cellular and humoral systems. Furthermore, nanopatch technology vaccination is needle-free, pain-free, cost-efficient, enhances the bioavailability of antigens, and facilitates site-specific delivery of antigens [10].

Nanomedicine and nanovaccinology consider complicated methods for the production of new drugs and vaccines, which need advanced technology machines and equipment, thus making their products very expensive [12]. Furthermore, since different sizes and shapes of nanomaterials are used in the manufacturing of nanomedicines and nanovaccines, the chemical composition of these nanomaterials is very difficult to alter and this may cause some cytotoxicity [12]. Furthermore, nanomedicines and nanovaccines are very small (nanoscale materials) and can be washed away from the body fast [9]. Some biodegradable polymers have limited applications in solid particulate vaccines, which aids in their entrapment to proteins and results in immunogenicity loss upon storage [9]. In addition, liposomal delivery systems exhibit a significant disadvantage in the formulation of nanovaccine that aggregates during its storage [9]. On other hand, the *in vivo* behavior of NPs in vaccine production is a big challenge in the new nanovaccine research and development, as there is a lack of fundamental understanding of how different nanomaterials behave in biological systems [10]. As a result, various nanomedicines and nanovaccine formulations, such as gold, calcium phosphate, and silica NPs, must be thoroughly evaluated before use, which takes additional time, effort, and raw materials.

2.4.3 Risks and Challenges

Surface engineering of NPs using chemical methods can change their biocompatibility potentials. These chemical transformations indicate the need for the development of novel tests/assays that are analytical in the prediction of target characteristics before their functionalization with desired proteins/antigens [10]. Likewise, the uniformity of nanomaterials and reproducibility in the experimental production of nanomedicines and nanovaccines need to be improved. Therefore, it is a considerable and critical standard for quality production of biogenic nanomaterials, where further uniform scaling-up of them to industrial scales is a big concern. VLPs have promising applications because of their easy engineering capabilities, superior flexibility, increased surface characteristics, and potential immunogenic features. Nonetheless, VLPs' ability to rapidly modify the viral proteins that are used in their creation poses a risk [10]. Other adjuvants/nanocarriers that are used in the formulation of core antigen for various types of nanovaccines can pose similar dangers. Direct animal models can be developed for preclinical assessment of such nanomedicines and nanovaccines [10].

2.5 Conclusions and Future Prospects

During the past decade, the improvement of nanomaterial-based therapeutic agents has been extensively studied, and these nanodelivery tools are very important for specific targeting of desired tissues/organs in the treatment of several deadly diseases. At present, many nanomaterials used for targeted drug delivery applications are prepared from lipids or polymers. The ability of nanomaterials to traverse physiological barriers due to their size, shape, porosity, charge, stability, and efficiency have been studied in nanomedicine and nanovaccine formulations for more efficient enhancement of immune responses at cellular and humoral levels. These novel nanomaterials possess many advantages such as high therapeutic plasmid biocompatibility and prolonged, slow antigen delivery to drastically improve immune responses. Although polymeric NPs reveal enormous advantages in the treatment of diseases, they also suffer from some disadvantages such as trouble in scaling up to industrial levels, large consumption of organic solvents for their fabrication, and other problems associated with cytotoxicity, biocompatibility, and immunogenicity. Conversely, lipid-based NPs display a good ability to traverse hard-to-reach regions without further surface modifications due to their chemical composition similarity to that of the cell membrane. Therefore, lipid-based nanodelivery tools are preferred for future generation therapeutics. Until now, therapeutic NPs are mainly developed for the prevention or treatment of a single disease only. But, researchers began combining different drugs and various NPs, so the therapeutic NPs future is guided along the direction of designing multitherapeutic NPs for the treatment of many diseases.

Although nanomaterial-based delivery tools considerably account for targeted therapy with their decreased side effects, enhanced efficacy, and good bioavailability, very little information exists about the clearance, metabolism, and toxicity of NPs. The majority of research publications reveal that NPs entrap medicinal drugs and vaccinations. Other medicinal investigations on enzymes, genes, and DNA/RNA, on the other hand, are scarce. The importance of published information on nanodelivery tools is frequently revealed with the number of patents filed but, only a few of these pass-through clinical trials to be commercially accessible in the market. This recommends that more investigations are needed in the future to further understand the fabrication, formulation, and toxicity of NPs. Furthermore, the cost of nanomedicines and nanovaccines manufacturing at larger industrial scales are other key issues that need to be addressed in near future. Detail understanding of the NPs characteristics, their interactions with the biological environment (targeting receptors), and deriving their exact cellular mechanisms of action in pathophysiological diseases will help in overcoming several limitations and thereby establishing new strategies for prevention, treatment, and diagnosis of many incurable diseases. Both nanomedicine and nanovaccinology will be the future of medical research, and nanomaterial-based therapeutics occupy the core of it. However, thorough groundwork needs to be done before reaping the success/prosperity of the field. Most significantly, detailed long-term toxicity/safety studies of NPs should be conducted during the clinical trials. In the future, discoveries of novel infection mechanisms and new therapeutics will direct to innovative paths of introducing more safer and effective nanomaterial-based therapeutics for the treatment of lethal infectious diseases.

Acknowledgments

The author is grateful to Abinnovus Consulting Pvt. Ltd, Technology Business Incubator, University of Madras, Guindy-Campus, India for providing the necessary facilities required for completion of the work.

References

1. Karthikeyan, S., Bhatlu, M.L.D., Sukanya, K., Jayan, N., Nanovaccination: Evolution and review. *J. Crit. Rev.*, 7, 7, 971–975, 2020.
2. Shafer, R.W., Rhee, S.Y., Pillay, D., Miller, V., Sandstrom, P., Schapiro, J.M., Kuritzkes, D.R., Bennett, D., HIV-1 protease and reverse transcriptase mutations for drug resistance surveillance. *AIDS (London, England)*, 21, 2, 215, 2007.
3. Singh, L., Kruger, H.G., Maguire, G.E., Govender, T., Parboosing, R., The role of nanotechnology in the treatment of viral infections. *Ther. Adv. Infect. Dis.*, 4, 4, 105–131, 2017.
4. Mao, L., Chen, Z., Wang, Y., Chen, C., Design and application of nanoparticles as vaccine adjuvants against human corona virus infection. *J. Inorg. Biochem.*, 219, 1114545, 2021.
5. Mehendale, R., Joshi, M., Patravale, V.B., Nanomedicines for treatment of viral diseases. *Crit. Rev.™ Ther. Drug Carrier Syst.*, 30, 1, 1–49, 2013.

6. Cosgrove, S.E., The relationship between antimicrobial resistance and patient outcomes: Mortality, length of hospital stay, and healthcare costs. *Clin. Infect. Dis.*, 42, Supplement_2, S82–S89, 2006.
7. Sulczewski, F.B., Liszbinski, R.B., Romão, P.R., Junior, L.C.R., Nanoparticle vaccines against viral infections. *Arch. Virol.*, 163, 9, 2313–2325, 2018.
8. Facciolà, A., Visalli, G., Laganà, P., La Fauci, V., Squeri, R., Pellicanò, G.F., Nunnari, G., Trovato, M., Di Pietro, A., The new era of vaccines: The nanovaccinology. *Eur. Rev. Med. Pharmacol. Sci.*, 23, 16, 7163–7182, 2019.
9. Zhao, L., Seth, A., Wibowo, N., Zhao, C.X., Mitter, N., Yu, C., Middelberg, A.P., Nanoparticle vaccines. *Vaccine*, 32, 3, 327–337, 2014.
10. Yadav, H.K., Dibi, M., Mohammad, A., Srouji, A.E., Nanovaccines formulation and applications-a review. *J. Drug Delivery Sci. Technol.*, 44, 380–3875, 2018.
11. Pezzotti, P., Bellino, S., Prestinaci, F., Iacchini, S., Lucaroni, F., Camoni, L., Barbieri, M.M., Ricciardi, W., Stefanelli, P., Rezza, G., The impact of immunization programs on 10 vaccine preventable diseases in Italy: 1900–2015. *Vaccine*, 36, 11, 1435–1443, 2018.
12. Li, S., Nakaya, H.I., Kazmin, D.A., Oh, J.Z., Pulendran, B., Systems biological approaches to measure and understand vaccine immunity in humans. *Semin. Immunol.*, 25, 3, 209–218, Academic Press, 2013.
13. Oberg, A.L., Kennedy, R.B., Li, P., Ovsyannikova, I.G., Poland, G.A., Systems biology approaches to new vaccine development. *Curr. Opin. Immunol.*, 23, 3, 436–443, 2011.
14. Nuismer, S.L., Althouse, B.M., May, R., Bull, J.J., Stromberg, S.P., Antia, R., Eradicating infectious disease using weakly transmissible vaccines. *Proc. R. Soc. B: Biol. Sci.*, 283, 1841, 20161903, 2016.
15. Sahoo, S.K., Parveen, S., Panda, J.J., The present and future of nanotechnology in human healthcare. *Nanomed.: Nanotechnol. Biol. Med.*, 3, 1, 20–31, 2007.
16. Bayda, S., Adeel, M., Tuccinardi, T., Cordani, M., Rizzolio, F., The history of nanoscience and nanotechnology: from chemical–physical applications to nanomedicine. *Molecules*, 25, 1, 112, 2020.
17. Feynman, R., There's plenty of room at the bottom. *Science*, 254, 1300–13015, 1991.
18. Taniguchi, N., On the Basic Concept of Nano-Technology. *Proceedings of the International Conference on Production Engineering*, Tokyo, Japan Society of Precision Engineering, 1974.
19. Petros, R.A. and DeSimone, J.M., Strategies in the design of nanoparticles for therapeutic applications. *Nat. Rev. Drug Discovery*, 9, 8, 615–627, 2010.
20. McNeil, S.E., Unique benefits of nanotechnology to drug delivery and diagnostics, in: *Characterization of Nanoparticles Intended for Drug Delivery*, pp. 3–8, Humana Press, Clifton, NJ, 2011.

21. Gupta, B.M., Dhawan, S.M., Ahmed, K.M., Mamdapur, G.M., Nanomedicine Research in India: A Bibliometric Assessment of Publications Output during 2002-20. *Int. J. Pharm. Investig.*, 11, 2, 143–153, 2021.
22. Bragazzi, N.L., Nanomedicine: Insights from a bibliometrics-based analysis of emerging publishing and research trends. *Medicina*, 55, 12, 785, 2019.
23. Rafiqi, S.I., Kumar, S., Zehra, A., Kumar, D., Jain, S., Sethi, K., Yadav, P.K., Nanovaccinology: Dawn of biomimetic vaccine carriers, *J. Entomol. Zool. Stud.*, 5, 2, 795–802, 2017.
24. Mahapatro, A. and Singh, D.K., Biodegradable nanoparticles are excellent vehicle for site directed *in-vivo* delivery of drugs and vaccines. *J. Nanobiotechnol.*, 9, 1, 1–11, 2011.
25. Xu, Q., Lv, Y., Dong, C., Sreeprased, T.S., Tian, A., Zhang, H., Tang, Y., Yu, Z., Li, N., Three-dimensional micro/nanoscale architectures: fabrication and applications. *Nanoscale*, 7, 25, 10883–10895, 2015.
26. Pulendran, B., Li, S., Nakaya, H.I., Systems vaccinology. *Immunity*, 33, 4, 516–529, 2010.
27. Kalkanidis, M., Pietersz, G.A., Xiang, S.D., Mottram, P.L., Crimeen-Irwin, B., Ardipradja, K., Plebanski, M., Methods for nano-particle based vaccine formulation and evaluation of their immunogenicity. *Methods*, 40, 1, 20–29, 2006.
28. Niikura, K., Matsunaga, T., Suzuki, T., Kobayashi, S., Yamaguchi, H., Orba, Y., Kawaguchi, A., Hasegawa, H., Kajino, K., Ninomiya, T., Ijiro, K., Gold nanoparticles as a vaccine platform: Influence of size and shape on immunological responses *in vitro* and *in vivo*. *ACS Nano*, 7, 5, 3926–3938, 2013.
29. Stone, J.W., Thornburg, N.J., Blum, D.L., Kuhn, S.J., Wright, D.W., Crowe Jr, J.E., Gold nanorod vaccine for respiratory syncytial virus. *Nanotechnology*, 24, 29, 295102, 2013.
30. Xu, L., Liu, Y., Chen, Z., Li, W., Liu, Y., Wang, L., Liu, Y., Wu, X., Ji, Y., Zhao, Y., Ma, L., Surface-engineered gold nanorods: Promising DNA vaccine adjuvant for HIV-1 treatment. *Nano Lett.*, 12, 4, 2003–2012, 2012.
31. Benezra, M., Penate-Medina, O., Zanzonico, P.B., Schaer, D., Ow, H., Burns, A., DeStanchina, E., Longo, V., Herz, E., Iyer, S., Wolchok, J., Multimodal silica nanoparticles are effective cancer-targeted probes in a model of human melanoma. *J. Clin. Invest.*, 121, 7, 2768–2780, 2011.
32. Cheng, K., El-Boubbou, K., Landry, C.C., Binding of HIV-1 gp120 glycoprotein to silica nanoparticles modified with CD4 glycoprotein and CD4 peptide fragments. *ACS Appl. Mater. Interfaces*, 4, 1, 235–243, 2012.
33. Bogala, M.R., Phyto-fabricated Metal Oxide Nanoparticles as Promising Antibacterial Agents, in: *Bio-Manufactured Nanomaterials*, pp. 279–297, Springer, Cham, 2021.
34. Irfan, M., Jeshurun, A., Baraneedharan, P., Reddy, B.M., A photoluminescence study of nitrogen-doped carbon quantum dots/hydroxyapatite (NCQDs/HAp) nanocomposites. *Mater. Technol.*, 36, 1–12, 2021.

35. Irfan, M., Suprajaa, P.S., Baraneedharan, P., Reddy, B.M., A comparative study of nanohydroxyapetite obtained from natural shells and wet chemical process. *J. Mater. Sci. Surf. Eng.*, 7, 938–9435, 2020.
36. Irfan, M., Suprajaa, P.S., Praveen, R., Reddy, B.M., Microwave-assisted one-step synthesis of nanohydroxyapetite from fish bones and mussel shells. *Mater. Lett.*, 282, 1286855, 2021.
37. Joyappa, D.H., Kumar, C.A., Banumathi, N., Reddy, G.R., Suryanarayana, V.V., Calcium phosphate nanoparticle prepared with foot and mouth disease virus P1-3CD gene construct protects mice and guinea pigs against the challenge virus. *Vet. Microbiol.*, 139, 1-2, 58–66, 2009.
38. Yetisgin, A.A., Cetinel, S., Zuvin, M., Kosar, A., Kutlu, O., Therapeutic nanoparticles and their targeted delivery applications. *Molecules*, 25, 9, 2193, 2020.
39. Peek, L.J., Middaugh, C.R., Berkland, C., Nanotechnology in vaccine delivery. *Adv. Drug Delivery Rev.*, 60, 8, 915–928, 2008.
40. Danhier, F., Ansorena, E., Silva, J.M., Coco, R., Le Breton, A., Préat, V., PLGA-based nanoparticles: an overview of biomedical applications. *J. Controlled Release*, 161, 2, 505–522, 2012.
41. Akagi, T., Baba, M., Akashi, M., Biodegradable nanoparticles as vaccine adjuvants and delivery systems: Regulation of immune responses by nanoparticle-based vaccine, in: *Polymers in Nanomedicine*, pp. 31–64, 2011.
42. Ferreira, S.A., Gama, F.M., Vilanova, M., Polymeric nanogels as vaccine delivery systems. *Nanomed.: Nanotechnol. Biol. Med.*, 9, 2, 159–173, 2013.
43. Nochi, T., Yuki, Y., Takahashi, H., Sawada, S.I., Mejima, M., Kohda, T., Harada, N., Kong, I.G., Sato, A., Kataoka, N., Tokuhara, D., Nanogel antigenic protein-delivery system for adjuvant-free intranasal vaccines. *Nat. Mater.*, 9, 7, 572–578, 2010.
44. Boas, U. and Heegaard, P.M., Dendrimers in drug research. *Chem. Soc. Rev.*, 33, 1, 43–63, 2004.
45. Koo, O.M., Rubinstein, I., Onyuksel, H., Role of nanotechnology in targeted drug delivery and imaging: a concise review. *Nanomed.: Nanotechnol. Biol. Med.*, 1, 3, 193–212, 2005.
46. Daraee, H., Etemadi, A., Kouhi, M., Alimirzalu, S., Akbarzadeh, A., Application of liposomes in medicine and drug delivery. *Artif. Cells Nanomed. Biotechnol.*, 44, 1, 381–391, 2016.
47. Watson, D.S., Endsley, A.N., Huang, L., Design considerations for liposomal vaccines: Influence of formulation parameters on antibody and cell-mediated immune responses to liposome associated antigens. *Vaccine*, 30, 13, 2256–2272, 2012.
48. Ahmad, Z., Shah, A., Siddiq, M., Kraatz, H.B., Polymeric micelles as drug delivery vehicles. *RSC Adv.*, 4, 33, 17028–17038, 2014.
49. Le Garrec, D., Ranger, M., Leroux, J.C., Micelles in anticancer drug delivery. *Am. J. Drug Deliv.*, 2, 1, 15–42, 2004.

50. Aucouturier, J., Dupuis, L., Deville, S., Ascarateil, S., Ganne, V., Montanide ISA 720 and 51: A new generation of water in oil emulsions as adjuvants for human vaccines. *Expert Rev. Vaccines*, 1, 1, 111–118, 2002.
51. Wang, T., Zou, M., Jiang, H., Ji, Z., Gao, P., Cheng, G., Synthesis of a novel kind of carbon nanoparticle with large mesopores and macropores and its application as an oral vaccine adjuvant. *Eur. J. Pharm. Sci.*, 44, 5, 653–659, 2011.
52. Solomonov, A. and Shimanovich, U., Self-assembly in protein-based bionanomaterials. *Isr. J. Chem.*, 60, 12, 1152–1170, 2020.
53. Homhuan, A., Prakongpan, S., Poomvises, P., Maas, R.A., Crommelin, D.J., Kersten, G.F., Jiskoot, W., Virosome and ISCOM vaccines against Newcastle disease: Preparation, characterization and immunogenicity. *Eur. J. Pharm. Sci.*, 22, 5, 459–468, 2004.
54. Zeltins, A., Construction and characterization of virus-like particles: A review. *Mol. Biotechnol.*, 53, 1, 92–107, 2013.
55. Davis, M.E., Chen, Z., Shin, D.M., Nanoparticle therapeutics: An emerging treatment modality for cancer, in: *Nanoscience and Technology: A Collection of Reviews from Nature Journals*, pp. 239–250, 2010.
56. Zaheer, T., Pal, K., Zaheer, I., Topical review on nano-vaccinology: Biochemical promises and key challenges. *Process Biochem.*, 100, 237–244, 2020.
57. Chidambaram, M., Manavalan, R., Kathiresan, K., Nanotherapeutics to overcome conventional cancer chemotherapy limitations. *J. Pharm. Pharm. Sci.*, 14, 1, 67–77, 2011.
58. Silverman, J.A. and Deitcher, S.R., Marqibo® (vincristine sulfate liposome injection) improves the pharmacokinetics and pharmacodynamics of vincristine. *Cancer Chemother. Pharmacol.*, 71, 3, 555–564, 2013.
59. Wohlfart, S., Gelperina, S., Kreuter, J., Transport of drugs across the blood–brain barrier by nanoparticles. *J. Controlled Release*, 161, 2, 264–273, 2012.
60. Bell, C., Anderson, J., Ganguly, T., Prescott, J., Capila, I., Lansing, J.C., Sachleben, R., Iyer, M., Fier, I., Roach, J., Storey, K., Development of Glatopa® (glatiramer acetate): The first FDA-approved generic disease-modifying therapy for relapsing forms of multiple sclerosis. *J. Pharm. Pract.*, 31, 5, 481–488, 2018.
61. Arzani, G., Haeri, A., Daeihamed, M., Bakhtiari-Kaboutaraki, H., Dadashzadeh, S., Niosomal carriers enhance oral bioavailability of carvedilol: Effects of bile salt-enriched vesicles and carrier surface charge. *Int. J. Nanomed.*, 10, 47975, 2015.
62. Phillips, M.A., Gran, M.L., Peppas, N.A., Targeted nanodelivery of drugs and diagnostics. *Nano Today*, 5, 2, 143–159, 2010.
63. Sharaf, M.G., Cetinel, S., Heckler, L., Damji, K., Unsworth, L., Montemagno, C., Nanotechnology-based approaches for ophthalmology applications: Therapeutic and diagnostic strategies. *Asia-Pac. J. Ophthal.*, 3, 3, 172–180, 2014.

64. Joseph, R.R. and Venkatraman, S.S., Drug delivery to the eye: What benefits do nanocarriers offer? *Nanomedicine*, 12, 6, 683–702, 2017.
65. Yhee, J.Y., Im, J., Nho, R.S., Advanced therapeutic strategies for chronic lung disease using nanoparticle-based drug delivery. *J. Clin. Med.*, 5, 9, 82, 2016.
66. Nasr, M., Najlah, M., D'Emanuele, A., Elhissi, A., PAMAM dendrimers as aerosol drug nanocarriers for pulmonary delivery via nebulization. *Int. J. Pharm.*, 461, 1-2, 242–250, 2014.
67. Gera, S., Sampathi, S., Dodoala, S., Role of nanoparticles in drug delivery and regenerative therapy for bone diseases. *Curr. Drug Deliv.*, 14, 7, 904–916, 2017.
68. Gonçalves, R.M., Pereira, A.C.L., Pereira, I.O., Oliveira, M.J., Barbosa, M.A., Macrophage response to chitosan/poly-(γ-glutamic acid) nanoparticles carrying an anti-inflammatory drug. *J. Mater. Sci.: Mater. Med.*, 26, 4, 167, 2015.
69. Dutta, T., Garg, M., Jain, N.K., Targeting of efavirenz loaded tuftsin conjugated poly (propyleneimine) dendrimers to HIV infected macrophages *in vitro*. *Eur. J. Pharm. Sci.*, 34, 2-3, 181–189, 2008.
70. Yudoh, K., Karasawa, R., Masuko, K., Kato, T., Water-soluble fullerene (C_{60}) inhibits the development of arthritis in the rat model of arthritis. *Int. J. Nanomed.*, 4, 2175, 2009.
71. Jain, K.K., *The Handbook of Nanomedicine*, Humana Press, New York, NY, 2017.
72. Yamaguchi, Y. and Igarashi, R., Nanotechnology for therapy of type 2 diabetes. *Nihon Rinsho. Japanese J. Clin. Med.*, 64, 2, 295–300, 2006.
73. Sprintz, M., Benedetti, C., Ferrari, M., Applied nanotechnology for the management of breakthrough cancer pain. *Minerva Anestesiol.*, 71, 7-8, 419–423, 2005.

3

Nanovaccinology and Superbugs

Sandhya Kalathilparambil Santhosh, Kaviya Parampath Kootery, Mridul Umesh, Preethi Mariam Alex, Meghna Mani, Adina Roy and Suma Sarojini*

Department of Life Sciences, CHRIST (Deemed to be University), Bangalore, India

Abstract

Superbugs pose a serious threat to humans as many of the currently available antibiotics are not effective in treating the diseases inflicted by these microbes. Among the different bacteria causing clinical infections, *Klebsiella pneumoniae, Escherichia coli, Serratia marcescens, Pseudomonas aeruginosa, Staphylococcus aureus, Proteus mirabilis,* and so on, are some of the most vicious ones emerging at an unprecedented rate with huge impact on public health. In this context, prophylactic measures for these diseases assume great significance and NVs indeed fit in as a promising measure. Sustained release, improved antigen stability, better immunogenicity, better access to lymph nodes and low minimum immunotoxicity translates to the better efficacy of nano-based vaccines. Lipid-based NP (nanoparticles), dendrimers, Polymeric NP, self-assembled peptide NP, virus like particles (VLPs), and so on, are the promising NV (nanovaccines) delivery approaches. Improvisations of NVs by decorating NP surfaces with ligands that target specific immune cells like the dendritic cells is also a promising approach to induce both T and B cell responses. The current review focuses on the breakthroughs in the NV domain with the challenges and opportunities of creating NVs to curb the menace of superbugs.

***Keywords*:** NVs, superbugs, multidrug resistance, gold NP, virus like particle (VLP)

**Corresponding author*: suma@christuniversity.in

Kaushik Pal (ed.) Nanovaccinology as Targeted Therapeutics, (53–76) © 2022 Scrivener Publishing LLC

3.1 Introduction

The discovery of antibiotics has undoubtedly revolutionized the field of healthcare and medicines by equipping humans to successfully battle against infectious agents, many of which had taken away lives of millions of humans in the past. However, sadly, the misuse and overuse of these wonder drugs have created the emergence and exponential increase of antibiotic-resistant microbes commonly referred to as superbugs [1]. The major superbugs posing grave concern in the healthcare sector belong to the ESKAPE group of organisms—*Enterococcus faecium, Staphylococcus aureus, Klebsiella pneumoniae, Acinetobacter baumannii, Pseudomonas aeruginosa,* and *Enterobacter* spp. [2]. The emergence of superbugs is majorly due to a repertoire of factors prevailing in our hospitals and environment. Anthropogenic contamination with residual antibiotics has also led to the conversion of environmental isolates into resistant strains and is thus visualized as a grave concern just like hospital acquired resistance patterns [3]. The nonjudicial antibiotic usage in agricultural formulation and their incorporation in animal feeds have clearly marked the increase in antibiotic resistance in microbes [4]. Self-medication tends to be one of the major factors responsible for emergence of antibiotic resistance. Resistance of antibiotics is a genetic phenomena in which the processes of natural selection allows the resistant bacteria harbouring plasmids responsible for antibiotic resistance to thrive and multiply in the environment leading to the formation of a family of superbugs making them champions of evolution [5].

There are multiple ways in which antibiotic resistance is initiated in microorganisms [6]. The most common pattern of resistance observed against β-lactams is through mutational alteration of their target protein in microbes [7]. Enzymatic inactivation of antibiotics by superbugs is majorly through the production of one or more of the hydrolytic enzymes, like β-lactamases, cephalosporinases, and esterase [8]. The tendency of pathogens to endow resistant genes from the environment and harbor them in their genome as evident from next-generation sequencing studies was reported to be one of the significant reasons for acceleration in the number and diversity of superbugs [9]. Another mechanism that the bacteria develops to circumvent the effect of antibiotics is bypassing the target molecule as observed in the case of vancomycin resistance [6]. Yet another interesting mechanism used by superbugs in their defence mechanism against antibiotics is the formation of biofilms. These are hydrated polymers produced by pathogenic bacteria, which makes the entry of cell wall targeting antibiotics impossible [10]. Other methods used by superbugs attributing their drug resistance include preventing drug access to targets, efflux of drugs using pumps and altering membrane permeability [6]. More than seven lakh people die every year globally due to drug-resistant superbugs and hence the World Health Organization has named antibiotic resistance as one of the gravest public health threats of the present century [11].

3.2 Need for Nanovaccines

Over the years scientists across the globe have tried to come up with better ways of combating diseases. The human and animal population have seen many deadly diseases, which have wiped out huge chunks of the population in many countries. Antimicrobial drugs and vaccines have been developed to circumvent this problem. The requirement for vaccines is very crucial not only because of the resistance that organisms develop against antibiotics but also because vaccines are a much better alternative when compared to conventional antibiotics. Through the process of spontaneous mutation, one in a billion bacteria can survive in the presence of an antibacterial drug. However, in the case of vaccines, the host system is trained to build an immune response even before the pathogen enters the host body. When bacteria enters the host body, they are neutralized at the beginning of the infection when their number is very low, maybe a few hundred or thousands. Hence, the mutation event of one-in-a-billion is very unlikely to occur [12].

However, some of the main shortcomings of conventional vaccines include fluctuating efficacies, low immunogenicity, and so on. The level of immunogenicity can be improved by modifying and controlling the vaccine formulation using NT [13]. The use of NT for developing vaccines has proven to be beneficial in several aspects. When compared with traditional vaccines, NVs have enhanced therapeutic effect, uniform distribution of the drug, lesser side effects, and so on [14]. NVs are mainly nanocarriers that are synthesized in various sizes, compositions, and surface properties [15]. Some nanocarriers have been designed in such a way that they can codeliver both the antigen and adjuvant at the same time [16].

The greatest advantage of NPs is their size. Because of their size of 1 to 100 nm for at least one dimension, they are similar to few cellular components and therefore can enter into living cells by the process of pinocytosis [17] and also reach cellular compartments more easily, thereby conferring targeted drug delivery. This also increases the cellular uptake of antigens and hence increases the efficiency of antigen recognition and presentation [18]. Moreover, with the emergence of multidrug-resistant (MDR) or extremely drug-resistant (XDR) organisms, like in the case of

Mycobacterium tuberculosis, there is an increasing challenge for scientists across the world to treat such diseases [19]. A promising alternative to reduce this menace is the use of NT in formulating and delivering drugs and vaccines. Moreover, it is also necessary to shift to such new technologies as there are many challenges in the conventional mode of drug delivery—stability issues, nontargeted approach, drug resistance issues, unequal drug distribution at the targeted site and long duration of therapy [20].

Attractive features of NVs, when compared to conventional vaccines, is the potential to overcome immune tolerance and eradicate the need for booster doses thereby decreasing the frequency of doses leading to increased patient compliance. Moreover, NV can induce both cell-mediated and antibody-mediated immunity. NVs are synthesized by incorporating pathogen-specific antigenic particles and synthetic or natural nanomaterials in an attempt to achieve a controlled immune response. Necessary components of pathogens, called subunits like peptides, polysaccharides, membranes, proteins, capsules, and toxins, are required to make the vaccine tunable and safer. When NPs are used with these, they can provide more stability with less proteasomal degradation of antigenic subunits [21].

Adjuvants, an important component of vaccines, produce coimmunostimulatory and immunomodulatory signals and tackles the issue of small subunits being less immunogenic. However, some of the conventional adjuvants cause side effects with individual-specific response, immune tolerance to target antigen, and unwanted reactions towards self-antigens. Hence biocompatible NP are used, which can be directly used as adjuvants and can be used in place of strong conventional adjuvants like Alum [21]. For subunit vaccines, NT plays an important role in providing multiple platforms to produce adjuvants—polymeric NPs, self-assembling peptides, liposomes, inorganic NPs, and so on [22]. Another interesting feature of NPs is their ability to mimic the features of pathogens like viruses. The poor immunogenicity of conventional vaccines can be improved by using NPs. For example, in peptide subunit vaccines, multiple peptide epitopes can be created in a repetitive pattern thereby mimicking the pathogen structure [23]. The new generation vaccines no longer focus on containing live or inactivated whole pathogens but rather contain pathogen subunits, and their immunogenicity is focused on specific antigenic epitopes [24]. Production of such subunits is easier than producing the whole live pathogens and is also highly immunogenic and safe. This goal also can be achieved using NVs. Polymeric NPs that have TLR ligands have the potential to induce robust immunity against the H1N1 influenza strain in

Rhesus macaques [25] and enhance humoral responses to malarial antigens in mice [26].

3.3 Types of Nanovaccines

NVs are based on the principle of using NPs made of proteins, lipids, metals, polymers, or even graphene as carriers to deliver the antigen into the host. The antigens are combined with the carrier NPs by bringing about certain surface modifications on the carriers or by encapsulation of the antigen [27]. Nanosized particles could also be viruses that can display the antigenic peptide on their surfaces Such genetically modified virus like particles are observed to be highly immunogenic as they showcase many features of pathogenic organisms, for example, shape, size and pathogen associated molecular patterns (PAMPS) [28].

3.3.1 Subunit Vaccines

Subunit (SU) vaccines consist of specific antigenic fragments that can elicit an immune response in the host and at the same time not cause an infection as the infectious organism or their entire nucleic acid is not being used [29]. However, SU vaccines are quite weak and therefore are most of the time combined with an adjuvant for a strong immune response. Carriers like polymers, chitosan and liposomes have been extensively used in the preparation of SUNVs. A relevant example of SUNV currently is a vaccine against SARS-COV-2. Of the several NVs that have been developed against SARS-COV-2 virus, using S1 SU, which is one part of the transmembrane spike glycoprotein, has given tremendous results. This component binds to the angiotensin-converting enzyme 2 (ACE-2) receptor in the host and activates the S2 subunit of the S protein to fuse the viral membrane with the host membrane. Cationic liposomes were used as carrier vehicles to deliver the S1 SU. At neutral pH the anionic S1 SU was adsorbed onto the cationic surface. The vaccine was found to activate both humoral and cell-mediated response in mice and sera from the vaccinated mice had the potential to curb virus infection in Vero cell lines [30].

Salmonella infection is a menace in the poultry industry. Extensive use of antibiotics in chickens have made it worse than good. Therefore, it was the need of the hour to come up with a vaccine against this superbug to protect chickens and thereby restrict zoonoses. A chitosan-based NV has been found to be very effective against *Salmonella enterica* serovar *enteritidis.* The amino and carboxyl groups of chitosan form hydrogen bonds with mucus glycoproteins due to which chitosan is able to adhere to the intestinal cells. The oral NV was prepared using outer membrane proteins (OMPs) and flagellin with chitosan and was seen to mitigate Salmonellosis in chicken [31].

3.3.2 Conjugate Vaccines

Conjugate vaccines came into existence in order to make the host react and produce antibodies to the otherwise weakly immunogenic substances, mainly capsular polysaccharides of several bacteria. To deal with meningococcus and pneumococcus, purified polysaccharides were used as vaccines. However, it showed only partial efficacy in adults and didn't show any response in infants for whom the vaccine was a requirement. It was in the 1980s, when John Robbins and Rachel Schneerson from Maryland and David Smith and Porter Anderson from New York, independently figured out that the immunogenicity of bacterial capsular polysaccharides increase manifold when covalently linked to a carrier protein. By using this technique, they were able to bring out a vaccine against *Haemophilus influenzae* that was very efficient in infants and children, thereby preventing meningitis in them [32]. Since then, a lot has progressed in the field of conjugate vaccines and the latest development in the NV domain is the use of Solid Lipid Nanoparticles (SLN) conjugated with alginate to prevent infections caused by *Pseudomonas aeruginosa*, a common causative agent for nosocomial infections. Over time, they have gained resistance to multiple antibiotics which is a matter of serious concern. Alginate antigen is a weak immunogen but is capable of producing antibodies that can kill the bacteria when it infects the host. Therefore, to increase the immunogenicity of alginate antigen in the host, alginate was conjugated with SLNs. Vaccinated mice showed better antibody titres to defend the organism when compared to the mice immunized with purified alginate alone [33].

3.3.3 RNA Vaccines

RNA vaccines come under the broad domain of vaccination called nucleic acid therapeutics. *In vitro* transcribed mRNA that translated into proteins, was an observation made in 1990 that definitely paved the way in discovering the importance of RNA vaccines. However, around that time DNA vaccines and protein-based therapeutics were in the limelight because of the apprehensions related to mRNA instability. However, the last decade has seen a radical development of mRNA vaccines because of its safety, efficacy and the ease at which it can be produced. mRNA could be easily degraded by the omnipresent ribonucleases. To overcome this challenge, several carrier proteins have been in use to deliver the mRNA efficiently into the cytosol of the cell. Once taken up by the cell, the mRNA undergoes translation and the resultant protein undergoes post translational modification that ensures correct folding of the protein. Further the mRNA is cleared from the system by a natural process [34].

Presently, the mRNA vaccines can be divided into two groups: conventional mRNA vaccine and self-amplifying mRNA vaccine. The conventional mRNA vaccine has the antigen ORF flanked by untranslated regions (UTRs) and a poly (A) tail added at the 3′ end. The self-amplifying mRNA vaccines involve the use of ss positive sense RNA viruses, wherein the structural genes of the viral genome are replaced by the gene of interest, ie., antigen. They are named self-amplifying vaccines because of their ability to direct self-replication by synthesizing RNA dependent RNA polymerase complexes that leads to production of multiple copies of the mRNA transcript and therefore high expression levels of the antigen, when taken up into the host cytosol. The self-amplifying mRNA vaccines have an edge over the conventional ones in this regard [35].

3.3.4 Reverse Vaccinology

Reverse vaccinology makes use of computational tools to identify antigens that can be used as vaccines. These should be however experimented with, in the laboratory before arriving at a conclusion regarding their immunogenicity. Only the initial anticipation is done using computational techniques [36]. It is quite impossible to achieve this without comparative genomics and structural biology. The whole genome database of several organisms helps us demarcate the less virulent forms of certain organisms from the hypervirulent ones by just spotting the unique, disease related genes [37]. The procedure revolves around sequencing the whole genome of pathogenic organisms and cloning each gene into a vector to study the proteins the gene codes for. For a long time, there were no vaccines available against *Neisseria meningitidis* serogroup B that causes meningitis in children. Attenuated vaccines were inefficient and therefore there had to be a breakthrough. All the proteins were assessed computationally to see if they could be potential antigens. Thus, about 350 genes that were screened to be surface proteins, were cloned into expression vectors and expressed in *E. coli*. The fractions that elicited an immune response in mice were studied in detail to analyse the immunogenicity of each protein. Of the 350 proteins that were analysed only 29

Table 3.1 Types of nanovaccines against superbugs.

Superbug species	Nanovaccine formulation	Type of vaccine	Reference
Campylobacter jejuni	Chitosan with DNA	Subunit	[39]
Escherichia coli	Gold nanoparticle combined with Entero Haemorrhagic *Escherichia coli* (EHEC) antigens	Subunit	[40]
Klebsiella pneumoniae	Outer membrane vesicles from carbapenem-resistant *Klebsiella pneumoniae* with Bovine Serum Albumin (BSA)	Conjugate	[41]
Mycobacterium tuberculosis	Chitosan nanoparticles with Mycobacterium lipids	Lipid based	[42]
Staphylococcus aureus	Extracellular vesicles coated with indocyanine green (ICG)-loaded magnetic mesoporous silica nanoparticles (MSN)	Multi-antigenic	[43]
Streptococcus pneumoniae	Trimethyl chitosan conjugated with B cell epitope and T cell epitope	Conjugate	[44]

proteins proved to be potential candidates [38]. Some of the NVs against superbugs are listed in Table 3.1.

3.3.5 Biomimetic Nanovaccines

3.3.5.1 Biomimetic Membranes

Biomimetic membranes are those that mimic biological membranes in structure and function. The physical properties like size, charge, permeability, flexibility, rigidity, and interaction with the surrounding environment makes these membranes a promising vaccine carrier. Biomimetic membrane materials can be natural ones or artificially engineered using modified proteins. NP doped membranes showed higher efficiency as

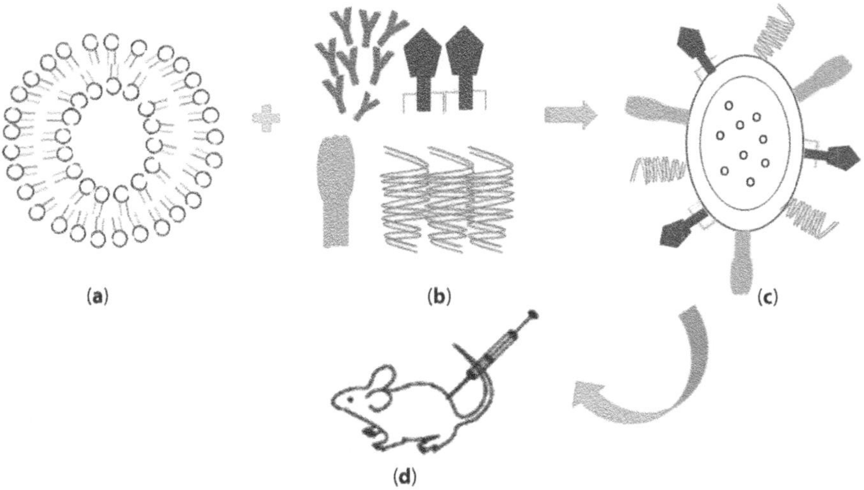

Figure 3.1 Schematic representation of biomimetic membranes and adjuvants as vaccines. (a) Biomimetic membranes. (b) Adjuvants like antigens, virus like proteins, toxoids and transmembrane proteins. (c) Biomimetic membrane-coated adjuvants. (d) Subcutaneous administration of biomimetic membrane vaccine.

vaccines. Cell membrane coated NPs are also used for drug delivery, imaging and photo therapies. NPs with reduced size and varied shapes can move through the epithelial membrane pores for site specific drug delivery. Membranes of RBCs, platelets, WBCs, cancer cells, stem cells, and bacterial outer membranes were coated with NPs of gold, iron oxide, silica, and nanogels. Cell membranes possessing cellular immunity, when doped with NPs, activate interferons and T cells for releasing cytokines and chemokines which in turn shows immune associated functions [45–48]). Biomimetic NVs help in the codelivery of antigens and immunomodulators together involving site-specific targeted delivery of the antigen or the drug. Biomimetic NVs with multiple immunoregulators increase the immune responses along with target specific delivery of antigen with no side effects to the adjacent cells [49]. Figure 3.1 depicts the usage of biomimetic membranes and adjuvants as vaccines.

3.3.5.2 Outer Membrane Vesicle Nanoparticles

Outer membrane vesicles (OMVs) are spherical liposomal membranes secreted by Gram negative bacteria having biologically active proteins. These proteins possess multiple functions implied in bacterial communication,

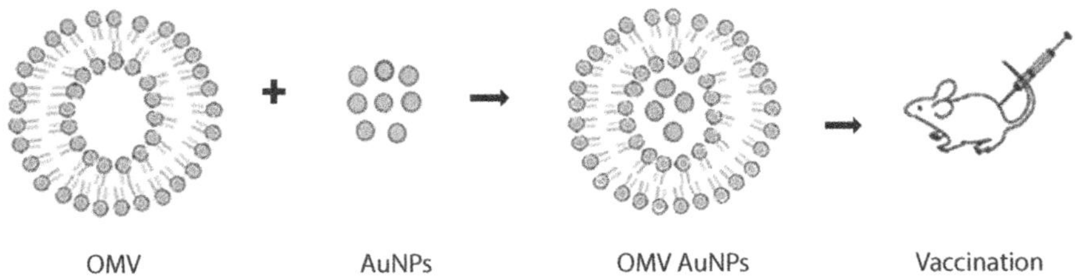

Figure 3.2 Schematic representation of outer membrane vesicle (OMV) coated AuNPs.

stress responses, nutrition acquisition, targeted enzyme delivery, and so on. OMVs were first discovered by Chatterjee and Das in 1967 from the cell wall of *Vibrio cholerae* [50]. OMVs fall in the 20 to 200 nm in size enabling them to diffuse into the lymph cells and induce antigen cells. OMVs are antigenic and are nonpathogenic making it a potential vaccine carrier. OMVs configure the surface antigens to elicit humoral response, T cell–mediated immune response and trigger innate immune response making them a potential vaccine candidate [51]. OMV-based vaccines were first developed against *Neisseria meningitidis* serogroup B, in 1987. OMVs can be separated from meningococcal bacteria [52]. Mutant derived OMV (mdOMV) is produced by disrupting the genes crosslinking outer membrane and peptidoglycan membrane of Gram negative bacteria. Disruption of the TolR gene of Gram negative bacteria leads to the high yield of mdOMV [53]. *In vivo* studies of OMV have shown interaction with different immune cells [54]. OMVs showed immune responses by inducing cytokines and chemokines in macrophages. Stability of the OMVs were maintained by electroporation of synthetic NPs in the inner hollow vesicle part. OMV of *Pseudomonas aeruginosa* were electroporated with AuNPs to create OMV NPs for drug delivery. Different antigen-loaded *E. coli* OMVs have been shown to induce the CXCL1 expression system which in turn increased the neutrophils in mouse models [55]. OMVs of *E. coli* treated with AuNPs have shown activation of dendritic cells when administered subcutaneously in mouse models [56]. Silica NPs with rifampicin coated OMVs in *E. coli* have depicted strong antibacterial activity [57]. Figure 3.2 depicts the of outer membrane vesicle (OMV) coated AuNPs.

3.3.6 Nanotoxoids

Nanotoxoids is a type of anti-virulence therapy. Pathogenic microbes secrete toxins, which play a major role in pathogenesis [58, 59]. Inactivated toxins known as toxoids act as antigens inducing positive immune responses.

Toxoid vaccines can help in reducing the virulence by incorporating suitable NPs along the membrane surface. Cell membrane doped NPs coated with toxin released by pathogens—nano toxoids—are used as efficient vaccines by inhibiting a pathogen from colonizing the host. Important examples of nano toxoid vaccines are tetanus toxoid and diphtheria toxoid where the toxins are inactivated and absorbed to aluminum adjuvants. At present, tetanus and diphtheria toxoid vaccines are administered intramuscularly. Aluminium hydroxide and aluminium phosphate are the adjuvants used in tetanus and diphtheria toxoid vaccine development [60, 61]. Oral administration of toxoid vaccines were developed by loading tetanus toxoid in chitosan NPs further stabilized using glutaraldehyde. A significant increase in IgG and IgA were noted in the toxoid-chitosan NP vaccine [62, 63].

3.3.7 Liposomes

Liposomes are one of the widely used artificial biodegradable vaccine carriers and drug delivery vehicles. Liposomes are unilamellar or multilamellar vesicles with phospholipids surrounding aqueous layers [64]. Liposomes are associated with endocytic pathways and deliver the vaccine adjuvants leading to cell-mediated immunization [65]. Micelles were developed by assembling a lipid polymer in aqueous layer with a hydrophobic lipid tail coupled to a polymer. The hydrophilic moieties bind to an aqueous layer, whereas hydrophobic moieties bind to phospholipid layers. Biodegradable phospholipids, like phosphatidylserine, phosphatidylcholine, cholesterol, and so on, were used to synthesize liposomes. Lipid-based surface engineering of PLGA NPs were used for drug and gene delivery applications [66]. Antigenic proteins were attached with the liposomes as they can bind to both hydrophilic and hydrophobic moieties as vaccine vehicles. Antigenic proteins incorporated with multilamellar vesicles have developed potent humoral and cellular immune responses [67]. Different methods including thin film hydration, micro emulsification, sonication and freeze thawing have been used for the preparation of liposomal NPs. Epaxal, Inflexal, and Mosquirix are three FDA approved vaccines comprising phosphatidylcholine membrane vesicle liposomes incorporating virus proteins. These protect antigens from enzymatic degradation and ensure targeted drug delivery by inducing cellular and humoral immunity [68].

3.3.8 Polymeric Nanoparticles

Self-assembled monomeric units of polymers with smaller size and properties were studied as vaccine transporters. Polymeric NPs have gained importance due to its biodegradability, ease in synthesis, reduced cytotoxicity, biocompatibility, and so on. Polysaccharide, a natural polymer with high biocompatibility and low cytotoxicity, acts as a pathogen associated with molecular patterns (PAMP) with enhanced immune response against antigens [69, 70]. Chitosan, a polysaccharide isolated from chitin, was the first polysaccharide used for antigen delivery. Cationic chitosan interacts with negatively charged antigens under functional conditions. Chitosan NPs conjugated with *Mycobacterium tuberculosis* lipids showed induced humoral and cellular immune responses [71]. PLA (Polylactic acid) or PLGA (Poly lactic-co-glycolic acid) is the commonly used polymeric vaccine. PLGA coated antigens showed high immunity by inducing cytokines in mycobacterial infection [72]. Naturally occurring bio polymers like inulin, alginate and pullans can also be used as vaccine adjuvants. Comparative study on administration of CPG (chemically synthesized DNA with unmethylated cytosine-phosphate-guanine) and CPG conjugated NPs showed increased dendritic cell activation and increased cellular immunity in CPG NPs.

Self-assembled NPs of specific size and stability are made using naturally occurring proteins. These NPs with size ranging from 10-150nm with diverse physiological properties and biomimetic shapes were used as vaccine carriers. Self-assembled NPs are made by the polymerization of protein monomers. Studies show that self-assembled protein NPs can activate the overall immune responses without the help of an adjuvant [73]. Ferritin, an iron storage protein with 12 nm size and an inner cavity, found in bacteria, plants and animals was explored as NV. An interesting property of ferritin molecules is its denaturation property in acidic condition at pH-2.5 and renaturation property in physiological pH of 7.5 [74]. Ferritin in artificial iron free condition is loaded with different species in its inner core region, and the outer surface can be genetically modified with different motifs.

3.3.9 Virus-Like Particle

Viruses are nanosized organisms ranging a size of 20 to 500 nm encircling the genetic material with an outer protein capsid layer. The absence of nucleic acid makes the virus-like particle (VLP) inactive, but at the same time the antigens in VLP can act as potential immune promoters [75]. Self-assembled viral capsid proteins known as VLPs lacking nucleic acid are also used as immune boosters. Drug molecules are infused in the pores of the surface of the capsid. Proteins isolated from influenza virus, bacteriophages, and flock house viruses were genetic engineered and successfully studied as vaccine carriers [76]. VLPs administered intramuscularly are recognized by antigen presenting cells which in turn induce MHC class II molecules and stimulate CD4+ T helper cells, further activating B-cells producing IgG antibodies.

3.3.10 Inorganic Nanoparticles

Inorganic materials having smaller particle size, stability, enhanced permeability, drug doping capacity, rapid drug releasing property, and so on, are considered ideal for drug delivery. Inorganic NPs are constructed with an outer organic# shell embedding an inner inorganic core [77]. Inorganic NPs are less expensive, reproducible, and safe, making them more advantageous. Compounds like gold, silica and carbon NPs were used for synthesizing inorganic NPs for vaccine delivery. Carbohydrate conjugated AuNPs is a promising vaccine for developing positive immunogenicity. Antigens coated with AuNPs induced immune responses against tuberculosis, foot and mouth disease, influenza and immunodeficiency virus [78]. Iron oxide NPs (IONP) were studied as vaccine adjuvants. Citrate coated manganese ferrite ($MnFe_2O_4$) NPs modified with Mycobacterium fusion proteins have shown elevated Th1 and CD8+ immune response. Mesoporous silica NPs functionalized with antigens were also studied as vaccine carriers [79].

3.4 Mechanism of Action of Nanovaccines

The therapeutic success of NVs can be attributed to their ability to induce effective immune responses through site-specific delivery of antigens, drugs, peptides, and genes *via* size modulation and association with immune regulatory factors [80]. They also offer improved *in vivo* and *in vitro* stability with minimal side effects [81]. Their high efficiency can be accredited to their particulate nature which increases the cross-presentation of peptides and also by playing an important role in the activity of antigen-presenting cells, which are the key mediators between the innate and adaptive immunity pathways [82]. The NPs are first dealt with by the macrophages of the immune system which can cause undesirable interactions such as immunostimulation or suppression leading to inflammatory reactions, autoimmune disorders, and increased host susceptibility to infections and cancer [80]. However, in the absence of immune recognition or when the NPs are recognized as self, they can be engineered to elicit an immune response by stimulation of antigen-presenting cells or antigen delivery to cellular compartments [83].

Our body is effectively and efficiently shielded from threats by foreign invaders by the rapid activity of the immune system of the body. The innate branch of the immune system issues quick and nonspecific removal of the foreign bodies, while the adaptive immune pathway generates focused responses against the specific antigen concerned [84]. Antigen-presenting cells such as macrophage and dendritic cells digest the antigenic proteins and present epitope peptide fragments on their surface after peptide loading onto MHC complexes [85, 86]. The activated APCs migrate to secondary lymphoid organs such as lymph nodes and spleen and interact with B cells and T cells of the adaptive immune system to elicit cellular or humoral immunity.The interactions between NVs and the immune system are dependent on NP characteristics such as charge, surface chemistry, shape, hydrophobic properties, protein binding to the NP surface, and administration routes. These factors govern the uptake of NPs by influencing NP interaction with the cell membrane and their translocation across physiological barriers. The NPs bind to the cell surface and are taken in by a specific endocytosis pathway [87].

The immune response associated with NPs involves antibodies generated by the NP themselves as well as the drug or antigen it is incorporated with [88]. Certain metals like silver, copper, zinc, and iron exhibit bactericidal and fungicidal properties in their NP form. In addition to combating bacteria themselves, their inert and nontoxic nature makes them highly efficient nano drug carriers for antimicrobial agents. However, immunization with gold NPs, cationic dendrimers, and carbon NPs failed to generate an immune response even when activated with potent adjuvants. NP-specific antibodies were observed when these NPs were conjugated with a carrier protein. Nonantigenic cationic polyamidoamine dendrimers produce dendrimer-specific antibodies when conjugated with a carrier protein such as bovine serum albumin. The development of antigenicity could be related to an increase in the size of the NPs when conjugated with the carrier protein [80].

Silver NPs have been shown to affect the replication ability of DNA and cause the inactivation of cellular proteins by binding to functional groups of proteins resulting in protein denaturation [89]. Reports suggest that the electrostatic attraction between negatively charged bacterial cells and positively charged NPs confer the bactericidal properties associated with silver NPs. The NPs interact with the structural elements of the bacterial cell membrane and disrupt its structural integrity resulting in degradation and cell death. *E. coli* treated with highly reactive metal oxide NPs exhibited the formation of irregularly shaped pits on the cell membrane surface which disturbed the membrane permeability due to progressive release of lipopolysaccharide molecules (LPS) which were responsible for providing an operational permeability barrier [90]. NPs have also shown antibacterial action by the production of reactive Nitrogen species which induces apoptosis [91].

Adjuvants are substances that are co-administered with the antigen to enhance the immune response. Aluminum is the most commonly used adjuvant for vaccine formulations. However, they fail to generate strong cell-mediated immunity and also possess the risk of inducing autoimmune disorders, long-term brain inflammation, and other adverse health issues. These drawbacks have called for the development of new adjuvants for successful vaccine delivery. The use of NPs as adjuvants have been studied extensively and many of these studies report the induction of similar or higher immune responses as compared to aluminum-containing adjuvants. NPs such as those of cobalt oxide were considered excellent vaccine adjuvants for their low *in vitro* toxicity and potent antibody responses [92].

Genetic and chemical engineering has made it possible to mount peptide-based epitopes on the surface of NPs. The adjuvenating effect of Polyacrylic acid-based polymers have been utilized by mixing them with protein antigen of interest to produce an immune response. Polyacrylate ester (PAE)-based dendritic polymer was chemically attached with *Streptococcus* specific peptide epitope J14, to produce repetitive antigen display on the surface of the polymer. Immunization of mice models was carried out subcutaneously and intranasally, both of which elicited an effective humoral response [93]. The immune system secretes cytokines in response to foreign substances and this constitutes an inflammatory response. The cytokines recruit effector immune cells which help in the clearance of the foreign material. Many NPs including gold colloids, carbon nanotubes, polymers, dendrimers, quantum dots, and silver NPs can induce an inflammatory response. However, this kind of response is dependent on factors such as surface charge, size, and composition of the NPs used [80].

Cationic NPs induce a stronger response as compared to negative or neutral particles. Cationic liposomes induce cytokine secretion in addition to dendritic cell surface marker expression which is vital for inflammatory responses [94]. Size is another important factor that determines the extent of the immune response - NPs of size between 100 and 500 nm induce a stronger response when compared to larger ones (>1000 nm). The smaller size makes it easier for these NPs to travel through the lymphatics as compared to larger particles that accumulate in the lymph node. NPs used in vaccine formulations are made in sizes comparable to that of pathogens so that they are easily recognized by the immune system [95].

3.5 Limitations of Nanovaccines

NVs and NP drug delivery systems are indeed practical approaches towards efficient disease treatment and in the field of precision medicine. However, one of the main limitations is the surface toxicity of the NPs. Because of their size, NPs can easily travel within the circulatory and lymphatic systems, causing damage to body tissues and organs. Based on the size, these particles can induce irreversible cell damage by oxidative stresses [96]. The construction of NPs, in general, and the building of NVs using these materials are complex processes as they must be done in highly sterile conditions. Various dermatological problems can arise as a result of the administration of NVs through intradermal injections. Oral administration of NVs can result in multiple gastrointestinal and respiratory problems [97]. Cardiovascular disorders have also been reported as a result of the parenteral route of administration of NVs. In addition to these factors, the penetration of these NPs into the blood-brain barrier can result in brain damage. Studies conducted in rats have demonstrated how the accumulation of NPs leads to vascular thrombosis [98]. When specific NPs remain in the body, it causes significant problems in the long run. A study on rats has shown that these remain in the body for two years and the saponin-based adjuvants can result in toxicity in the organism's body [88]. Another major limitation is concerning the stability of NVs. Liposome storage becomes a significant disadvantage as it leads to aggregation and structural destabilization. Another challenge is the scaling up of NVs [99]. It is often difficult to construct such complex structures in batches as multiple loading of molecules such as adjuvants and antigens in a single nanoplatform, and producing these compounds in batches tends to be a tedious and complex process [100].

Moreover, since the development of NVs is a new domain, these do not have an enduring safety profile and hence there are regulatory concerns related to the production and distribution of NVs. Various environmental factors with respect to the use of NVs have not been thoroughly analysed. Nano-based-carrier systems and vaccine delivery must be investigated with respect to interaction with physical factors such as air and water, biodegradation, bioaccumulation, and interaction of NPs with various environmental contaminants. Another factor to be considered is the possible exposure to humans during the manufacture of NVs and the risks associated with it. Various ethical, legal and social issues have also been brought up with respect to the use and manufacture of NVs in various developed countries as compared to underdeveloped countries [101].

3.6 Conclusion

Superbugs are no longer just laboratory threats but have turned to be a global concern leading to accelerated death toll among susceptible populations. The after effects of these issues are aggravated in case of conditions like natural calamities, civil war, and famine. WHO has clearly warned the seriousness of handling emergence of antibiotic resistance with utmost importance post antibiotic era. If we fail to take quick action there could be prolonged hospitalization and death of immunocompromised people. The whole idea behind NVs is relevant in the current times as several bacteria are developing resistance against a wide spectrum of antibiotics. More than bacteria developing resistance towards antibiotics, the major concern is the rate at which they are developing resistance. Sometimes, a drug becomes ineffective within six months of coming on to the market and at times even before coming to the market. Prophylaxis is always better than therapy and hence efficient vaccines could be better life savers than drugs. Nanovaccines by way of their numerous positive virtues like small size, more surface area strong immune response, controlled antigen presentation, high antigen loading, higher immunogenicity and better retention in lymph nodes are a potential tool to combat threats posed by superbugs, but more research has to be conducted to fully understand its advantages and limitations.

Acknowledgment

The authors are grateful to the faculty of the Department of Life Sciences, CHRIST (Deemed to be University), Bangalore, for the support extended for the successful completion of this work.

References

1. Walsh, C.T., Fisher, S.L., Park, I.S., Prahalad, M., Wu, Z., Bacterial resistance to vancomycin: Five genes and one missing hydrogen bond tell the story. *Chem. Biol.*, 3, 21–28, 1996.
2. Rice, L.B., Federal funding for the study of antimicrobial Resistance in nosocomial pathogens: No ESKAPE. *J. Infect. Dis.*, 197, 1079–1081, 2008.
3. Gillings, M.R., Evolutionary consequences of antibiotic use for the resistome, mobilome and microbial pangenome. *Front. Microbiol.*, 4, 4, 2013.

4. Adegoke, A.A., Faleye, A.C., Singh, G., Stenström, T.A., Antibiotic resistant Superbugs: Assessment of the interrelationship of occurrence in Clinical settings and environmental niches. *Molecules*, Basel, Switzerland, *22*, 1, 29, 2016. https://doi.org/10.3390/molecules22010029.
5. de la Cruz, F. and Davies, J., Horizontal gene transfer and the origin of species: lessons from bacteria. *Trends Microbiol.*, *8*, 128–133, 2000.
6. Baral, B. and Mozafari, M.R., Strategic moves of "superbugs" Against available chemical scaffolds: Signaling, regulation, and challenges. *ACS Pharmacol. Transl. Sci.*, *3*, 373–400, 2020.
7. Buchanan, C.E. and Strominger, J.L., Altered penicillin-binding components in penicillin-resistant mutants of Bacillus subtilis. *Proc. Natl. Acad. Sci. U. S.A.*, *73*, 1816–1820, 1976.
8. Wright, G., Bacterial resistance to antibiotics: Enzymatic degradation and modification. *Adv. Drug Delivery Rev.*, *57*, 1451–1470, 2005.
9. Wiley, *Antibiotics and Bacterial Resistance*, John Wiley & Sons, 2013.
10. Koo, H., Allan, R.N., Howlin, R.P., Stoodley, P., Hall-Stoodley, L., Targeting microbial biofilms: Current and prospective therapeutic strategies. *Nat. Rev. Microbiol.*, *15*, 740–755, 2017.
11. World Health Organization (WHO), *Antimicrobial resistance: Global report on surveillance*, Geneva, WHO Press, 2014.
12. Rappuoli, R., Bloom, D.E., Black, S., Deploy vaccines to fight superbugs. *Nature*, *552*, 165–167, 2017.
13. Kim, M.-G., Park, J.Y., Shon, Y., Kim, G., Shim, G., Oh, Y.K., Nanotechnology and vaccine development. *Asian J. Pharm. Sci.*, *9*, 5, 227–235, 2014.
14. Minakshi, P., Gosh, M., Brar, B., Kumar, R., Lambe, U.P., Ranjan, K., Manoj, J., Prasad, G., Nano-antimicrobials: A new paradigm for combating mycobacterial resistance. *Current Pharmaceutical Design*, *25*, 13, 1554–1579, 2019. https://doi.org/10.2174/1381612825666190620094041
15. Peek, L.J., Middaugh, C.R., Berkland, C., Nanotechnology in vaccine delivery. *Advanced Drug Delivery Reviews*, *60*, 8, 915–928, 2008. https://doi.org/10.1016/j.addr.2007.05.017.
16. Fischer, N.O., Rasley, A., Corzett, M., Hwang, M.H., Hoeprich, P.D., Blanchette, C.D., Colocalized delivery of adjuvant and antigen using nanolipoprotein particles enhances the immune response to recombinant Antigens. *J. Am. Chem. Soc.*, *135*, 2044–2047, 2013.
17. Moghimi, S.M., Hunter, A.C., Murray, J.C., Nanomedicine: Current status and future prospects. *FASEB J.*, *19*, 311–330, 2005.
18. Facciola, A., Visalli, G., Lagana, A., La Fauci, V., Squeri, R., Pellicano, G.F., Nunnari, G., Trovato, M., Pietro, A.D., The new era of vaccines: The "nanovaccinology". *Eur. Rev. Med. Pharmacol. Sci.*, *23*, 7163–7182, 2019.
19. Sarkar, S. and Suresh, M.R., An overview of tuberculosis chemotherapy – A literature review. *J. Pharm. Pharm. Sci.*, *14*, 148–61, 2011.

20. Singh, J., Garg, T., Rath, G., Goyal, A.K., Advances in nanotechnology-based carrier systems for targeted delivery of bioactive drug molecules with special emphasis on immunotherapy in drug resistant tuberculosis – A critical review. *Drug Delivery, 23*, 1676–1698, 2015.
21. Bhardwaj, P., Bhatia, E., Sharma, S., Ahamad, N., Banerjee, R., Advancements in prophylactic and therapeutic nanovaccines. *Acta Biomaterialia, 108*, 1–21, 2020. https://doi.org/10.1016/j.actbio.2020.03.020.
22. Skwarczynski, M. and Toth, I., Peptide-based subunit nanovaccines. *Curr. Drug Deliv., 8*, 282–289, 2011.
23. Fujita, Y. and Taguchi, H., Current status of multiple antigen-presenting peptide vaccine systems: Application of organic and inorganic nanoparticles. *Chem. Cent. J., 5*, 48–0, 2001.
24. Mamo, T. and Poland, G.A., Nanovaccinology: The next generation of vaccines meets 21st century materials science and engineering. *Elsevier. 30*, 47 6609–6611, 2012. https://doi.org/10.1016/j.vaccine.2012.08.023.
25. Kasturi, S.P., Skountzou, I., Albrecht, R.A., Koutsonanos, D., Hua, T., Nakaya, H.I., *et al.*, Programming the magnitude and persistence of antibody responses with innate immunity. *Nature, 470*, 543–7, 2011.
26. Moon, J.J., Suh, H., Li, A.V., Ockenhouse, C.F., Yadava, A., Irvine, D.J., Enhancing humoral responses to a malaria antigen with nanoparticle vaccines that expand Tfh cells and promote germinal center induction. *Proc. Natl. Acad. Sci., 109*, 1080–5, 2010.
27. Rosales-Mendoz, S. and Gonzalez-Ortega, O., *Nanovaccines: An innovative technology to fight human and animal diseases*, Springer International Publishing, Switzerland, 2019.
28. Liu, Z.-H., Xu, H.-L., Han, G.-W., Tao, L.-N., Lu, Y., Zheng, S.-Y., Fang, W.-H., & He, F. Self-assembling nanovaccine enhances protective efficacy against CSFV in pigs. *Frontiers in Immunology, 12*, 689187, 2021. https://doi.org/10.3389/fimmu.2021.689187
29. Wang, N., Shang, J., Jiang, S., Du, L., Subunit vaccines against emerging pathogenic human coronaviruses. *Front. Microbiol., 11*, 298, 2020.
30. Liu, L., Liu, Z., Chen, H., Liu, H., Gao, Q., Cong, F., Gao, G., Chen, Y., Subunit nanovaccine with potent cellular and mucosal immunity for COVID-19. *ACS Appl. Bio Mater., 3*, 5633–5638, 2020.
31. Renu, S., Markazi, A.D., Dhakal, S., Shaan Lakshmanappa, Y., Shanmugasundaram, R., Selvaraj, R.K., Renukaradhya, G.J., Oral deliverable mucoadhesive, chitosan-salmonella subunit nanovaccine for layer chickens. *Int. J. Nanomed., 15*, 761–777, 2020.
32. Rappuoli, R., De Gregorio, E., Costantino, P., On the mechanisms of conjugate vaccines. *Proc. Natl. Acad. Sci., 116*, 14–16, 2019.
33. Afshari, H., Maleki, M., Hakimian, M., Tanha, R.A., Salouti, M., Immunogenicity evaluating the SLNs-alginate conjugate against pseudomonas aeruginosa. *J. Immunol. Methods, 488*, 112938, 2021.

34. Pardi, N., Hogan, M.J., Porter, F.W., Weissman, D., mRNA vaccines—A new era in vaccinology. *Nat. Rev. Drug Discovery, 17*, 261–279, 2018.
35. Zhang, C., Maruggi, G., Shan, H., Li, J., Advances in mRNA vaccines for infectious diseases. *Front. Immunol., 10*, 594, 2019.
36. Moxon, R., Reche, P.A., Rappuoli, R., Editorial: Reverse Vaccinology. *Front. Immunol.*, 10, 2776, 2019.
37. Motin, V. L., & Torres, A. G. Molecular approaches to bacterial vaccines, in: *Vaccines for Biodefense and Emerging and Neglected Diseases*, pp. 63–76. Academic Press, Amsterdam. 2009. https://doi.org/10.1016/B978-0-12-369408-9.00006-8.
38. Clark, D.P. and Pazdernik, N.J., Immune Technology, in: *Biotechnology*, pp. 181–217, Academic Cell, Elsevier, USA, 2016.
39. Huang, J., Yin, Y.-X., Pan, Z., Zhang, G., Zhu, A., Liu, X., & Jiao, X. Intranasal immunization with chitosan/pCAGGS-*fla* a nanoparticles Inhibits Campylobacter jejuni in a White Leghorn Model. *Journal of Biomedicine and Biotechnology, 2010*, 1–8, 2010. https://doi.org/10.1155/2010/589476.
40. Sanchez-Villamil, J.I., Tapia, D., Torres, A.G., Development of a gold nanoparticle vaccine against enterohemorrhagic escherichia coli O157:H7. *mBio*, 10, 78, 2019.
41. Wu, G., Ji, H., Guo, X., Li, Y., Ren, T., Dong, H., Liu, J., Liu, Y., Shi, X., He, B., Nanoparticle reinforced bacterial outer-membrane vesicles effectively prevent fatal infection of carbapenem-resistant Klebsiella pneumoniae. *Nanomed.: Nanotechnol. Biol. Med., 24*, 102148, 2020.
42. Das, I., Padhi, A., Mukherjee, S., Dash, D.P., Kar, S., Sonawane, A., Biocompatible chitosan nanoparticles as an efficient delivery vehicle for mycobacterium tuberculosis lipids to induce potent cytokines and antibody response through activation of gammadelta T cells in mice. *Nanotechnology*, 28, 323, 2017.
43. Chen, G., Bai, Y., Li, Z., Wang, F., Fan, X., Zhou, X., Bacterial extracellular vesicle-coated multi-antigenic nanovaccines protect against drug-resistant *Staphylococcus aureus* infection by modulating antigen processing and presentation pathways. *Theranostics, 10*, 7131–7149, 2020.
44. Nevagi, R.J., Khalil, Z.G., Hussein, W.M., Powell, J., Batzloff, M.R., Capon, R.J., Good, M.F., Skwarczynski, M., Toth, I., Polyglutamic acid-trimethyl chitosan-based intranasal peptide nano-vaccine induces potent immune responses against group A streptococcus. *Acta Biomater., 80*, 278–287, 2018.
45. Fang, R.H., Kroll, A.V., Gao, W., Zhang, L., Cell membrane coating nanotechnology. *Adv. Mater., 30*, 1706759, 2018.
46. Vijayan, V., Uthaman, S., Park, I.-K., Cell membrane coated nanoparticles: An emerging biomimetic nanoplatform for targeted bioimaging and therapy, in: *Biomimetic Medical Materials*, pp. 45–59, 2018.
47. Pasto, A., Giordano, F., Evangelopoulos, M., Amadori, A., Tasciotti, E., Cell membrane protein functionalization of nanoparticles as a new tumor-targeting strategy. *Clin. Transl. Med.*, 8, 1–9, 2019.

48. Liu, W.L., Zou, M.Z., Qin, S.Y., Cheng, Y.J., Ma, Y.H., Sun, Y.X., Zhang, X.Z., Recent advances of cell membrane-coated nanomaterials for biomedical applications. *Adv. Funct. Mater.*, 30, 2003559, 2020.
49. D'Amico, C., Fontana, F., Cheng, R., Santos, H.A., Development of vaccine formulations: Past, present, and future. *Drug Deliv. Transl. Res.*, *11*, 353–72, 2021.
50. Tan, K., Li, R., Huang, X., Liu, Q., Outer membrane vesicles: Current status and future direction of these novel vaccine adjuvants. *Front. Microbiol.*, *9*, 783, 2018.
51. Kaparakis-Liaskos, M. and Ferrero, R.L., Immune modulation by bacterial outer membrane vesicles. *Nat. Rev. Immunol.*, *15*, 375–87, 2015.
52. Holst, J., Martin, D., Arnold, R., Huergo, C.C., Oster, P., O'Hallahan, J. *et al.*, Properties and clinical performance of vaccines containing outer membrane vesicles from *Neisseria meningitidis*. *Vaccine*, *27*, B3–B12, 2009.
53. Gnopo, Y.M., Watkins, H.C., Stevenson, T.C., DeLisa, M.P., Putnam, D., Designer outer membrane vesicles as immunomodulatory systems–Reprogramming bacteria for vaccine delivery. *Adv. Drug Delivery Rev.*, *114*, 132–42, 2017.
54. Zhu, Z., Antenucci, F., Villumsen, K.R., Bojesen, A.M., Bacterial outer membrane vesicles as a versatile tool in vaccine research and the fight against antimicrobial resistance. *Mbio*, *12*, 01707–21, 2021.
55. Lee, J., Yoon, Y.J., Kim, J.H., Dinh, N.T.H., Go, G., Tae, S. *et al.*, Outer membrane vesicles derived from Escherichia coli regulate neutrophil migration by induction of endothelial IL-8. *Front. Microbiol.*, *9*, 2268, 2018.
56. Gao, W., Fang, R.H., Thamphiwatana, S., Luk, B.T., Li, J., Angsantikul, P. *et al.*, Modulating antibacterial immunity via bacterial membrane-coated nanoparticles. *Nano Lett.*, *15*, 1403–9, 2015.
57. Wu, S., Huang, Y., Yan, J., Li, Y., Wang, J., Yang, Y.Y. *et al.*, Bacterial outer membrane-coated mesoporous silica nanoparticles for targeted delivery of antibiotic rifampicin against gram-negative bacterial infection *In Vivo*. *Adv. Funct. Mater.*, *31*, 2103442, 2021.
58. Wei, X., Ran, D., Campeau, A., Xiao, C., Zhou, J., Dehaini, D. *et al.*, Multi Antigenic nanotoxoids for antivirulence vaccination against antibiotic-resistant gram-negative bacteria. *Nano Lett.*, *19*, 4760–9, 2019.
59. Guo, Z., Kubiatowicz, L.J., Fang, R.H., Zhang, L., Nanotoxoids: Biomimetic Nanoparticle Vaccines against Infections. *Adv. Ther.*, 4, 2100072, 2021.
60. Liang, Z., Yang, Y., Yu, G., Zhu, H., Xia, X., Chen, C. *et al.*, Engineering Aluminum Hydroxyphosphate Nanoparticles with well-controlled surface property to enhance humoral immune responses as vaccine adjuvants. *Biomaterials*, 275, 120960, 2021.
61. Azuar, A., Li, Z., Shibu, M.A., Zhao, L., Luo, Y., Shalash, A.O. *et al.*, Poly (hydrophobic amino acid)-based self-adjuvanting nanoparticles for group A streptococcus vaccine Delivery. *J. Med. Chem.*, *64*, 2648–58, 2021.

62. Mohammed, M.A., Syeda, J., Wasan, K.M., Wasan, E.K., An overview of chitosan nanoparticles and its application in non-parenteral drug delivery. *Pharmaceutics*, *9*, 53, 2017.
63. Kumar, S. and Ramaswamy, N., Chitosan microspheres as potential vaccine delivery systems. *Int. J. Drug Deliv.*, *3*, 43–50, 2011.
64. Large, D.E., Abdelmessih, R.G., Fink, E., Auguste, D.T., Liposome composition in drug delivery design, synthesis, characterization, and clinical application. *Adv. Drug Deliv. Rev.*, 176, 113851, 2021.
65. Rao, M., Peachman, K.K., Alving, C.R., Liposome formulations as adjuvants for vaccines, in: *Nanoparticles for Rational Vaccine Design. Current Topics in Microbiology and Immunology*, H.S. Gill and R.W. Compans (Eds.), p. 433, Springer, Cham, 2021.
66. Vartak, A. and Sucheck, S.J., Recent advances in subunit vaccine carriers. *Vaccines*, *4*, 12, 2016.
67. Magar, K.T., Boafo, G.F., Li, X., Chen, Z., He, W., Liposome-based delivery of biological drugs. *Chin. Chem. Lett.*, 12, 1054, 2021.
68. Kim, E.-M. and Jeong, H.-J., Liposomes: Biomedical applications. *Chonnam Med. J.*, *57*, 27, 2021.
69. Spirescu, V.A., Chircov, C., Grumezescu, A.M., Andronescu, E., Polymeric nanoparticles for antimicrobial Therapies: An up-to-date overview. *Polymers*, *13*, 724, 2021.
70. Makabenta, J.M.V., Nabawy, A., Li, C.-H., Schmidt-Malan, S., Patel, R., Rotello, V.M., Nanomaterial-based therapeutics for antibiotic-resistant bacterial infections. *Nat. Rev. Microbiol.*, *19*, 23–36, 2021.
71. Khan, A. and Alamry, K.A., Recent advances of emerging green chitosan-based biomaterials with potential biomedical applications: A review. *Carbohydr. Res.*, 506, 108368, 2021.
72. Polla Ravi, S., Shamiya, Y., Chakraborty, A., Elias, C., & Paul, A. Biomaterials, biological molecules, and polymers in developing vaccines. *Trends in Pharmacological Sciences*, *42*, 10, 813–828, 2021. https://doi.org/10.1016/j.tips.2021.07.006.
73. Pan, J. and Cui, Z., Self-assembled nanoparticles: Exciting platforms for vaccination. *Biotechnol. J.*, *15*, 2000087, 2020.
74. Lin, X., Xie, J., Niu, G., Zhang, F., Gao, H., Yang, M. *et al.*, Chimeric ferritin nanocages for multiple function loading and multimodal imaging. *Nano Lett.*, *11*, 814–9, 2011.
75. Cimica, V. and Galarza, J.M., Adjuvant formulations for virus-like particle (VLP) based vaccines. *Clin. Immunol.*, *183*, 99–108, 2017.
76. Donaldson, B., Lateef, Z., Walker, G. F., Young, S. L., & Ward, V. K. Virus-like particle vaccines: Immunology and formulation for clinical translation. *Expert Review of Vaccines*, 17, 9, 833–849, 2018. https://doi.org/10.1080/14760584.2018.1516552.
77. Poon, C. and Patel, A.A., Organic and inorganic nanoparticle vaccines for prevention of infectious diseases. *Nano Express*, 1, 1, 01200, 2020.

78. Mateu Ferrando, R., Lay, L., & Polito, L., Gold nanoparticle-based platforms for vaccine development. *Drug Discovery Today: Technologies*, 38, 57–67, 2020. https://doi.org/10.1016/j.ddtec.2021.02.001
79. Liu, G., Zhu, M., Zhao, X., Nie, G., Nanotechnology-empowered vaccine delivery for enhancing CD8+ T cells-mediated cellular immunity. *Adv. Drug Delivery Rev.*, 176, 113889, 2021.
80. Zolnik, B.S., González-Fernández, A., Sadrieh, N., Dobrovolskaia, M.A., Minireview: Nanoparticles and the Immune System. *Endocrinology, 151*, 458–465, 2010.
81. Roopngam, P.E., Liposome and polymer-based nanomaterials for vaccine applications. *Nanomed. J.*, 6, 1–10, 2019.
82. Iwasaki, A. and Medzhitov, R., Regulation of adaptive Immunity by the innate immune system. *Science, 327*, 291–295, 2010.
83. Aggarwal, P., Hall, J.B., McLeland, C.B., Dobrovolskaia, M.A., McNeil, S.E., Nanoparticle interaction with plasma proteins as it relates to particle biodistribution, biocompatibility, and therapeutic efficacy. *Adv. Drug Delivery Rev., 61*, 428–437, 2009.
84. Zhou, J., Kroll, A.V., Holay, M., Fang, R.H., Zhang, L., Biomimetic nanotechnology toward personalized vaccines. *Adv. Mater., 32*, 190–1255, 2019.
85. Unanue, E.R., Antigen-presenting function of the macrophage. *Annu. Rev. Immunol., 2*, 395–428, 1984.
86. Banchereau, J. and Palucka, A.K., Dendritic cells as therapeutic vaccines against cancer. *Nat. Rev. Immunol., 5*, 296–306, 2005.
87. Saptarshi, S. R., Duschl, A., & Lopata, A. L. Interaction of nanoparticles with proteins: Relation to bio-reactivity of the nanoparticle. *Journal of Nanobiotechnology, 11*, 1, 26, 2013. https://doi.org/10.1186/1477-3155-11-26.
88. Zaman, M., Good, M.F., Toth, I., Nanovaccines and their mode of action. *Methods*, 60, 226–231, 2013.
89. Pelgrift, R.Y. and Friedman, A.J., Nanotechnology as a therapeutic tool to combat microbial resistance. *Adv. Drug Delivery Rev., 65*, 1803–1815, 2013.
90. Rai, M., Deshmukh, S., Ingle, A., Gade, A., Silver nanoparticles: The powerful nanoweapon against multidrug-resistant bacteria. *J. Appl. Microbiol., 112*, 841–852, 2012.
91. Morones, J.R., Elechiguerra, J.L., Camacho, A., Holt, K., Kouri, J.B., Ramírez, J.T., Yacaman, M.J., The bactericidal effect of silver nanoparticles. *Nanotechnology, 16*, 2346–2353, 2005.
92. Dobrovolskaia, M.A., Aggarwal, P., Hall, J.B., McNeil, S.E., Preclinical studies to understand nanoparticle interaction with the immune system and its potential effects on nanoparticle biodistribution. *Mol. Pharmaceutics, 5*, 487–495, 2008.
93. Skwarczynski, M., Zaman, M., Urbani, C., Lin, I.C., Jia, Z., Batzloff, M., Good, M., Monteiro, M., Toth, I., Polyacrylate dendrimer nanoparticles: A self-adjuvanting vaccine delivery system. *Angew. Chem. Int. Ed., 49*, 5742–5745, 2010.

94. Aggarwal, P., Hall, J.B., McLeland, C.B., Dobrovolskaia, M.A., McNeil, S.E., Nanoparticle interaction with plasma proteins as it relates to particle biodistribution, biocompatibility and therapeutic efficacy. *Adv. Drug Delivery Rev.*, 61, 428–437, 2009.
95. Lutsiak, M.E.C., Kwon, G.S., Samuel, J., Biodegradable nanoparticle delivery of a Th2-biased peptide for induction of Th1 immune responses. *J. Pharm. Pharmacol.*, *58*, 739–747, 2006.
96. Choi, Y.S., Lee, M.Y., David, A.E., Park, Y.S., Nanoparticles for gene delivery: Therapeutic and toxic effects. *Mol. Cell. Toxicol.*, *10*, 1–8, 2014.
97. Marasini, N., Skwarczynski, M., Toth, I., Oral delivery of nanoparticle-based vaccines. *Expert Rev. Vaccines*, *13*, 1361–1376, 2014.
98. Shahbazi, M.A. and Santos, H.A., Revolutionary impact of nanovaccines on immunotherapy. *New Horiz. Transl. Med.*, *2*, 44–50, 2015.
99. Sercombe, L., Veerati, T., Moheimani, F., Wu, S.Y., Sood, A.K., Hua, S., Advances and challenges of liposome assisted drug delivery. *Front. Pharmacol.*, *6*, 1–13, 2018.
100. Arms, L., Smith, D.W., Flynn, J., Palmer, W., Martin, A., Woldu, A., Hua, S., Advantages and limitations of current techniques for analyzing the biodistribution of nanoparticles. *Front. Pharmacol.*, *9*, 1–17, 2018.
101. Karandikar, S., Mirani, A., Waybhase, V., Patravale, V.B., Patankar, S., Chapter 10 - Nanovaccines for oral delivery-formulation strategies and challenges, in: *Micro and Nano Technologies, Nanostructures for Oral Medicine*, pp. 263–293, 2017.

4

Current Research Trends on SARS-CoV2 Virus Against Nanovaccine Formulation

Pushpalatha C.[1*], Chhaya Kumar[1], Sowmya S.V.[2], Dominic Augustine[2], Elizabeth Abbu Varghese[1] and Jithya Suresh[1]

[1]*Department of Pedodontics & Preventive Dentistry, Faculty of Dental Sciences, M.S. Ramaiah University of Applied Sciences, MSR Nagar, Bengaluru Karnataka, India*

[2]*Department of Oral Pathology and Microbiology, Faculty of Dental Sciences, M.S. Ramaiah University of Applied Sciences, MSR Nagar, Bengaluru, Karnataka, India*

Abstract

The field of vaccination has advanced by leaps and bounds; however, effective and novel vaccines are yet to be developed, especially for rapidly spreading coronavirus disease 2019 (COVID-19)/SARS-CoV2. Many vaccines are created using conventional approaches to eradicate COVID-2019, which is presently a global threat. Even vaccines using nanotechnology are also in the race. Nanotechnology has accelerated the evolution of newer vaccines that are safe and highly effective in eradicating the SARS-CoV2. Nanovaccines (NVs) were developed recently where new drugs can be accommodated through nanoparticle (NP) carriers. The similar nanosize between the nano-scaled materials and pathogens ensures optimal trigger response of the immune system, resulting in satisfactory cellular and humoral immunity responses. Targeted delivery of NPs results in enhanced antibody response, improved stability coupled with longer duration drug release, and prolonged immunogenic memory. This chapter highlights recently developed antiviral nanovaccines against COVID-19. Although the development of NVs is in the infancy stage and few are in the early clinical phases, we firmly believe the newer generation of NVs have greater possibility of treatment and prevention of bacterial and viral infections.

***Keywords*:** COVID-19, nanovaccines, biomimetic nanovaccines, nanotechnology

**Corresponding author*: drpushpalatha29@gmail.com

Kaushik Pal (ed) Nanovaccinology as Targeted Therapeutics, (77–94) © 2022 Scrivener Publishing LLC

4.1 Introduction

COVID-19 was announced as a pandemic disease by WHO on March 11, 2020, based on the database of 5.5 million confirmed cases and recorded death of 346,000 people around the world. SARS-CoV2 is a causative organism for this pandemic COVID-19, which is a Coronaviridae species that are grouped into various genera α, β, γ, and δ with RNA genomes viruses [1]. For the prevention and protection from further spread, various approaches are being explored one of them being vaccination, which can be done at a large scale. Using traditional and nanotechnological approaches, multiple vaccines can be developed, which are effective against coronavirus. Numerous clinical trials are in progress for vaccine development mainly focusing on nucleic acid as compared with protein based because of their easier production. Presently, the most recent vaccine is RNA based, which targets the spike (S) protein. With the increasing demand for vaccination, there are more advanced vaccines coming up which are based on target-specific epitopes primarily to reduce the possibility of inducing undesired immune responses and also to produce vaccines, which are economic, safe, and reachable to all population. Nanotechnology can exhibit a significant role in this aspect where it has been proven successful in the earlier instances, such as for use in the form of biomarkers and biosensors. Procedures using nanodiagnostic tools are carried out in nanoscale measures, so that it is easy to use, accessible, stable and highly sensitive. In context of nanovaccines, the most acceptable approach till date has been the macromolecular complexes formed by the structural viral proteins known as the virus-like particles (VLPs), which is noninfective but mimics the virus without the presence of genomes [2, 3]. There is no literature that illustrates the effective use of nanotechnology against SARS-CoV2, especially since it being a rapid-onset new illness. The present chapter will aid in understanding SARS-CoV2 pathophysiology and newer developed nanovaccine against SARS-CoV2 using nanotechnology approach.

4.2 COVID-19/SARS-CoV2 Pathophysiology

Coronavirus are RNA viruses, that infect humans and other animals, such as dogs, cats, chicken, and so on. Coronavirus infections also cause respiratory, neurological, and gastrointestinal problems as well. In clinical practice, the common coronaviruses causing common cold symptoms, especially in immunocompromised individuals, are OC43, 229E, HKU1, and NL63.

SARS-CoV-2, a recently documented virus, possessing distinctive spikes measuring between 9 and 12 nm with a diameter of 60 to 140 nm, gives a solar corona appearance to the virions. This virus has spread worldwide in the last two decades. Genetic recombination and diversity has allowed the virus to adapt to the environment, enabling them to enter the new host system easily. Bats are thought to be a SARS-CoV2 natural reservoir, whereas humans gets infected through an intermediary host, the pangolin [4].

4.3 Development of Nanovaccines Against SARS-CoV2

The nanotechnology field is very helpful in solving the problems related to the pandemic and can also decrease the medical fraternity load. Nanotechnology offers a dominant platform to combat against COVID-19/SARS-CoV2 by developing different generations of nanovaccines comprising of nanoparticles that can activate protective immunity and attack virus specific proteins. The nanoparticles enhances antigen stability, immunogenicity and exhibits targeted drug delivery. The innovative nanoparticles denoted as 1c-SApNPs aids the immune system to produce rapid antibodies thus deactivating the coronavirus, and help protect the original virus. The system needs special nanoparticles surface properties in association with virus surface proteins, hence this system has difficulty in producing viral proteins in a larger scale, which is scalable and economical. To overcome these shortcomings, nanovaccines containing messenger RNA (mRNA) was developed, which offers artificial mRNA of the virus to the host. Moderna, a clinical-stage biotechnology firm, was the first to develop a mRNA-based vaccination against SARS-CoV2. National Institutes of Health encapsulated this mRNA vaccine with lipid NANOparticle, since mRNA molecule was instable. Novavax, a late-stage biotechnology firm, created the NVX-CoV2373 coronavirus vaccine, which is stable and with the potential of the highest neutralizing antibodies. Nanovaccines, composed of gold, chitosan, and poly(lactic-co-glycolic acid), have also been exploited. A liposome-based nanovaccine was another approach, which targets basically nonstructural polyprotein 1a (pp1a) [5]. Sekimukai *et al.*, combined gold nanoparticles with the S protein of SARS-CoV1 and on immunization of the mice and at a 2 week interval demonstrated excellent IgG response. Nsp10 of human SARS-CoV2 was also used to develop a self assembly SARS CoV2 vaccine that helped be effective against pulmonary fibrosis. Ufovax Company patented 1c-SApNP vaccine, a self-assembling

Table 4.1 WHO-approved SARS-CoV2 vaccines.

Manufacturer	Vaccine
Moderna	mRNA-1273
Pfizer/BioNTech	BNT162b2
Janssen	Ad26.COV2.S
Oxford/AstraZeneca	AZD1222
Serum Institute of India	Covishield
Bharat Biotech	Covaxin
Sinopharm (Beijing)	BBIBP-CorV
Sinovac	CoronaVac

protein, to combat coronaviruses and had the potential to enhance immune response and neutralize antibody titer against the virus. The combination of nanoparticles and cationic liposomes can be used as the carriers for the delivery of DNA vaccines [7]. To deliver SARS-CoV2 mRNA vaccines, the combination of liposomes, dendrimers/polysaccharide particles, and cationic nanoemulsions is also used [8]. Even Bacteriophage P22 capsid, cowpea mosaic viruses, and ferritin nanocages are utilized to deliver vaccine [9]. The above mentioned literature shows that the amalgamation of nanotechnology with existing vaccines helped to develop a strong vaccine against SARS CoV2, having a potent immune-stimulating effect. The 8 SARS-CoV2 vaccines approved by WHO updated as per November 2021 and vaccines that are in Phase 4 clincial trials are shown in Tables 4.1 and 4.2.

4.4 Biomimetic Nanovaccines Against SARS-CoV2

Biomimetic nanovaccines are composed of biomimetic carrier along with therapeutic molecules which is target specific. The main benefits of biomimetic nanovaccines are that it can keep the germinal center and B-cells within the body itself, which helps antiviral neutralizing antibody release against viruses, it has the potential make the humoral immune response stronger, and it can act as carrier for antigens, adjuvants, and

Table 4.2 SARS-CoV2 vaccines in Phase 4 clinical trials.

Clinical trial registration	Platform of vaccine development	Vaccine candidate	Number of doses	Schedule	Route of administration	Developers	Phase
NCT05057169	Inactivated virus	CoronaVac; inactivated SARS-CoV-2 vaccine (vero cell)	2	Day 0 + 14	IM	Sinovac Research and Development Co., Ltd	Phase 4
NCT04863638	Inactivated virus	Inactivated SARS-CoV-2 vaccine (Vero cell), vaccine name BBIBP-CorV	2	Day 0 + 21	IM	Sinopharm + China National Biotec Group Co + Beijing Institute of Biological Products	Phase 4
NCT04760132	Viral vector (Non-replicating)	ChAdOx1-S-(AZD1222)	1-2	Day 0 + 28	IM	AstraZeneca + University of Oxford	Phase 4
NCT04775069 NCT04914832	Viral vector (Non-replicating)	Covishield	1-2	Day 0 + 28	IM	AstraZeneca + University of Oxford	Phase 4

(Continued)

Table 4.2 SARS-CoV2 vaccines in Phase 4 clinical trials. (Continued)

Clinical trial registration	Platform of vaccine development	Vaccine candidate	Number of doses	Schedule	Route of administration	Developers	Phase
NCT05057897	Viral vector (Non-replicating)	Vaxzevria	1-2	Day 0 + 28	IM	AstraZeneca + University of Oxford	Phase 4
NCT04892459	Viral vector (Non-replicating)	Recombinant novel coronavirus vaccine (Adenovirus type 5 vector)	1	Day 0	IM	CanSino Biological Inc./Beijing Institute of Biotechnology	Phase 4
NCT05037266	Viral vector (Non-replicating)	Ad26.COV2.S	1-2	Day 0 or Day 0 + 56	IM	Janssen Pharmaceutical	Phase 4
NCT05047718	RNA based vaccine	mRNA-1273	2	Day 0 + 28	IM	Moderna + National Institute of Allergy and Infectious Diseases (NIAID)	Phase 4

(Continued)

Table 4.2 SARS-CoV2 vaccines in Phase 4 clinical trials. (Continued)

Clinical trial registration	Platform of vaccine development	Vaccine candidate	Number of doses	Schedule	Route of administration	Developers	Phase
NCT05057182	RNA based vaccine	BNT162b2 (3 LNP-mRNAs), also known as “Comirnaty”	2	Day 0 + 21	IM	Pfizer/BioNTech + Fosum Pharma	Phase 4
NCT04878211, NCT04869358	RNA based vaccine	mRNA-1273.351 LNP based mRNA vaccine	3	Day 0 or Day 0 + 28 or Day 56	IM	Moderna + National Institute of Allergy and Infectious Diseases (NIAID)	Phase 4

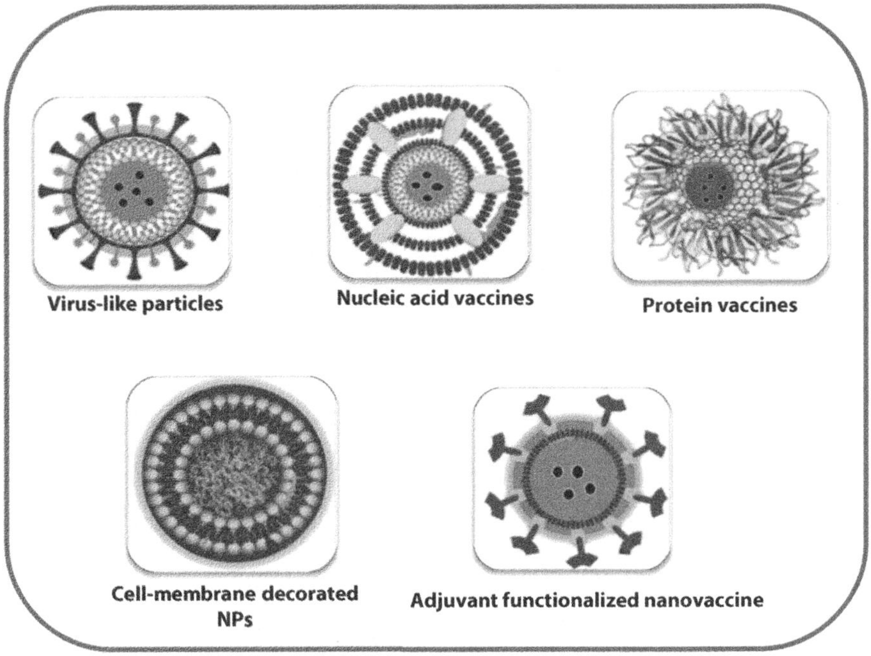

Figure 4.1 Types of biomimetic nanovaccines [10].

drug molecules. The different types of biomimetic nanovaccines available are virus-like particles, nucleic acid vaccines, protein vaccines, cell-membrane decorated NPs, and antibody/adjuvant functionalized nanovaccine as shown in Figure 4.1.

4.4.1 Virus-Like Particles

As viruses have the ablity to provoke a strong immune response, they've been in the limelight to develop a vaccine that can show the same properties. These viruses, like particles, mimic the virus in structure, form, and size which is essential for vaccination. Important feature of this particle is that it is non-infectious without any nucleic acids. This technology being manufactured in a heterologous host systems, is one of the manufacturing challenges. Several viruses, like particle-based vaccines, are developed and are in the clinical trial stage [11]. Among them, some have been licensed and marketed. Heterologous expression system has also helped to produce virus-like particles that have the capability to express one or many SARS-CoV2 structural proteins [12].

4.4.2 Nucleic Acids Vaccines

To fight coronavirus, vaccinations based on nucleic acids such as DNA or RNA was created using the nanotechnology method. A nanotechnology method. During cell internalization, nucleic acids enclosed in a lipid coat transforms into a specific to the specific viral spike protein. This foreign protein delivers signals to the host immune system to engulf it by the antigen-presenting cells. The engulfed cell then activates T and B cells, resulting in immunity. Vaccines based on nucleic acids are safe, have low reactogenicity, and are simple to design and manufacture. These vaccinations are simple to design and do not require a lengthy production procedure because they are developed based on nanotechnology. Many biotech firms are well known for their competence in delivering mRNA therapies to specific locations utilizing various mRNA delivery formulations. Various formulations can be created, depending on the therapeutic use and delivery method. Based on mRNA therapeutics and delivery routes, the various formulations are lipid nanoparticles (LNPs), lipoplexes, and polyplexes. In LNP formulation, mRNAs is encapsulated by LNPs. The external surfaces of LNPs can be modified for target delivery using different types of proteins or chemicals. The target antigens are expressed by the mRNAs that are encased in LNPs and transported into the host cells. The mRNA is incorporated in the lipid bilayer in the lipoplexes formulation. The negatively surface-charged mRNA and cationic lipids can be used to modify the dimension and surface charge of lipoplexes. The lipoplexes formulation stimulates the immune system by delivering mRNA to target-specific cells, particularly to the dendritic cells. The polyplexes formulation is a polymeric nuclei acid complex prepared with different types of nuclei acid and several cationic polymers. The polyplexes formulation can be formed into different shapes and sizes with different modifications on the surface; hence, this formulation can be used for different applications. LNPs prevent nucleic acids degradation in nucleic acid-based vaccines when administered to the host. Research evidence demonstrates favorable results for vaccines of the nucleic acids [13, 14]. Moderna on March 16, 2020, introduced mRNA-1273 vaccine in the United States, which first passed the human trials against SARS-CoV2. It was reported to be safe and exhibited maximum neutralizing antibody levels. Pfizer Inc. on May 5, 2020, announced SARS-CoV-2 RNA vaccine, which was also safe with a potential of four mRNAs encoding for target antigens. Inovio Pharmaceuticals introduced DNA vaccines on April 6, 2020, after a successful phase I clinical trial while Entos Pharmaceuticals, Inc. came up with DNA vaccines that exhibited high stability when compared with mRNA vaccines.

4.4.3 Protein Vaccines

Novavax is a recombinant protein nanoparticle vaccine used to prevent SARS-CoV2. Phase I clinical trial was performed using either MATRIX-M adjuvant or without it. The adjuvant will help in reducing number of antigens essential for vaccination. Clover Biopharmaceuticals also evaluated SCB2019, a recombinant SARS-CoV2 trimeric S protein subunit vaccine (NCT04405908) in human for the first time. Peptide-based vaccines are also formulated to deliver suitable nanocarrier by nucleic acid vaccine. This vaccine contains B- and T-cell epitopes, which are active against SARS-CoV2 [15].

4.5 Translatable Subunit Nanovaccine Against SARS-CoV2

Vaccines containing whole S protein or S1/S2 subunits with adjuvants are the SARS-CoV2 subunit vaccine. Novavax, a front-runner among developers, started a Phase I/II study as early as May 25, 2020. Protein nanoparticles can also be used as subunit vaccinations (VLPs). Recombinant expression may be used to make VLP vaccines. The combination of protein nanoparticles and fermentation or molecular farming provides monodisperse vaccine. Medicago and iBio, for example, use *Nicotiana benthamiana* to manufacture VLPs, while AdaptVac/ExpreS2ion uses an insect cell expression method to produce VLPs. The spike protein receptor-binding domain (RBD) and manganese nanoadjuvant (MnARK) form a novel nanovaccine that promotes humoral and cellular responses. RBD gets exposed during the binding process between new coronaviruses and host cells, and it is quickly identified by the host immune, thus triggering immunological process. According to studies, RBD has attained importance recently, in generating an antinovel coronavirus that had the ability to neutralize antibodies in both, animal models and humans. The mice vaccinated with MnARK vaccine demonstrated better neutralizing efficiency against the pseudo virus infection (270-fold) and live coronavirus (> 8-fold) even at a five-fold lower antigen dosage and with fewer injections than the Alum-adsorbed RBD vaccine (Alu-RBD) inoculated animals. The findings emphasize the relevance of MnARK adjuvant in the development of newer vaccines and offer a logical method for developing protective vaccines by increasing cellular internalization and immune-related pathway activation [16–18].

4.6 Separable Microneedle Patch Nanovaccine

A microneedle-based DNA vaccine has been introduced that could express SN-proteins in APCs and that trigger an immune response to

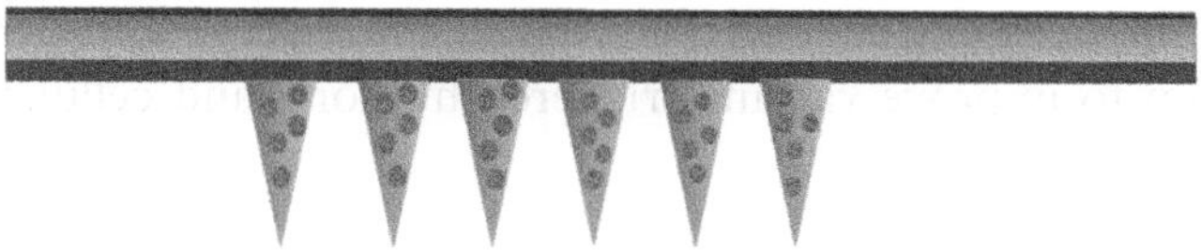

Figure 4.2 Schematic representation of separable microneedle patch [19].

prevent SARS-CoV2 virus infection (Figure 4.2). The DA-LPEI polymer may encapsulate the immune adjuvant which is hydrophobic (R848) and allows escape of DNA vaccines from endo/lysosomes with minimal cytotoxicity. To carry DNA vaccines into the intradermal layer in an APC-rich region, a detachable microneedle patch was used. The backing layer may be readily removed from the patches using PNIPAM-thermal B's responsiveness, and the microneedle can be left in the intradermal layer for several days. As a result, DLP-RS or DLP-RN nanovaccines administered intradermally will be effectively stimulating the humoral and cellular immune responses. This research might pave the way for the development of a potential SARS-CoV2 pandemic vaccine that is both thermally stable and simple to use [19].

4.7 Polymer-Based Nanovaccines

Polylactide-co-glycolide (PLGA) polymer-based nanosystems are the most popular form observed in literature. Enzymes in lactic acid and glycolic acid monomers help in the metabolism of PLGA in the human body. The PLGA formulations that are used as vaccine are nanoparticles, nanoemulsions, nanospheres, micelles, and (nano/hydro) gels. The physicochemical properties, the thermodynamic stability and the solubility of PLGA nanosystems can be fine-tuned widely. PLGA can also be coupled with polyethylene glycol (PEG) or polyetherimide to produce block copolymers that self-assemble into polymeric micelles, and the resultant micellar nanoparticles can include hydrophobic compounds, as well as hydrophobic peptide antigens or proteins [20]. Alginate-poly(ethylenimine) (PEI) is a bioreducible polymer material self-assembled into nanogel formulation for antigen loading and delivery vehicle that significantly improves vaccine-elicited humoral and cellular immune responses [21]. This nanoplatform enhances vaccine-induced antibody secretion and $CD8^{+}$ T cell–mediated tumor cell lysis. For this reason, this polymer vehicle could serve as a potent adjuvant system to improve vaccine-triggered humoral and cellular immune responses.

4.8 Pharmaceutical Challenges of SARS-CoV2 Nanovaccines

The rapid increase in the SARS-CoV2 cases has raised concern in vaccine production and delivery. Even though a successful vaccination has been created, the cost, formulation, and scale-up manufacturing must be considered. Economic differences between nations will influence large manufacturing and international supply of SARS-CoV2 vaccines. When need exceeds the distribution, poor nations are at a problem in bidding for the required vaccine. As a result, it is essential to think about technologies and platforms that are appropriate for developing countries. Production of recombinant proteins may be done in numerous platforms having both profit and loss in terms of yield, safety, economical, adaptable, fast supply, and regulatory compliance. Traditional pharmaceutical manufacturing techniques employing bioreactors and cultures of mammalian, bacterial, or yeast cell are well established, but these platforms are costly, and human pathogen contamination can stymie output. Innovative production methods that can fulfil global demand and distribution in the event of an outbreak have recently been successfully introduced. The challenges of vaccine administration during worldwide pandemic must be considered while choosing vaccine platforms. Several vaccine formulations must be kept refrigerated at all times. The need for a cold chain makes worldwide supply logically challenging, if not impossible, for underdeveloped and emerging countries with tropical temperatures. The dependency on refrigerated shipping of solution-based vaccinations has been one of the most significant problems. According to the WHO, 2.8 million vaccinations were lost mainly because of cold chain failures in five countries, and less than 10% of countries followed WHO guidelines for storing vaccines. The lyophilized vaccines may be kept at room temperature, but it is difficult to manufacture and has healthcare workers issues. Stable nanocontainers extracted from plant viruses and bacteriophages are used to safeguard genomic cargo in different environmental circumstances, resulting in a highly appropriate nanotechnology platform. For example Cowpea mosaic virus in a buffered solution is stable at ambient temperature for at least one hour at temperatures above 60°C and pH values between 3.5 and

9.0. Access to healthcare professionals (HCP) is also required for effective vaccination campaigns, which is difficult in lack of resources or in developing countries with larger population under usual situation but becomes even more complex during a worldwide pandemic when the healthcare system is already drained [9].

4.9 Future Prospects of SARS-CoV2 Nanovaccines

Nanotechnology's application in COVID-19/SARS-CoV2 therapies and vaccine development is not restricted to traditional therapeutic and vaccine designs. Other methods, such as advanced nanomaterials and biomimetic technologies, have a strong chance of being used in a SARS-CoV2–like epidemic. Szunerits and colleagues looked at the possibility of using functionalized carbon quantum dots (CQDs) to prevent infection by the human coronavirus (HCoV-229E). Pathogens can be fooled and trapped using cell membranes that imitate nano decoys. Liposomal formulations, reconstituted lipoproteins, and cell-membrane nanostructures are among the biomimetic nano decoys [22].

Other studies on vaccine development, report the development of nanomicroparticle-based next-generation vaccines that utilizes engineered nanoparticles (NPs) delivery system [23]. This type of vaccine is advantageous over conventional method by producing maximum CD8+ T cell response and acts as an appropriate carriers for peptides, mRNA, DNA, and adjuvants for the next-generation vaccine development. Covalent conjugation techniques have also been examined where proteins or peptide antigens are grafted onto nanoparticles or other molecules to develop subunit nanovaccines [24]. Rapaka *et al.* examined the adjuvants application in next-generation vaccines to promote T-cell responses in case of infectious disease [25]. Walkowski *et al.* reviewed the use of intranasal vaccine delivery for a respiratory tract infection like a pneumococcal illness [26].

4.10 Challenges and Limitations

In the fields of immunization, molecular diagnostics, and therapy, nanomedicine provides various options for combating coronaviral infections. Nonetheless, despite these efforts, safely translating NPs from the laboratory to the clinic remains a major challenge. From studying a viral genomic and proteomic composition through clinical translation, the major obstacles and roadblocks were met at various phases. While the genomic and proteomic components of SARS-CoV2 were quickly discovered to aid in the design and development of NP-based methods to combat the virus, the virus's high mutation rate and resulting genetic variety remained a key barrier to effective therapy. Viruses lack therapeutic targets that can be easily addressed without harming the host cells. SARS-CoV2 is an emerging disease with a scarcity of animal models for preclinical research. In addition, each virus behaves differently in various hosts, and the host response to SARS-CoV2 is currently being studied. As a result, extending the range for NP-based immunization, diagnostics, or therapy against other viruses remains a challenge. Importantly, given the rapid pace of viral spread and the frustratingly lengthy medication development process, novel nanomedicines of high quality, safety, and accessibility to all countries at a fair cost are urgently needed [9]. There is currently a dearth of understanding of NPs biological behaviour in relation to *in vivo* dispersion, at organ and cellular part. The effect of long-term NPs exposure on the human body is not still clear. The NPs can cause persistent inflammatory responses when it is used as adjuvants. Another threat associated with NPs are that they aggregate and can block the arteries leading to thrombosis in the host. The key obstacles mentioned in the case of vaccines is the hurry to test a vaccine but maintaining safety and efficacy in the animals tested and the further licence needed for clinical trials. The postvaccination, Antibody-dependent enhancement (ADE) antibodies activate the Fc receptor pathway, increasing the viral infectivity. An increase of the virus while entering and its duplication is the hallmark of ADE [27]. This can be the major issue while developing SARS CoV2 vaccines. Theoretically, ADE has the potential to increase viral infections or it can also induce immunopathology. This was observed during the development of vaccine against Dengue, Zika, and Ebola viruses [28–30]. ADE is now linked to both the β coronavirus and the SARS-CoV2 pandemic [31–33]. ADE is still a major concern in the SARS-CoV2 vaccine development [34]. Mutation frequency is another problem associated with vaccine development. The mutation rate of SARS-CoV2 is greater than DNA viruses, which can be linked to dissimilarity in the genes coding for the spike glycoprotein's RBD. As a result, when designing a COVID-19 vaccine, the mutation factor should be taken into consideration [35]. Combining the components of ADE and gene mutation with nanotechnology, SARS CoV, and MERS CoV vaccines might aid in SARS-CoV2 vaccine repurposing. The approved and patented vaccine candidates have to be verified at several stages before being marketed and given to the general public.

4.11 Conclusion and Outlook

The outbreak of the COVID-19/SARS-CoV2 pandemic has claimed a huge number of lives all around the globe. In an effort to find a cure to this deadly disease, research in large numbers is going on to find an effective vaccine to vaccinate the population all across the globe. While many vaccines are already in the pipeline, many are in the clinical trial, in phase I, there are as many as 16 vaccine candidates and some even in phase II and III. Universities and many manufacturing companies are putting lot of efforts to combat SARS-CoV2, still there is no specific therapy identified. Some vaccines are developed using a nanotechnological approach which is also in the trial phase and their success is based on the same. A vaccine developed with a nanotechnological approach has many advantages because it can mimic the actual virus and thus can induce a better immune response and also a single vaccine consist of a multiple mRNAs to defend against different variants. These viruses are intelligent "tricky" nanoparticles capable of entering human host cells, replicating their genetic part and then comes out as a new infectious viral nanoparticles. To prevent viruses from replicating, gene silencing techniques like RNA interference can be used to switch off the genes required for viral survival. We can achieve this by converting infectious into noninfectious viruses and using them to transmit silencing genes to cells along the same virus's path. As a result, effective vaccination techniques based on biomimetic nanotechnology can be used to assist and address variety of coronavirus outbreak challenges.

References

1. Su, S., Wong, G., Shi, W., Liu, J., Lai, A.C., Zhou, J., Liu, W., Bi, Y., Gao, G.F., Epidemiology, genetic recombination, and pathogenesis of coronaviruses. *Trends Microbiol.*, 24, 6, 490–502, 2016 Jun 1.
2. Chauveau, L., Bridgeman, A., Tan, T.K., Beveridge, R., Frost, J., Pedroza-Pacheco, I., Partridge, T., Borrow, P., Drakesmith, H., Townsend, A., Rehwinkel, J., cGAMP loading enhances the immunogenicity of VLP vaccines. *bioRxiv*, 1–50, 2020 Jan 1.
3. Campos, E.V., Pereira, A.E., De Oliveira, J.L., Carvalho, L.B., Guilger-Casagrande, M., De Lima, R., Fraceto, L.F., How can nanotechnology help to combat COVID-19? Opportunities and urgent need. *J. Nanobiotechnology.*, 18, 1, 1–23, 2020 Dec.
4. Zhao, J., Cui, W., Tian, B.P., The potential intermediate hosts for SARS-CoV-2. *Front. Microbiol.*, 11, 2400, 2020 Sep 30.

5. Iyer, S., Yadav, R., Agarwal, S., Tripathi, S., Agarwal, R., Bioengineering Strategies for Developing Vaccines against Respiratory Viral Diseases. *Clin. Microbiol. Rev.*, 35, 1, e00123-21, 2021 Nov 17.
6. Sekimukai, H., Iwata-Yoshikawa, N., Fukushi, S., Tani, H., Kataoka, M., Suzuki, T., Hasegawa, H., Niikura, K., Arai, K., Nagata, N., Gold nanoparticle-adjuvanted S protein induces a strong antigen-specific IgG response against severe acute respiratory syndrome-related coronavirus infection, but fails to induce protective antibodies and limit eosinophilic infiltration in lungs. *Microbiol. Immunol.*, 64, 1, 33–51, 2020 Jan.
7. Lim, M., Badruddoza, A.Z., Firdous, J., Azad, M., Mannan, A., Al-Hilal, T.A., Cho, C.S., Islam, M.A., Engineered nanodelivery systems to improve DNA vaccine technologies. *Pharmaceutics.*, 12, 1, 30, 2020 Jan.
8. Zeng C., Zhang C., Walker P.G., Dong Y. Formulation and delivery technologies for mRNA vaccines. iCurrent topics in microbiology and immunology. Springer, Berlin, Heidelberg, 2020, https://doi.org/10.1007/82_2020_217
9. Shin, M.D., Shukla, S., Chung, Y.H., Beiss, V., Chan, S.K., Ortega-Rivera, O.A., Wirth, D.M., Chen, A., Sack, M., Pokorski, J.K., Steinmetz, N.F., COVID-19 vaccine development and a potential nanomaterial path forward. *Nat. Nanotechnol.*, 15, 8, 646–55, 2020 Aug.
10. Vijayan, V., Mohapatra, A., Uthaman, S., Park, I.K., Recent advances in nanovaccines using biomimetic immunomodulatory materials. *Pharmaceutics*, 11, 10, 534, 2019 Oct.
11. Chroboczek J., Szurgot I., Szolajska E., Virus-like particles as vaccine. *Acta Biochim Pol.*, 61, 3, 531– 539, 2014.
12. Mortola, E. and Roy, P., Efficient assembly and release of SARS coronavirus-like particles by a heterologous expression system. *FEBS Lett.*, 576, 1-2, 174–8, 2004 Oct 8.
13. Feldman, R.A., Fuhr, R., Smolenov, I., Ribeiro, A.M., Panther, L., Watson, M., Senn, J.J., Smith, M., Almarsson, Ö., Pujar, H.S., Laska, M.E., mRNA vaccines against H10N8 and H7N9 influenza viruses of pandemic potential are immunogenic and well tolerated in healthy adults in phase 1 randomized clinical trials. *Vaccine*, 37, 25, 3326–34, 2019 May 31.
14. Jagger, B.W., Dowd, K.A., Chen, R.E., Desai, P., Foreman, B., Burgomaster, K.E., Himansu, S., Kong, W.P., Graham, B.S., Pierson, T.C., Diamond, M.S., Protective efficacy of nucleic acid vaccines against transmission of zika virus during pregnancy in mice. *J. Infect. Dis.*, 220, 10, 1577–88, 2019 Oct 8.
15. Chen, Z., Ruan, P., Wang, L., Nie, X., Ma, X., Tan, Y., T and B cell epitope analysis of SARS-CoV-2 S protein based on immunoinformatics and experimental research. *J. Cell. Mol. Med.*, 25, 2, 1274–89, 2021 Jan.
16. Wang, Y., Xie, Y., Luo, J., Guo, M., Hu, X., Chen, X., Chen, Z., Lu, X., Mao, L., Zhang, K., Wei, L., Engineering a self-navigated MnARK nanovaccine for inducing potent protective immunity against novel coronavirus. *Nano Today*, 38, 101139, 2021 Jun 1.

17. Saunders, K.O., Lee, E., Parks, R., Martinez, D.R., Li, D., Chen, H., Edwards, R.J., Gobeil, S., Barr, M., Mansouri, K., Alam, S.M., Neutralizing antibody vaccine for pandemic and pre-emergent coronaviruses. *Nature*, 10, 1–7, 2021 May.
18. Liu C., Zhou Q., Li Y., *et al.* Research and development on Therapeutic agents and vaccines for COVID-19 and related human coronavirus diseases. *ACS Cent Sci.*, 6, 3, 315–331, 2020.
19. Yin, Y., Su, W., Zhang, J., Huang, W., Li, X., Ma, H., Tan, M., Song, H., Cao, G., Yu, S., Yu, D., Separable microneedle patch to protect and deliver DNA nanovaccines against COVID-19. *ACS Nano*, 15, 9, 14347–59, 2021 Sep 2.
20. Pippa, N., Gazouli, M., Pispas, S., Recent advances and future perspectives in polymer-based nanovaccines. *Vaccines*, 9, 6, 558, 2021 Jun.
21. Li, P., Luo, Z., Liu, P., Gao, N., Zhang, Y., Pan, H., Liu, L., Wang, C., Cai, L., Ma, Y., Bioreducible alginate-poly (ethylenimine) nanogels as an antigen-delivery system robustly enhance vaccine-elicited humoral and cellular immune responses. *J. Controlled Release*, 168, 3, 271–9, 2013 Jun 28.
22. Szunerits, S., Barras, A., Khanal, M., Pagneux, Q., Boukherroub, R., Nanostructures for the inhibition of viral infections. *Molecules*, 20, 8, 14051–81, 2015 Aug.
23. Cappellano, G., Comi, C., Chiocchetti, A., Dianzani, U., Exploiting PLGA-based biocompatible nanoparticles for next-generation tolerogenic vaccines against autoimmune disease. *Int. J. Mol. Sci.*, 20, 1, 204, 2019 Jan.
24. Lu, L., Duong, V.T., Shalash, A.O., Skwarczynski, M., Toth, I., Chemical conjugation strategies for the development of protein-based subunit nanovaccines. *Vaccines*, 9, 6, 563, 2021 Jun.
25. Rapaka,R. R., Hammershaimb, E. A., Neuzil, K. M., Are some COVID-19 vaccines Better Than others? Interpreting and comparing estimates of efficacy in vaccine trials, *Clinical Infectious Diseases*, 74, 2, 352–358, 15 January 2022.
26. Walkowski, S., Singh, M., Puertas, J., Pate, M., Goodrum, K., Benencia, F., Osteopathic manipulative therapy induces early plasma cytokine release and mobilization of a population of blood dendritic cells. *PLoS One*, 9, 3, e90132, 2014 Mar 10.
27. Tirado, S.M. and Yoon, K.J., Antibody-dependent enhancement of virus infection and disease. *Viral Immunol.*, 16, 1, 69–86, 2003 Apr 1.
28. Katzelnick, L.C., Gresh, L., Halloran, M.E., Mercado, J.C., Kuan, G., Gordon, A., Balmaseda, A., Harris, E., Antibody-dependent enhancement of severe dengue disease in humans. *Science*, 358, 6365, 929–32, 2017 Nov 17.
29. Khandia, R., Munjal, A., Dhama, K., Karthik, K., Tiwari, R., Malik, Y.S., Singh, R.K., Chaicumpa, W., Modulation of dengue/zika virus pathogenicity by antibody-dependent enhancement and strategies to protect against enhancement in zika virus infection. *Front. Immunol.*, 9, 597, 2018 Apr 23.
30. Bardina, S.V., Bunduc, P., Tripathi, S., Duehr, J., Frere, J.J., Brown, J.A., Nachbagauer, R., Foster, G.A., Krysztof, D., Tortorella, D., Stramer, S.L.,

Enhancement of Zika virus pathogenesis by preexisting antiflavivirus immunity. *Science*, 356, 6334, 175–80, 2017 Apr 14.
31. Wan, Y., Shang, J., Sun, S., Tai, W., Chen, J., Geng, Q., He, L., Chen, Y., Wu, J., Shi, Z., Zhou, Y., Molecular mechanism for antibody-dependent enhancement of coronavirus entry. *J. Virol.*, 94, 5, e02015–19, 2020 Mar 1.
32. Wang, S.F., Tseng, S.P., Yen, C.H., Yang, J.Y., Tsao, C.H., Shen, C.W., Chen, K.H., Liu, F.T., Liu, W.T., Chen, Y.M., Huang, J.C., Antibody-dependent SARS coronavirus infection is mediated by antibodies against spike proteins. *Biochem. Biophys. Res. Commun.*, 451, 2, 208–14, 2014 Aug 22.
33. Tetro, J.A., Is COVID-19 receiving ADE from other coronaviruses? *Microbes Infect.*, 22, 2, 72–3, 2020 Mar 1.
34. Arvin, A.M., Fink, K., Schmid, M.A., Cathcart, A., Spreafico, R., Havenar-Daughton, C., Lanzavecchia, A., Corti, D., Virgin, H.W., A perspective on potential antibody-dependent enhancement of SARS-CoV-2. *Nature*, 584, 7821, 353–63, 2020 Aug.
35. Zhou, P., Yang, X.L., Wang, X.G., Hu, B., Zhang, L., Zhang, W., Si, H.R., Zhu, Y., Li, B., Huang, C.L., Chen, H.D., A pneumonia outbreak associated with a new coronavirus of probable bat origin. *Nature*, 579, 7798, 270–3, 2020 Mar.

5

Nanovaccinology Against Infectious Disease

S. Chakroborty[1]* and P. Panda[2]

[1]Department of Basic Sciences, IITM, IES University, Bhopal, Madhya Pradesh, India
[2]Department of Chemistry, Ravenshaw University, Cuttack, Odisha, India

Abstract
Nowadays, the whole world is under the threat of infectious diseases that affect people of developed and developing countries. Although vaccine invention reached its optimum level, there are still limitations because of high cost and lack of proper treatment. In this regard, nanotechnology offers a broad scope, and it has tremendous medical applications against all types of infectious diseases. As compared with organic molecules as vaccines, nanoparticles as the carriers have a huge demand in the market because of its simple and cost-effective strategies of preparation. Also, because of its low particle size and high surface to volume ratio, it can be highly specific for target drug delivery. It stabilizes the antigen and also in turn increases the immunogenicity of the body. There are various types of nanocarriers that include synthetic and biological polymeric nanoparticles, inorganic nanomaterials, liposomes, emulsions, nanobeads, emlusions, and so on. These adjuvants were found to be highly active and selective toward the selective biological target. Because of their high permeability, less side effect, less toxicity, long-term stability, and target-specific interaction ability, these have a huge demand to treat both infectious and non-infectious diseases. In this chapter, we are particularly emphasizing the importance of nanovaccines against various infectious diseases, such as bacterial diseases, viral diseases, cancer, parasite-born diseases, and autoimmune disorders.

***Keywords*:** Nanovaccinology, liposomes, nanoparticles, nanocarriers, cancer, bacterial disease, viral disease

**Corresponding author*: subhendu.cy@gmail.com

Kaushik Pal (ed.) Nanovaccinology as Targeted Therapeutics, (95–114) © 2022 Scrivener Publishing LLC

5.1 Introduction

Nowadays, the whole world is under the control of a number of different types of terrible infectious diseases, like cancer, tumor, malaria, parasite-born diseases, bacterial and viral infections, different types of autoimmune disorders, and so on. These deadly poisonous diseases are becoming a burden both on the economy of the both developed and developing countries. It is not only affecting the healthy lifestyle of peoples but also causes high levels of morbidity and mortality [1–3]. Therefore, in the current scenario, making a healthy lifestyle by defeating these poisonous diseases is a major concern of scientific community. Although a number of preventive measures are available to tackle the situation, there is still some sort of limitations. The available treatments against these diseases are highly costly, toxic, and many of the treatments available still cannot be reached by the people because of their ignorance. Therefore, now is the time to create public awareness among the peoples about these diseases and their preventive measures. The current situation demand is to prepare more potent, cost-effective, less toxic, and target-specific drug, which can reach all types of people (people in remote areas) even if they are socially and economically backward. In this regard, nanaoscience and its application give a new direction to research. The study of naoscience is always enthusiastic for material chemist because of its vast range of applications. Nanotechnology has a great demand in all sectors of life, most importantly in medical science [4–6]. Currently, the most emerging application of nanoscience is the vaccination by using nanoparticle-based vaccines. Preparations of nanovaccines using different types of safe, biocompatible, less toxic, and cost-effective nanocarriers constitute the forefront of medicinal chemistry research. Nanovaccines can also cross the blood brain barrier through various delivery pathways, including oral, intravenous, intranasal, transdermal, and so on. The nanovaccines should be designed in such a way that it must be stable, water-soluble, after target binding, it should have specific mechanism of action and should be inert toward other biological part. In general, target-specific antigens were loaded over specific nanocarriers (mimicking process). Similarly, there are also different types of nanocarriers, which include liposomes, emulsions, nanobeads, carbon nanotubes, inorganic nanomaterials, biological polymeric nanoparticles, and so on [7, 8]. The nanovaccines have a special tendency to train the immune system against the diseases, i.e., they were designed in such a way that whenever they get inserted inside the body cells, they will interact with the specific proteins and lipids present in the cell membrane and penetrate inside the cell. After penetration, they will stabilize the immune system of the body by the activation of the T cells, cytokines (CDs), and permit for the maturation of dendritic cells (DCs) to fight against specific diseases. Many of the developed nanovaccines have already been used for the treatment of different infectious, as well as noninfectious, diseases and also a plenty more are there under clinical trial for different therapeutical purpose [9, 10].

5.2 Nanovaccinology Against Bacterial Disease

PLGA nanoparticle, used as nanocarriers of lipopolysaccharide *Brucella melitensis* antigen to the immune system, was prepared to fight against *Brucella* infection. The as-prepared nanovaccine displayed antibacterial efficiency by the active delivery of LPS antigen to the target-specific site, enhances the production of immunoglobulines, thereby promoting the efficiency of *Brucella* bacteria removal [11].

Xyloglycan-based naovaccine was prepared by using a proficient, environmentally friendly, and industrially scalable methodology (supercritical fluid technology) against brucellosis. The nanovaccine was loaded with lipopolysaccharides as antigen derived from S19 (*B. abortus*) and quillaja saponin as the immunocarrier. The vaccine was found to be effective to bring out cell-mediated and humoral immunogenicity in female Balb/c mice. Intranasal delivery of the prepared nanovaccine was found to be more effective because it results in improved levels of production of mucosal IgG and IgA as compared with the aqueous solution of quillaja saponin and solublilized lipopolysaccharides. The formation of high levels of IgG helps in boosting the cells and increases their immunogenicity (Figures 5.1, 5.2, and 5.3) [12].

A hybrid nanovaccine consisting of PLGA NPs encapsulated with OPS and LPS antigens was prepared to enhance the formation of immunoglobulins against Brucella. The mice cells were treated separately with different doses of OPS-PLGA, LPS-PLGA, OPS, LPS, PBS, and PLGA, and their effects were studied through opsonophagocytosis assay. It was noticed that comparative to OPS-PLGA nanovaccine, LPS-PLGA–based nanovaccine was more against brucellosis and more immunogenicity. The developed nanovaccine was found to be an active candidate against both animal and human cells producing more immunogenic response (immunoglobulins) against Brucella bacterial infection (Figure 5.4) [13].

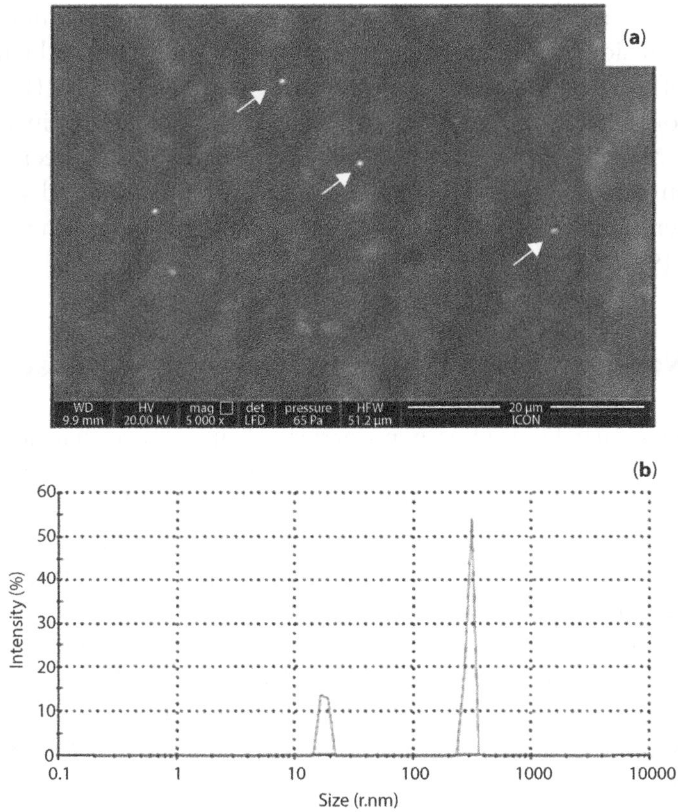

Figure 5.1 (a) FE-SEM image, and (b) dynamic light scattering data of the nanovaccine. Figure reproduced with permission from Ref. [12].

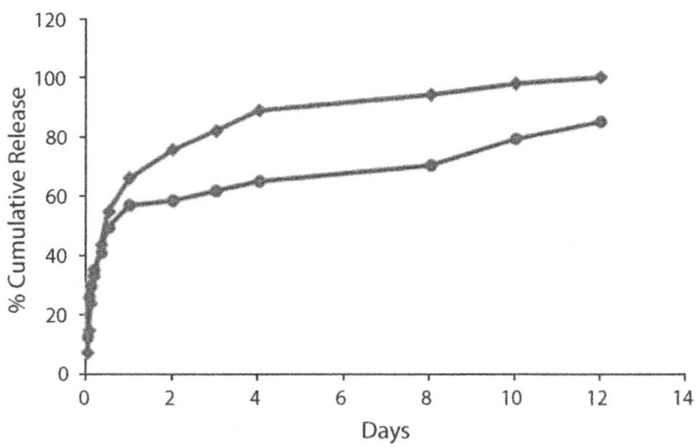

Figure 5.2 *In vitro* cumulative release of lipopolysaccharides (antigen) (blue) and quillaja saponin (immunoadjuvant) (red) from nanovaccine. Figure reproduced with permission from Ref. [12].

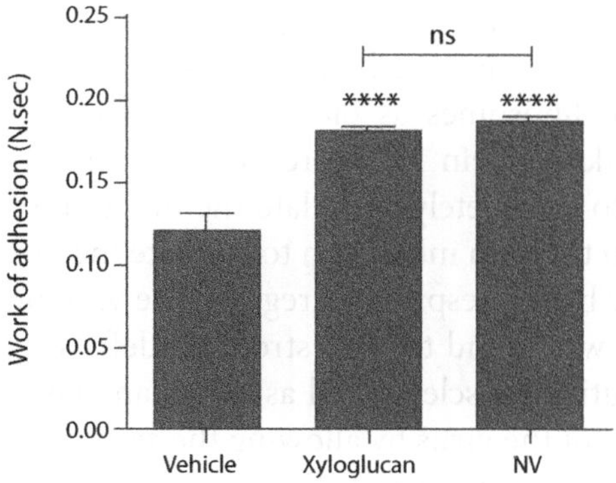

Figure 5.3 Mucoadhesion exhibited by the nanovaccine (NV) in comparison to xyloglucan. Values are expressed as mean ± SD. One way ANOVA with Bonferroni correction was applied to test significance of the results (****P < .0001, ns—not significant). Figure reproduced with permission from Ref. [12].

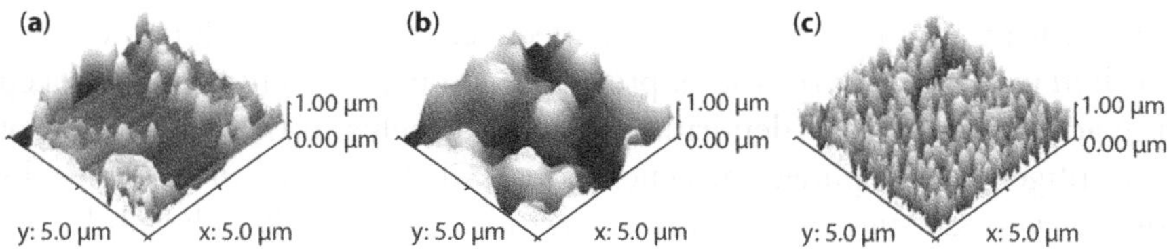

Figure 5.4 AFM microscope three-dimensional images: (a) PLGA (Uncoated nanoparticles), (b) LPS-PLGA (lipopolysaccharide antigen-coated nanoparticles) and (c) OPS-PLGA (Oligopolysaccharide antigen coated nanoparticles). Figure reproduced with permission from Ref. [13].

5.3 Nanovaccinology Against Viral Disease

A BP_{26}-M_{2e}–based nanobarrel was developed as nanovaccine for the treatment of viral infection caused by influenza virus. The hybrid nanovaccine showed greater potentiality as compared to the physical mixture of soluble BP26 and M2e including/excluding adjuvant alum. The BP_{26}-M_{2e} nanobarrels showed potent antiviral properties by the generation of antibody anti-M2e after binding with the virus infected cells. These nanovaccines were found to be more effective against mice cell lines affected by influenza virus in the absence of adjuvant also by the activation of T cells thereby enhanced the performance of the immune system [14].

In order to fight against COVID-19, the viral infection generally occurred at the respiratory tract, a bionic-virus nanovaccine was developed which will enhance the mucosal immunity through nasal delivery.

The nanovaccine was developed though mimicking process i.e. composed of poly(I:C)viral genes prepared via mimicking viral genetic material as immunoadjuvant, liposomes as bio-PS (biomimetic pulmonary surfactant) and the spike protein as the receptor binding domain for SARS-CoV-2 in order to completely stimulate the function of coronavirus. The vaccine was taken through inhalation to emulate the progression of SARS-CoV-2 infectivity by the respiratory region. The vaccine with bionic virus like morphology was found to have strongest defensive outcomes against mucosal than routine muscle as well as subcutaneous injection. It caused the neutralization of the virus by allowing the secretion of immunoglobulin A and prevents it to enter inside the body *via* the respiratory zone [15].

A virus mimicked nanovaccine was prepared for tumor immunotherapy by activating the immunogenic response. The designed was composed of CpG ODN (nucleic acids), tumor associated proteins (antigens) nAvidin (neutravidin). The dye molecules were used to synthesize nanoparticles of comparable size to viruses so that the vaccine will be traced by the virus more easily. The authors studied the effectiveness of the developed vaccine both *in vivo* and *in vitro*. The as-prepared nanoparticles efficiently induced the activation of DCs (dendritic cells) which helps in the penetration of the antigen and amplified the generation of CD (cytokine) *in vitro*. Results of *in vivo* study suggested that, the vaccine targeted the lymph cells by the formation of tumor antigen-specific CD8, induced the activation of T cells as well as Th1-biased immunogenic responses inside the cell. Using the concept of recognisation, the nanovaccine considerably targeted the tumor causing cells and inhibited the development of overexpression of antigens in tumor causing cells by extending the time of attachment to the receptor site of tumor bearing mice [16].

In this study the authors isolated three different IAV (Influenza A virus) M2e proteins from swine, human and avian and injected it to C-terminal of Cap protein to form universal influenza nanovaccines. The different immunoprotective effects observed were investigated upon the mice cell lines. The M2e proteins which were bounded tightly by the nanoparticles displayed more effectiveness against IAV [17].

A nanovaccine is made by the coordination of spike protein with metal (Mn)-nanoadjuvant known as MnARK to fight against viral infections. The nanovaccine was designed in such a way that after get injected in to the cell it causes neutralization of the viral strains. The developed vaccine was found to be nearly 270-fold active towards pseudo virus and >8-fold activeness against corona virus *in vitro* as compared to that of Alu-RBD. The nanoadjuvant caused the active delivery of the MnARK to lymph nodes and causes activation of the immune cells like DCs, CDs and T cells [18].

A nanovaccine was designed against HBV (hepatitis B virus) by the combination of chitosan, heparin, hepatitis B virus surface antigen (rHB-sAg) or core antigen (rHBcAg). The prepared nanovaccine showed excellent target-specific drug delivery and also their administration activated the BMDCs (bone marrow-derived dendritic cells) present at different lymph nodes (LNs) with prolonged retention time [19].

CS NPs-KAg nanaovaccine was prepared against influenza virus by the loading of chitosan NPs over influenza virus (KAg) as antigen using poly (I:C) as adjuvant. The developed CS NPs-KAg and CS NPs-poly(I:C) were found to bear a surface charge of +30.7 mV and +25.1 mV. The nanovaccine CS NPs-KAg was co-administered as intranasal mist by mixing it with CS NPs-poly(I:C) (chitosan nanovaccine). Nanovaccines were found as the successive inhibitors of H1N2-OH10 (homologous) and H1N1-OH7 (heterologous) viral strains in animals as compared to the solution of only soluble form of poly(I:C) taken as standard. Also, chitosan nanovaccine works by the activation of DCs and T cells in the tracheobronchial lymph nodes thereby enhancing the immunogenic responses against viral diseases [20].

5.4 Nanovaccinology Against Cancer

Hybrid nanovesicles of DOX-LINV were prepared by the loading of doxorubicin (DOX) over fused liposomes (LIPs) containing tumor-derived nanovesicles, which was further used in immunochemotherapeutics for the treatment of tumor. The developed nanovesicles of DOX-LINV showed excellent target specificity and drug deliverability. The antitumor drug DOX carried by the nanovesicles was successfully delivered at the specified tumor tissue and also causes death of the tumor cells by the activation of dendritic cells therby increasing the cell immunogenicity. The developed nanovesicles were found to be quite effective against lung cancer, breast cancer, murine melanoma and activates the immune cells by simultaneous inhibition of tumor causing microenvironment. The antitumor efficacy of the nanovesicles against the mice tumor cells was found to be 33.3%, which suggest that this can be further act as potential drug candidate for successful immunochemotheraphy purpose [21].

A biocompatible nanovaccine was developed by the co-ordination of Ca-metal with bisphosphonates (a type of orthopaedics drug) by the loading of peptide antigens for boosting innate and adaptive immunity. Peptides increase the hydrophilicity of the nanocarrier and also provide stability to the carried antitumor drug and helps for specific drug delivery at TLR4 receptor cells which are generally found to be overexpressed in tumor cells. The mechanism of developed nanovaccine suggested that the nanocarriers showed antitumor ability by the activation of the DCs and T cells. It was also been observed that 50% of the tumor cell disappeared by the application of this nanovaccine [22].

An anticancer nanovaccine consisting of MnO_2, OVA (ovalbumin), and OMPN (polydopamine) was developed by following a facile one-pot protocol. Polydopamine was found to exhibit superior anticancer potential against orthotopic melanoma cells and also prevented liver tumor metastasis in mice. After the nanovaccine was injected, the dendritic cells (DCs) were fund to be highly active at lymph nodes, thereby enhancing the immune response. These results indicated that the nanovaccine OMPN can be used for the suppression of tumor metastasis and can also act as a target-specific, multipurposeful nanovaccine for cancer prevention, and therapy [23].

In malignant melanoma therapy, combining a Mn porphyrin-based metal-organic frameworks (Mn-MOF) with a CpG and OVA-overexpressing melanoma B16 cell cell membranes helps to enhance the potency of the anti–PD-1 antibody. Because of the alleviation of tumour hypoxia, it was discovered that the newly developed nanovaccine had excellent tumour killing efficiency. As a result of the SDT effects, the nanovaccine was able to cause immunogenic cell death. Tumor associated antigens derived *in situ* from both OVA and SDT demonstrated a vaccine-like effect by activating T cells and maturing DCs. A new nanovaccine based on a CpG-adsorbed Mn-MOF was discovered that could be used for sonodynamic therapy (SDT) by combining an immune adjuvant CpG with a Mn-MOF to coat cell membranes derived from melanoma B16 cells. Because of the alleviation of tumour hypoxia, it was discovered that the newly developed nanovaccine had excellent tumor killing efficiency. As a result of the SDT effects, the nanovaccine was able to cause immunogenic cell death. Tumor-associated antigens derived *in situ* from both OVA and SDT demonstrated a vaccine-like effect by activating T cells and maturing DCs [24].

A Man-PLL-RT–based nanovaccine was prepared by the combination of mannose receptor-mediated nanovaccine and PD-L1 gene (ability of stimulating the immuno system and has auto-killing ability) against tumor. It was capable of encapsulating ovalbumin (OVA) antigen and CpG (cytosine-phosphate-guanine) as adjuvant through electrostatic interaction. The +vely charged Man-PLL-RT/OVA/CpG nanovaccine inhibited the growth of the tumor environment in the B16F10 melanoma-bearing mice by the activation of DCs and T cells (Scheme 5.1) [25].

A safe, potent, and effective nanovaccine was developed by the fusion of OMVs and TCMs derived from bacterial and tumor cell membranes

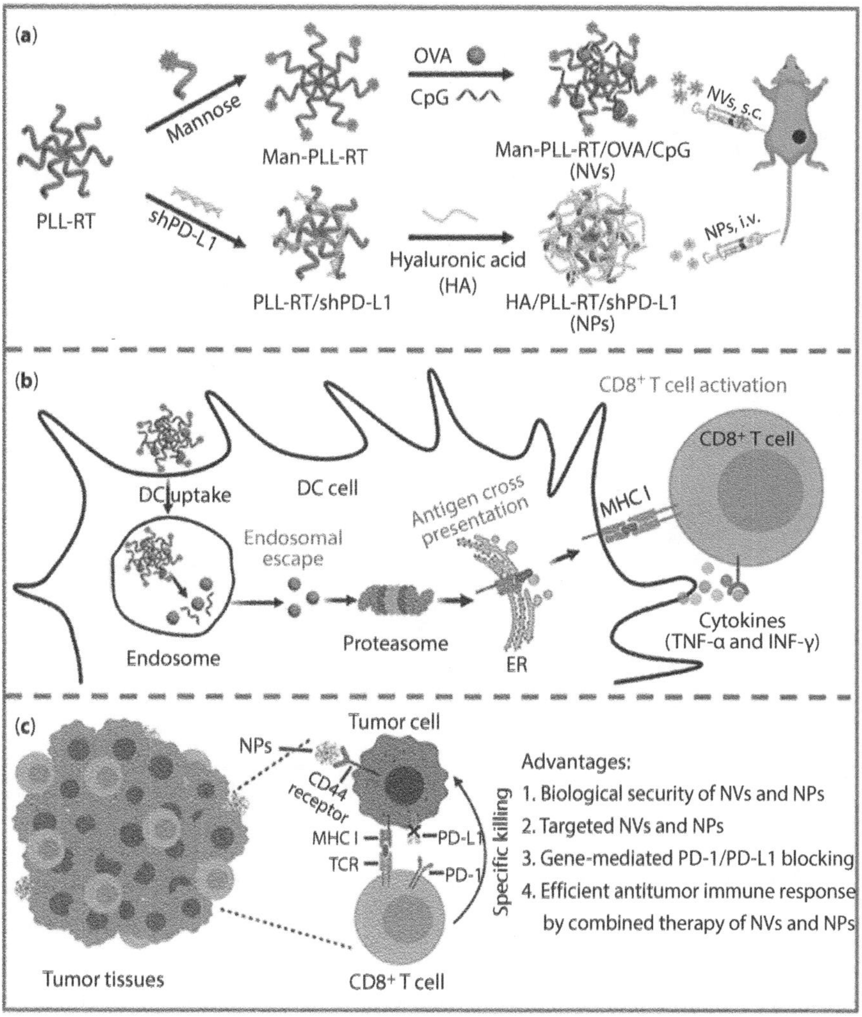

Scheme 5.1 Combining mannose receptor-mediated nanovaccines and gene-regulated PD-L1 blockade for boosting cancer immunotherapy. (a) Preparation of targeted Man-PLL-RT/OVA/CpG nanovaccines (NVs) and HA/PLL-RT/shPD-L1 nanoparticles (NPs). (b) Activation of NVs. (c) PD-1/PD-L1 blockade and antitumor immune responses. Figure reproduced with permission from Ref. [25].

called BTs. The adjuvalent BTs have the high ability to target DCs and helps in the full maturation of DCs. The TCMs in BTs have the ability to train the immune system to produce multiantigenic antitumor immunity. Nanovaccines composed of BTs@PLGA as low as 1 μg of OMVs was found to be very effective against tumor and eradicate up to 30% of tumor in mice

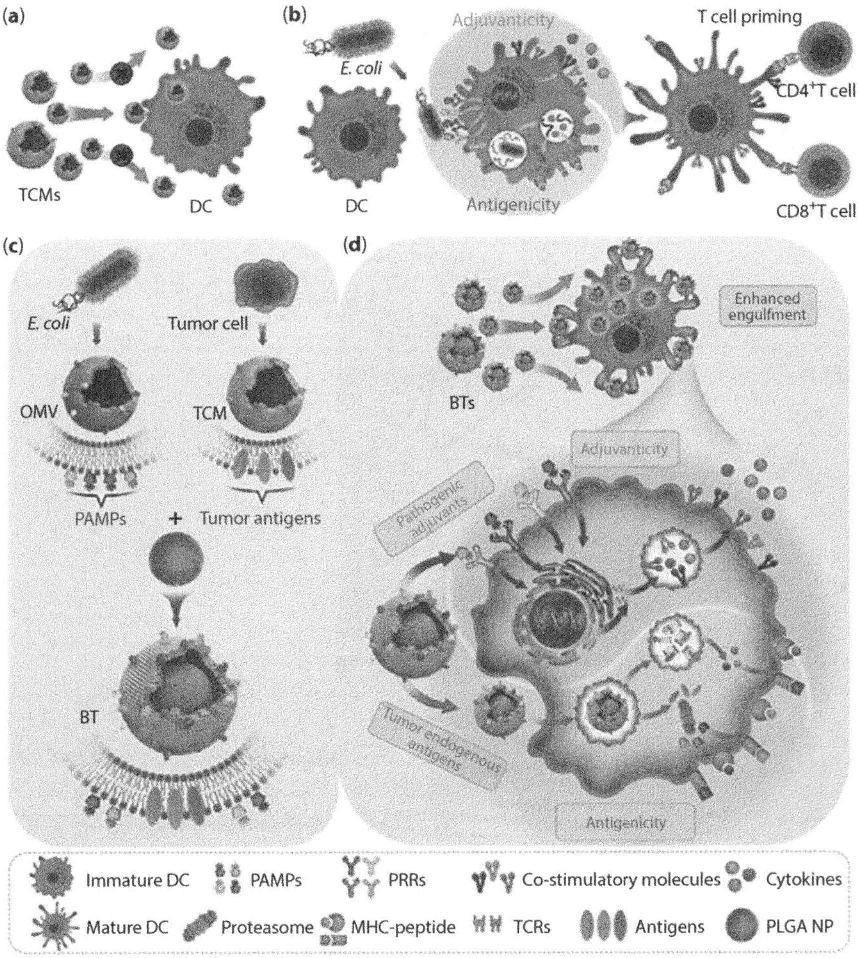

Scheme 5.2 Schematic showing BTs as nanovaccines for cancer immunotherapy. (a) TCMs could not be efficiently detected and phagocytosed by DCs due to the absence of danger signals. (b) In nature, bacteria containing several kinds of PAMPs and bacterial antigens are recognized and internalized by DCs based on the interaction of PAMPs on bacteria and PRRs on DCs. The bacteria simultaneously provide adjuvanticity and antigenicity to stimulate the maturation of DCs (up-regulated expression of co-stimulatory molecules and secretion of pro-inflammatory cytokines) and the presentation of bacterial antigens by DCs. The DCs can potently trigger the bacteria-specific T cell responses. (c) Preparation of BTs. TCMs, OMVs, and PLGA NPs were mixed, sonicated, and repeatedly extruded to prepare BTs. The BTs thus inherit multiple PAMPs from bacteria and diverse tumor endogenous antigens from tumor cells. (d) Due to the presence of PAMPs, BTs could be efficiently recognized and uptaken by DCs, enabling the co-delivery of tumor antigens and adjuvants to DCs. The multiple pathogenic PAMPs of BTs could induce the full maturation of DCs by simultaneously targeting various PRRs. Meanwhile, the diverse tumor endogenous antigens of BTs could be processed and presented. The mature DCs presenting tumor antigens could elicit robust tumor antigen-specific T cell responses for tumor eradication. Figure reproduced with permission from Ref. [26].

cells (B16F10) over 100 days. PLGA as the active drug delivery candidate has already been admitted by FDA and also the applications of BTs to make the cells tumor free are under clinical trial (Scheme 5.2) [26].

CT-LDH and CO-LDH–based nanovaccines were prepared, and their effectiveness was studied against B16F10 tumor cells in mouse models. The efficacy of the nanovaccine against the tumor-specific area was decided by their way of injection inside the cells, i.e., through intravenous (IV), subcutaneous (SC) or by grouping, i.e., IV + IV, SC + IV, IV + SC, and SC + SC. Among the four different strategies of injection of vaccine, the IV + SC combination was found as the most efficient pathway for vaccination to induce fast, effective, and long-lasting antitumor responses, which is generally sufficient to inhibit the expansion of early stage tumor (>75–90%) and also delays the regrowth of advanced state tumors (Scheme 5.3) [27].

Taking the advantage of biomimetic process, an antitumor nanovaccine (CM-CaPyro) was developed by the combination of tumor cell antigens

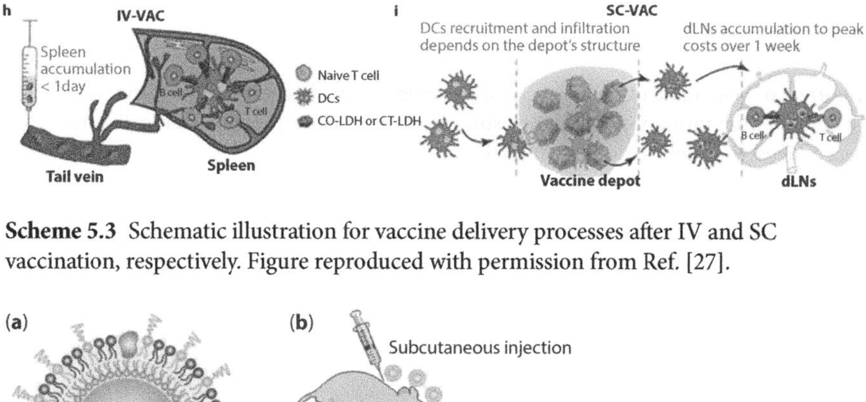

Scheme 5.3 Schematic illustration for vaccine delivery processes after IV and SC vaccination, respectively. Figure reproduced with permission from Ref. [27].

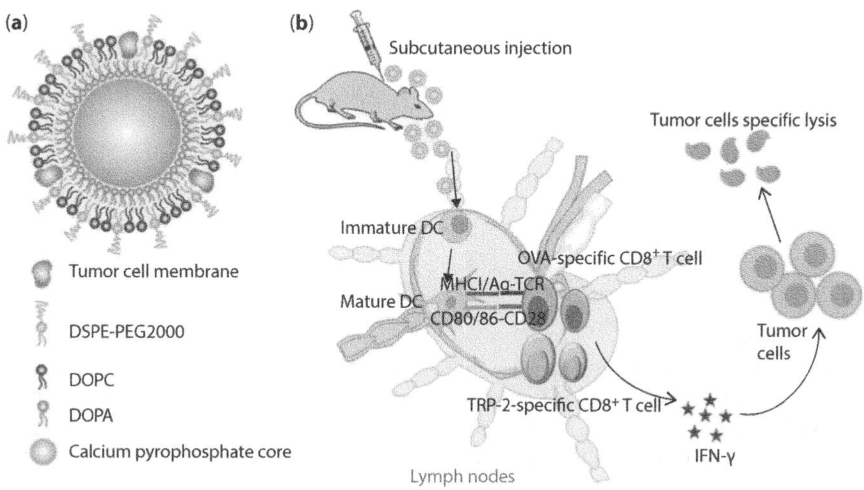

Figure 5.5 Schematic illustration to show the structure of (a) tumor CM@CaPyro NGs and (b) their functions to induce antitumor immunity as a nanovaccine. Figure reproduced with permission from Ref. [28].

(B16-OVA) and biocompatible nanocarriers/adjuvant as calcium pyrophosphate, which has greater immune potentiating effect. The nanocarriers were coated with B16-OVA protins and lipids tumor cell membranes, so that they can be specifically identified by the tumor causing cells and will serve as tumor-specific antigens. The nanovaccine works by the promoter of maturation and activation of DCs and T cells. These results suggested

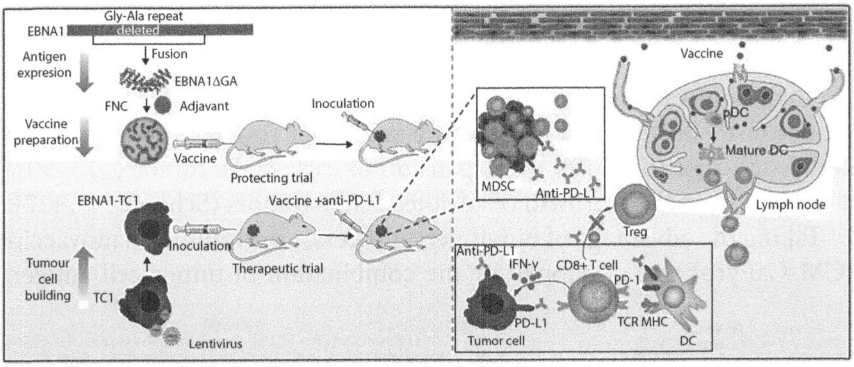

Figure 5.6 Schematic of the tannic acid-formulated nanovaccine and the process of combination immunotherapy consisting of immune checkpoint blockade. Figure reproduced with permission from Ref. [29].

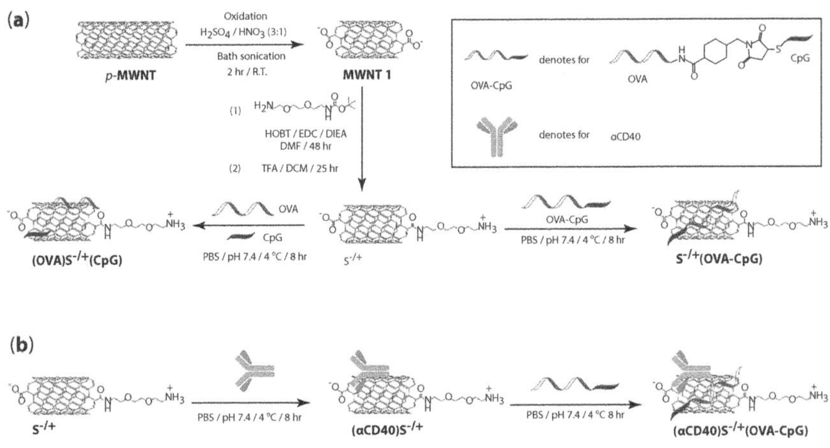

Scheme 5.4 Synthesis of the conjugates. (a) Synthesis of (OVA)S/þ(CpG) or S/þ(OVACpG) conjugates. pMWNT was oxidized using acidic mixture yielding MWNT. The carboxylic acid moieties of MWNT were reacted with Bocprotected amineterminated spacer via amide coupling reaction yielding S/þ. (OVA)S/þ(CpG) was synthesized by the imultaneous addition of OVA and CpG to S/þ, while S/þ(OVACpG) was synthesized by reacting the OVACpG with S/þ. (b) Synthesis of (aCD40)S/þ(OVACpG). aCD40 was irst conjugated with S/þ yielding (aCD40)S/þ that following conjugation with OVACpG yielded (aCD40) S/þ(OVACpG). Figure reproduced with permission from Ref. [30].

that the developed vaccine can be used as an excellent agent in tumor therapy (Figure 5.5) [28].

A nanovaccine was prepared against EBV-associated tumors by taking tannic acid (TA) as antigen and IFN-α/CpG as adjuvants. The antigen and

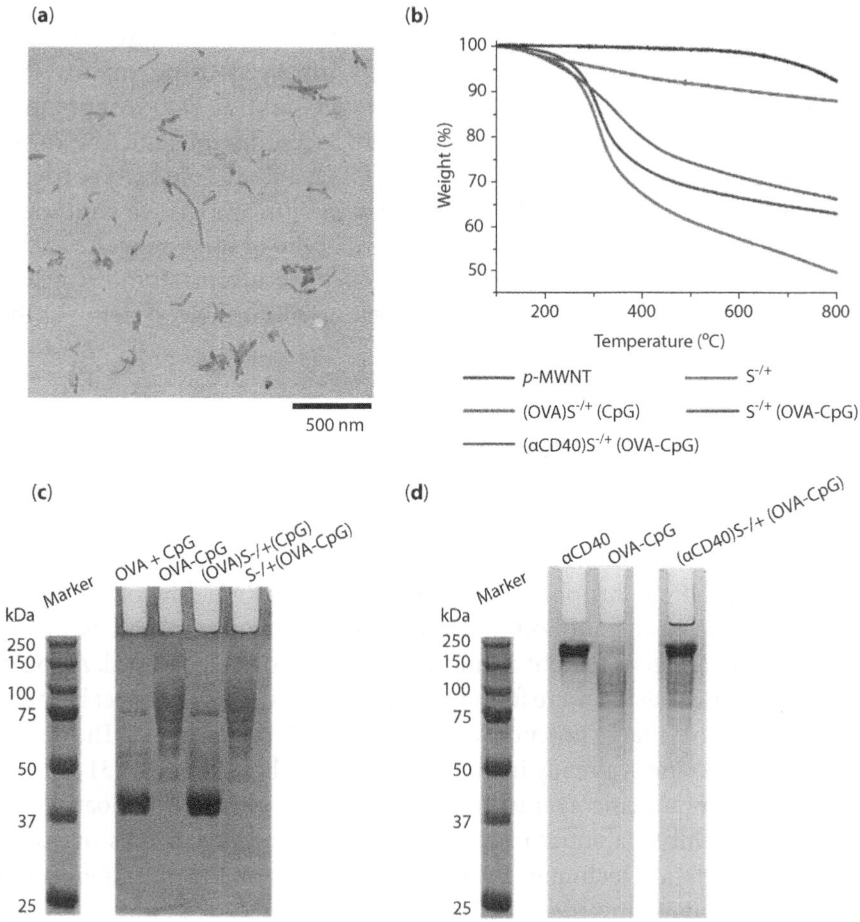

Figure 5.7 Characterization of the conjugates. (a) Representative TEM image of an aqueous dispersion of S/þ. (b) Thermogravimetric profiles. S/þ or the conjugates, of know weights, were subjected to increasing temperatures and the weight loss was measured at the increased temperature. (c) PAGE of (OVA)S/þ(CpG) or S/þ(OVACpG). Free OVA, or OVA contained in the conjugates, each at 10 mg OVA, were loaded in the appropriate lane of 10% native, nonreducing gel. (d) PAGE of (aCD40)S/þ(OVACpG). OVACpG conjugate containing 3 mg OVA, 10 mg of aCD40 or (aCD40)S/þ(OVACpG) containing 3 mg OVA and 10 mg aCD40 were loaded in the appropriate lane of 10% native, nonreducing gel. Bands were detected by gel staining with Coomassie Brilliant blue. Figure reproduced with permission from Ref. [30].

the adjuvants were combined together through H-bonding interaction to form well-shaped nanoparticles through flash nanocomplexation process. The adjuvant CpG induced strong immune activation in the lymph nodes and exhibited inhibition of tumor growth cells. TA-CpG-anti–PD-L1 results a marked decrease in the size of the tumor size by the maturation of the DCs and T cells. The developed nanovaccine provided a valuable strategy for treating patients with EBV-positive tumours (Figure 5.6) [29].

A nanovaccine against anticancer was prepared using multiwalled carbon-nanotubes (MWNT) loaded with CpG and αCD40 as immuno-adjuvants and OVA as the antigen (Scheme 5.4). Immunogenic responses observed by the delivery of each of OVA, CPG, and αCD40 by incorporation of MWNT was recorded. The results of *in vitro* and *in vivo* anticancer study against C57BL and B16F10 melanoma cells of mice suggested that, the as-prepared nanovaccine was quite effective against tumor-causing cells. The nanovaccine works by the activation of immuno system *via* the activation of T cells (Figure 5.7) [30].

5.5 Nanovaccinology Against Parasite-Born Disease

A safe, potent, and effective nanovaccine was developed against malaria parasite by the combination of *Plasmodium falciparum* CHrPfs25 as antigen and Au-NPs as nanocarrier. The nanovaccine worked by blocking the transmission causing antibodies and increases the immunogenicity by the activation of antigens to fight against different parasites. In general, Au NPs, having spherical shape, were found to have more pronounced effect because of high negative charge potential as compared with other shapes. The developed nnaovaccine is already in phase I clinical trial (Figure 5.8) [31].

A new nanovaccine against leishmaniasis was prepared by loading of SODB1 (Leishmania superoxide dismutase) over chitosan NPs by using ionotropic gelation techique. The effect on the NPs on the immune system was studied by taking the BALB/c cell lines of mice. The mice cell lines were injected by SODB1 and PBS (phosphate buffer saline), as well as SLA (soluble leishmania antigens) and CFA (complete Freund's adjuvant) were also injected into it. The nanovaccines significantly enhanced the immunogenicity by the production of IgG2a in mice from TH_1 cells, which was very effective toward the eradication of leishmania [32].

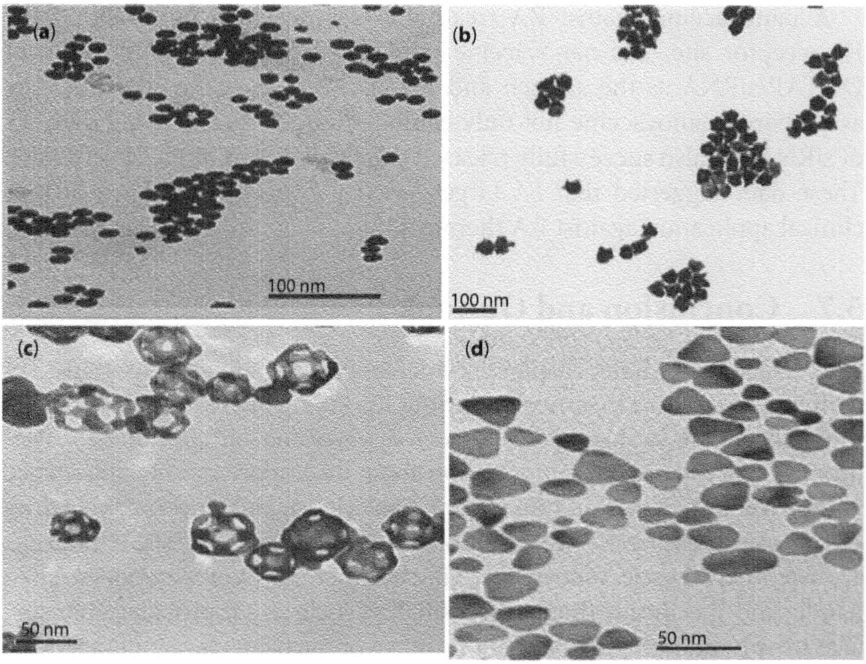

Figure 5.8 Characterization of Gold nanoparticles (GN-particles). Transmission Electron Microscopy (TEM) images of GN-particles of different shapes. (a) Spherical (GNP); (b) Star (GNS); (c) Cage (GNC); (d) Nanoprism (NPR). Figure reproduced with permission from Ref. [31].

5.6 Nanovaccinology Against Autoimmune Disorders

FA-PEG-DEAE/siRNA–based nanovaccine was developed for the treatment of arthritis. The nanovaccine targeted the receptors present on the cell membrane and made specified drug delivery. The developed medicine has no toxic side effects and significantly reduces cytokine release. With the sophisticated treatment, no hazardous side effects and a notable reduction in the production of cytokines, joint synovial fluid conc. of TNF-α, and bone loss have been diminished [33].

A PLGA-PEI/COX2 siRNA-based nanovaccine was designed against RA therapy by the combination of PEI-PLGA as the nanocarrier and siRNA-COX2 as antigen. The as-prepared nanovaccine showed high effectiveness against the diseases by significantly lowering the overexpression of C28/I2 protein and other interrelated apoptotic issues [34].

A nanovaccine against RA treatment was designed by targeting the FA receptor site. The nanovaccine was designed by the composition of DOTAP/siRNA as the antigen and FA-PEG-PLGA as the adjuvant. The as-prepared nanovaccine not only exhibited target-specific drug delivery of siRNA but also successfully released the carried drug at the specific site. These data suggested that FA target-based naovaccine can have further clinical application against RA therapy [35].

5.7 Conclusion and Outlook

In conclusion, this book chapter provides an outlook about the usefulness of nanovaccines for the treatment of various life killing diseases, such as cancer, tumor, bacterial, viral and parasite-born diseases and autoimmune diseases. Moreover, it also provides information about the importance of nanoscience in the invention of various safe, potent, stable, inert, and biocompatible drug discoveries. Comparative to traditional way of drug synthesis, nanodrugs are safe to synthesize, follows cost-effective method of preparation, easy to handle and specifically due to their small particle size it provides high surface to volume ratio. Therefore, a number of particles can simultaneously make interaction with the specific target which in turn makes these molecules more effective. Also it has fewer side effects because the nanocarriers are merged by target-specific antigens, therefore after getting injected inside the cells, the target-specific proteins will be overexpressed and taking the advantage of their desperateness (based upon plug and play principle), the nanocarrier will attach to the specific site and work by inhibiting the specific diseases by the activation of immuno system. Therefore, we thought that this chapter will help the medicinal chemists to take idea about the designing of specific nanovaccines which will provide very fast response against the specific disease, should have high half-life, stable and biocompatible.

Acknowledgments

SC is grateful to the IITM, IES University, Bhopal, India.

References

1. Fries, C.N., Curvino, E.J., Chen, J.L., Permar, S.R., Fouda, G.G., Collier, J.H., Advances in nanomaterial vaccine strategies to address infectious diseases impacting global health. *Nat. Nanotechnol.*, *16*, 1–14, 2021.

2. Sangiao, E.T., Holban, A.M., Gestal, M.C., Advanced nanobiomaterials: vaccines, diagnosis and treatment of infectious diseases, *Molecules, 21*, 867, 2016.
3. Poon, C. and Patel, A.A., Organic and inorganic nanoparticle vaccines for prevention of infectious diseases, *Nano Express, 1*, 012001, 2020.
4. Yang, G., Chen, S., Zhang, J., Bioinspired and Biomimetic Nanotherapies for the Treatment of Infectious Diseases, *Front. Pharmacol., 10*, 751, 2019.
5. Kirtane, A.R., Verma, M., Karandikar, P., Furin, J., Langer, R., Traverso, G., Nanotechnology approaches for global infectious diseases, *Nat. Nanotechnology, 16*, 369–384, 2021.
6. Qasim, M., Lim, D.J., Park, H., Na, D., Nanotechnology for diagnosis and treatment of infectious diseases, *J. Nanosci. Nanotechnol., 14*, 7374–7387, 2014.
7. Zhao, L., Seth, A., Wibowo, N., Zhao, C.X., Mitter, N., Yu, C., Middelberg, A.P.J., Nanoparticle vaccines, *Vaccine, 32*, 327–337, 2014.
8. Pati, R., Shevtsov, M., Sonawane, A., Nanoparticle Vaccines Against Infectious Diseases, *Front. Immunol., 9*, 2224, 2018.
9. Reljic, R. and Fernández, Á. G., Nanoparticle vaccines against infectious diseases, *Front. Immunol., 10*, 2615, 2019.
10. Butkovich, N., Li, E., Ramirez, A., Burkhardt, A.M., Wang, S.W., Advancements in protein nanoparticle vaccine platforms to combat infectious disease, *Wires Nanomed. Nanobiotechnol., 13*, e1681, 2021.
11. Malekia, M. and Salouti, M., Immunization effect of lipopolysaccharide antigen in conjugation with PLGA nanoparticles as a nanovaccine against Brucella melitensis infection, *Biologicals, 72*, 10–17, 2021.
12. Vyas, S., Dhoble, S., Ghodake, V., Patravale, V., Xyloglucan based mucosal nanovaccine for immunological protection against brucellosis developed by supercritical fluid technology, *Int. J. Pharm.: X, 2*, 100053, 2020.
13. Afshari, H., Maleki, M., Salouti, M., Immunological effects of two new nanovaccines against Brucella based on OPS and LPS antigens conjugated with PLGA nanoparticles, *Eur. Polym. J., 139*, 110021, 2020.
14. Kang, S., Kim, Y., Shin, Y., Song, J.J., Jon, S., Antigen-presenting, self-assembled protein nanobarrels as an adjuvant-free vaccine platform against influenza virus, *ACS Nano, 15*, 10722–10732, 2021.
15. Zheng, B., Peng, W., Guo, M., Huang, M., Gu, Y., Wang, T., Ni, G., Ming, D., Inhalable nanovaccine with biomimetic coronavirus structure to trigger mucosal immunity of respiratory tract against COVID-19, *Chem. Eng. J., 418*, 129392, 2021.
16. Lu, Z., Zhang, Y., Wang, Y., Tan, G.H., Huang, F.Y., Cao, R., He, N., Zhang, L., A biotin-avidin-system-based virus-mimicking nanovaccine for tumor immunotherapy, *J. Controlled Release, 332*, 245–259, 2021.
17. Ding, P., Zhang, G., Chen, Y., Liu, H., Liu, Y., Ji, R., Wang, Y., Li, G., Wang, A., Reasonable permutation of M2e enhances the effect of universal influenza nanovaccine, *Int. J. Biol. Macromol., 173*, 244–250, 2021.

18. Wang, Y., Xie, Y., Luo, J., Guo, M., Hu, X., Chen, X., Chen, Z., Lu, X., Mao, L., Zhang, K., Wei, L., Ma, Y., Wang, R., Zhou, J., He, C., Zhang, Y., Chen, S., Sheni, L., Chend, Y., Qiu, N., Liu, Y., Cu, Y., Li, G., Liu, Y., Chen, C., Engineering a self-navigated MnARK nanovaccine for inducing potent protective immunity against novel coronavirus, *Nano Today*, *38*, 101139, 2021.
19. Qi, D., Chen, Y., Liu, L., Engineered therapeutic nanovaccine against chronic hepatitis B virus infection, *Biomaterials*, *269*, 120674, 2021.
20. Renu, S., Ruiz, N.F., Ghimire, S., Han, Y., Schrock, J., Dhakal, S., Patil, V., Krakowk, S., Renukaradhya, G.J., Poly(I:C) augments inactivated influenza virus-chitosan nanovaccine induced cell mediated immune response in pigs vaccinated intranasally, *Vet. Microbiol.*, *242*, 108611, 2020.
21. Hu, M., Zhang, J., Kong, L., Yu, Y., Hu, Q., Yang, T., Wang, Y., Tu, K., Qiao, Q., Qin, X., Zhang, Z., Immunogenic hybrid nanovesicles of liposomes and tumor-derived nanovesicles for cancer immunochemotherapy. immunogenic hybrid nanovesicles of liposomes and tumor-derived nanovesicles for cancer immunochemotherapy, *ACS Nano*, *15*, 3123–3138, 2021.
22. Qin, M., Li, M., Song, G., Yang, C., Wu, P., Dai, W., Zhang, H., Wang, X., Wang, Y., Zhou, D., He, B., Zhang, Q., Boosting innate and adaptive antitumor immunity via a biocompatible and carrier-free nanovaccine engineered by the bisphosphonates-metal coordination, *Nano Today*, *37*, 101097, 2021.
23. Xi, B., Li, D., Xu, H., Zhou, X., Xu, X., Qian, Y., Yu, F., Hu, H., Zhou, Z., Liu, X., Gao, J., Slater, N.K.H., Shen, Y., Tang, J., An MRI-trackable therapeutic nanovaccine preventing cancer liver metastasis, *Biomaterials*, *274*, 120893, 2021.
24. Zhan, G., Xu, Q., Zhang, Z., Wei, Z., Yong, T., Bie, N., Zhang, X., Li, X., Li, J., Gan, L., Yang, X., Biomimetic sonodynamic therapy-nanovaccine integration platform potentiates Anti-PD-1 therapy in hypoxic tumors, *Nano Today*, *38*, 101195, 2021.
25. Chen, J., Fang, H., Hu, Y., Wu, J., Zhang, S., Feng, Y., Lin, L., Tian, H., Chen, X., Combining mannose receptor mediated nanovaccines and gene regulated PD-L1 blockade for boosting cancer immunotherapy, *Bioact. Mater.*, 7, 167–180, 2022.
26. Lia, M., Zhou, H., Jiang, W., Yang, C., Miao, H., Wang, Y., Nanovaccines integrating endogenous antigens and pathogenic adjuvants elicit potent antitumor immunity, *Nano Today*, *35*, 101007, 2020.
27. Zhang, L.X., Suna, X.M., Jia, Y.B., Liu, X.G., Dong, M., Xu, Z.P., Liu, R.T., Nanovaccine's rapid induction of anti-tumor immunity significantly improves malignant cancer immunotherapy, *Nano Today*, *35*, 100923, 2020.
28. Li, M., Qin, M., Song, G., Deng, H., Wang, D., Wang, X., Dai, W., He, B., Zhang, H., Zhang, Q., A biomimetic antitumor nanovaccine based on biocompatible calcium pyrophosphate and tumor cell membrane antigens, *Asian J. Pharm. Sci.*, *16*, 97–109, 2021.

29. Liu, H., Chen, H., Liu, Z., Le, Z., Nie, T., Qiao, D., Su, Y., Mai, H., Chen, Y., Liu, L., Therapeutic nanovaccines sensitize EBV-associated tumors to checkpoint blockade therapy, *Biomaterials, 255*, 120158, 2020.
30. Hassan, H.A.F.M., Smyth, L., Wang, J.T.W., Costa, P.M., Ratnasothy, K., Diebold, S.S., Lombardi, G., Al-Jamal, K.T., Dual stimulation of antigen presenting cells using carbon nanotube-based vaccine delivery system for cancer immunotherapy, *Biomaterials, 104*, 310–322, 2016.
31. Kumara, R., Ray, P.C., Datta, D., Bansala, G.P., Angov, E., Kumar, N., Nanovaccines for malaria using Plasmodium falciparum antigen Pfs25 attached gold nanoparticles, *Vaccine, 33*, 5064–5071, 2015.
32. Danesh-Bahreini, M.A., Shokri, J., Samiei, A., Kamali-Sarvestani, E., Barzegar-Jalali, M., Mohammadi-Samani, S., Nanovaccine for leishmaniasis: preparation of chitosan nanoparticles containing Leishmania superoxide dismutase and evaluation of its immunogenicity in BALB/c mice, *Int. J. Nanomed.*, *6*, 835–842, 2011.
33. Shi, Q., Rondon-Cavanzo, E.P., Dalla-Picola, I.P., Tiera, M.J., Zhang, X., Dai, K., Benabdoune, H.A., Benderdour, M., Fernandes, J.C., *In vivo* therapeutic efficacy of TNFα silencing by folate-PEG-chitosan-DEAE/siRNA nanoparticles in arthritic mice, Int., J., *Nanomedicine, 13*, 387–402, 2018.
34. Park, J.S., Yang, H.N., Jeon, S.Y., Woo, D.G., Kim, M.S., Park, K.H., The use of anti-COX2 siRNA coated onto PLGA nanoparticles loading dexamethasone in the treatment of rheumatoid arthritis, *Biomaterials, 33*, 8600–8612, 2012.
35. Sun, X., Dong, S., Li, X., Yu, K., Sun, F., Lee, R.J., Li, Y., Teng, L., Delivery of siRNA using folate receptor-targeted pH-sensitive polymeric nanoparticles for rheumatoid arthritis therapy, *Nanomedicine, 20*, 102017, 2019.

6

Preclinical and Commercial Trials of Cancer Diagnosis via Nano-Imaging and Nanovaccinology

Sowmya S.V.[1], Pushpalatha C.[2*], Dominic Augustine[1], Sibikar P.[2], Bharkhavy K.V.[2] and Elizabeth Abbu Varghese[2]

[1]*Department of Oral Pathology and Microbiology, Faculty of Dental Sciences, M.S. Ramaiah University of Applied Sciences, MSR Nagar, Bengaluru, Karnataka, India*

[2]*Department of Pedodontics & Preventive Dentistry, Faculty of Dental Sciences, M.S. Ramaiah University of Applied Sciences, MSR Nagar, Bengaluru, Karnataka, India*

Abstract

Biomedical imaging using nanotechnology is emerging as a significant tool for the diagnosis, assessment of the treatment progress, and prediction of the outcome of cancer. Although nanoparticle-based imaging probes possess great advantages, researches are facing many challenges in their use for clinical applications. Nanovaccines are evolving as a boon for cancer patients that may be an adjuvant and an alternative to conventional cancer therapy. Anti-cancer nanovaccines stimulate specific immune responses and preferably target only the cancer cells. The therapeutic efficacy using nanovaccines is significantly enhanced compared to traditional formulations. Recent developments in the field of nanovaccinology employ STING activating nanovaccines, neoantigens, aAPCs, mRNA, and combination therapy involving nanovaccines. They have a role in modulating the innate immunity, reduce autoimmune reactions, utilize immunostimulatory properties of mRNA and stimulate T-and B-cell immune responses. This chapter focuses on the current preclinical and clinical trials in nanoimaging and nanovaccines that are applicable to cancer immunotherapy. The recent advances in anti-cancer nanovaccines using nanocarriers that is a breakthrough in delivery is expected to play a vital role in improving the stability and immunogenicity of antigens. The future

**Corresponding author*: drpushpalatha29@gmail.com

Kaushik Pal (ed.) Nanovaccinology as Targeted Therapeutics, (115–130) © 2022 Scrivener Publishing LLC

in management of cancer patients appears to be promising with the advances in nanoimaging and nanovaccinology trends under trials.

Keywords: Anti-cancer vaccines, immunotherapy, nanoimaging, nanovaccines, nanovaccinology

6.1 Introduction

The development of nanoparticles (NPs)-based imaging techniques has been a breakthrough in the field of biomedical imaging of cancer [1]. NPs not only have a diagnostic role but also contribute significantly toward therapeutics and theranostics in cancer. The use of NPs in diagnostics has enhanced the most relied upon imaging techniques, such as optical imaging, positron emission tomography, and magnetic resonance imaging. Therapeutic NPs function by enhancing the uptake and release of pharmacologically active agents at the site of cancer and improving the efficiency of nanovaccines. The NPs that possess both diagnostic and therapeutic properties have theranostic applications and can be used for personalized nanomedicine-based approaches. Recently, multimodal imaging techniques that takes advantage of a combination of imaging techniques are employed for appropriate diagnostics [2].

Nanooncology is attracting researchers and clinicians to bring about a change in the treatment modalities so as to make use of the benefits of newer drug delivery systems. They accelerate the effect of chemotherapy in cancer. This is achieved by targeting the tumor site either with specific ligands, cytotoxic agents, imaging probes or antibodies [3]. Early detection of cancer is the key to successful treatment [4]. However, the current methods are not satisfactory because of their inherent limitations. The advantages of nanotechnology in oncology for the identification of biomarkers and *in vivo* imaging are increased sensitivity and specificity [5].

This chapter highlights nanoparticles used for different nanoimaging techniques in cancer. The nanodevices with different NPs that play a major role in cancer diagnosis, response to treatment, and assessment of prognosis have been explained. The challenges that the researchers and clinicians encounter to apply these techniques to clinical setup have been discussed. The benefits, composition, and mechanism of action of nanovaccines in cancer immunotherapy have been appraised. The trials that are ongoing and future work that can be done in this field have also been reviewed.

6.2 Role of Nano-Imaging in Cancer Diagnosis, Progression, and Treatment

Molecular biology depends on imaging for cancer diagnosis, assessment of progression, and outcome of treatment. Imaging provides the clinicians or researchers to get a detailed view of the changes in cells and tissues and predict the biological outcome of cancer. Advanced imaging techniques helps us to visualize the biological specimens from all aspects with specificity. This enables to reveal all minute pathologies that have encroached the cellular machinery. Nanotechnology in molecular imaging has its application in ultrasonography, computed tomography, optical, nuclear and magnetic resonance imaging [6, 7].

Nanoparticles are used in nanodevices that are taken up by the cancer cells prefentially and are retained within them. The different sizes of nanoparticles permit them to be included in any of the imaging nanodevices, such as probes, contrast agents, or multifunctional reagents for *in vivo* imaging [3]. The target-specific and highly sensitive nanodevices can identify any cancer-related molecular changes that occur in even a minor population of cells [8, 9].

The diagnosis of cancer makes use of gold nanoparticles (NPs), quantum dots, magnetic NPs, magnetic iron oxide NPs, carbon nanotubes, and nanowires in the nanodevices. They may also be combined with drugs and other targeting molecules [10].

6.2.1 Gold Nanoparticles

The size-dependent optical property of gold nanoparticles permits absorption and scattering of light from wavelengths of visible to infrared regions that is necessary for *in vivo* imaging. Gold nanoparticles as carriers have been modified by the addition of multimodal Gd dendrimer or glucosamine to enhance their contrast and increase their affinity to cancer cells. Gold nanoparticles possess high x-ray absorption coefficient. Tumor imaging is effective using computed tomography–enhanced permeability and retention effect. The specific targeting ability is enhanced by the conjugation of gold NPs with polyethylene glycol chains and biomarkers, such as epidermal growth factor-2 [1, 5].

6.2.2 Quantum Dots

Quantum dots (QDs) are nanoprobes with good imaging properties for assessing the specificity of tumor targets of *in vitro* and *in vivo* cancer cells. These are evolving as efficient imaging tools for the diagnosis of cancer. They possess signal brightness, size-tunable light emission, increased fluorescence signal, and emission of various fluorescence colors. QDs detect cancer biomarkers with decreased detection time [1].

6.2.3 Carbon Nanotubes

Carbon nanotubes are used to develop DNA biosensors currently. Various types of carbon nanotube-based biosensors are available, such as in association with field-effect transistor and dendrimers. The former is used for the identification of biomarkers related to lung cancer, whereas the latter are used in MRI to view many diseases.

6.2.4 Nanowires

Various biomarkers are detected using nanowires of silicon, gold, and conducting polymers. Nanowire-based imaging technology involves conventional high-resolution and analytical electron microscopy methods. Nanowire-related structures depend on TEM and STEM imaging and analysis for further developments.

6.2.5 Cantilevers and Nanopores

Nanoscale cantilevers and nanopores are part of biosensors that can be coated with antibodies capable of binding to specific antigenic sites on cancer cells. This results in a physical change that can be monitored in real time. These agents permit rapid diagnosis and are highly sensitive for detection of biomarkers on cancer cells.

6.2.6 Other Types of Nanoparticles

The use of magnetic, silica, and metal NPs have evolved into cancer biomarker detection. Image enhancement and optical differentiation of leukemic cells are brought about by silica NPs incapacitated with fluorescence resonance energy transfer dyes. Target-specific MRI contrast agents are developed with the use of precursor NPs, such as super paramagnetic iron oxide. These nanoparticles are biodegradable, less toxic, and have long blood retention time [1, 5].

6.3 Challenges in the Translation of Nanotechnology-Based Imaging Methods Into Clinical Application

Nanotechnology-based imaging in cancer diagnosis and therapeutics is quite a challenging arena to be translated into clinical practice. Current clinical practice involves tumor imaging methods that comprise of computed tomography, ultrasound, endoscopy, MRI with modifications, such as gadolinium-enhanced, diffusion-weighted, elastography, spectroscopy, and cholangiography. However, these techniques pose many limitations. There could be decreased sensitivity, suboptimal image resolution, radiation exposure, signal specificity, toxicity of contrast agents like gadolinium, and compromised depth penetration. The use of nanomaterials in imaging could probably overcome some of these drawbacks [1].

The translational barriers of the NP-based imaging agents used include toxicity, stability of manufacturing methods, characterization predictability in preclinical animal models *in vivo*, favorable biodistribution, commercial incentives, less return on investment, regulatory frameworks, reducing batch to batch variation, scale-up of production, and so on. The failures in clinical trials are mainly attributed to tumor heterogeneity and poor understanding of the effect of NP-based agents on biological tissues. The difficulties encountered with the clinical translation are overcome by the addition of lipids to the NP agents and enhancing signal-to-noise and contrast-to-noise ratios. There is limited access to the NP-based imaging agents that has wide application in diagnosis, monitoring the progress of treatment, predicting the outcome, and as supplementary diagnostics during treatment procedures [11]. These applications outnumber the drawbacks of use of NP-based contrast and imaging agents and provides a hope for better-quality patient care.

6.4 Nanovaccines for Cancer Immunotherapy

The emerging field in nanotechnology is focusing on the use of vaccines with nanoparticles that have direct effect to the site of origin of the disease or infection in the body unlike conventional drugs that are non-specific. Vaccine systems have been developed by the incorporation of components that possess properties contributing to vaccine efficacy. As a combined product, these nanovaccines will provide an additive or synergistic immune response [12, 13]. Vaccines used for cancer immunotherapy act as an adjuvant or alternative to traditional cancer therapies. The mechanism

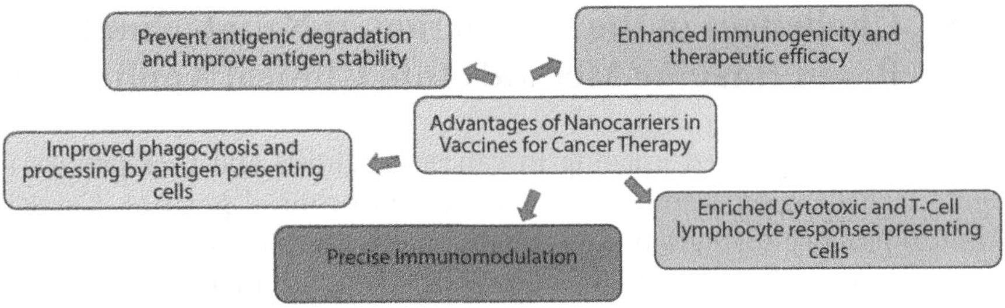

Figure 6.1 Advantages of nanocarriers in vaccines for cancer therapy.

by which these vaccines act is by the stimulation of anticancer immune response, immune memory for the prevention of recurrence, and induction of tumor cells specific killing. Nanovaccines against cancer have been developed with delivery vehicles, such as nanoparticles, to facilitate antigen delivery and the action of antigen-presenting cells for antigen presentation [14]. The advantages of nanocarriers in nanovaccines for cancer therapy are depicted in Figure 6.1.

Nanocarriers can be synthetic, semi-biogenic, and biogenic types that carry subunit vaccine components. They are tumor-associated antigens (TAAs)/neoantigens made of peptides or mRNA, and immunostimulatory adjuvants.

6.4.1 Composition of Nanovaccines in Cancer Therapy

6.4.1.1 Antigens

Tumor cells have endogenous antigens that fail to exhibit immune responses of therapeutic significance. Therefore, exogenous cancer-specific antigens will be introduced that have the capacity to initiate antigen-specific anticancer immune responses that mediates cancer immunotherapy.

6.4.1.1.1 Tumor-Associated Antigens (TAAs)

They are expressed by both cancerous and non-cancerous cells. Cancer-testis antigens are TAAs that are specifically expressed in cancer cells and germline tissues possessing immunological characteristics. However, they do not get expressed in normal adult cells. Melanoma-associated antigens-A for New York's esophageal squamous cell carcinoma 1, LAGE-1, and TTK protein kinase, have been explored to be a part of cancer vaccines. HER-2/neu, an oncoprotein expressed in breast and ovarian cancers also have been studied extensively as TAAs.

6.4.1.1.2 Neoantigens

Neoantigens are the result of genetic mutations or abnormal gene expression and are only expressed in cancer cells. Stimulation of anti-cancer immune responses using neoantigen vaccines happens by their recognition as non-self and therefore escaping from the central immune tolerance.

6.4.1.2 Immunostimulatory Adjuvants

Adjuvants that stimulate the immune system can be of two classes. Vaccine delivery systems contribute to preventive and defensive functions by presenting antigens to the immune system. They comprise of mineral salts, liposomes, emulsions, and virosomes. Immunostimulatory molecular adjuvants that include toll-like receptor (TLR) agonists, STING agonists, costimulatory ligands, and cytokines. They activate immune cells, such as APCs, leading to the potentiation of the antigen-specific immune responses.

6.4.1.3 Nanocarriers

Delivery of subunit vaccines using NPs has a lot of scope to be investigated. Various nanomaterials have been studied for vaccine delivery in cancer immunotherapy. The carriers for nanovaccine development have been discussed in the following section.

6.4.1.3.1 Biogenenic Nanocarriers

Nanomaterials obtained from biological tissues are biogenic nanocarriers that possess low toxicity, high biocompatibility and degradability. Exosomes and outer membrane vesicles (OMVs) are some of the biogenic nanocarriers. T and B lymphocytes, cancer cells and APCs secrete exosomes that can be immunosuppressive or immunostimulatory [15]. The cancer cells and dendritic cells derived exosomes containing MHC/epitope molecular complexes for T cell activation has immunotherapeutic potential. Outer membrane vesicles also play a role in immunotherapy by trafficking DNA, RNA, proteins, endotoxins, and allied virulence molecules in bacterial cells and are recently being engineered to display HPV16 and is used in cancer vaccines.

6.4.1.3.2 Non-Biogenic Nanocarriers

These are semisynthetic nanocarriers that are a combination of biogenic and synthetic components. They are engineered to get properties of easy and reproducible manufacturing in addition to biocompatibility and low toxicity. The types of semisynthetic nanocarriers are virus-like particles, cell membrane-coated type, and endogenous protein-based variants [16].

6.4.1.3.3 Synthetic Nanocarriers

They are made of polymers, liposomes, and inorganic nanoparticles suitable for delivery of vaccine in cancer immunotherapy. Polylactide-co-glycolide polymer-based nanoparticle is biodegradable and its size, solubility, and stability can be modified. Antigen-loaded polymer nanovaccines are effective in inducing T-cell immune response. Liposome-encapsulated mRNAs have high immunogenicity of antigens. For instance, the ovalbumin-encoding plasmid DNA showed a high T-cell response compared with plasmid DNA alone when delivered by liposomes. Inorganic nanocarriers cause suppression of tumor growth based on their antigenicity. For example, spherical nucleic acids with gold nanoparticles have been used to deliver cancer vaccines with increased immunomodulatory potential.

6.5 Functionalities of Nanocarriers for the Delivery of Cancer Vaccines

With increase in importance of nanotechnology in vaccine development, there is a need to increase the successful vaccine delivery of antigens and adjuvants to improve the antigenic stability and immunogenicity [17]. The pathways involved in cancer immunotherapy are summarized in Figure 6.2.

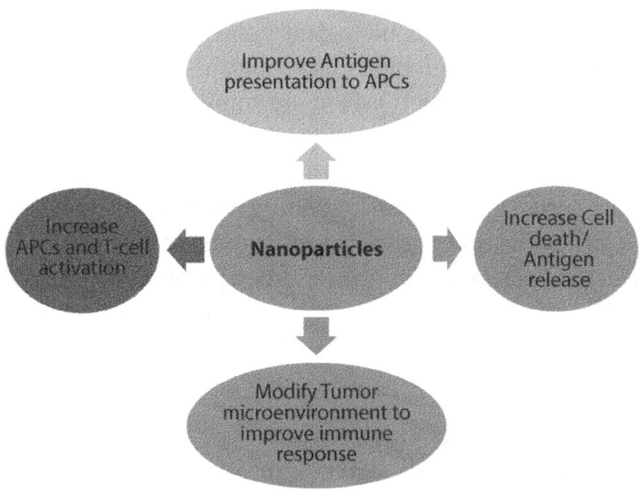

Figure 6.2 Pathways in cancer immunotherapy.

The functionalities of nanocarriers for the delivery of cancer vaccines are as follows.

6.5.1 Efficient Delivery of Vaccines by Nanocarriers

The design of NPs should favor direct delivery to lymph nodes or spleen for efficient immunomodulation. Specificity to immune cells can be enhanced by the modification of nanocarriers.

6.5.2 Co-Delivery of Antigens and Adjuvants via Nanocarriers

Co-delivery of antigen and adjuvant molecules can be done so as to elicit CD4 or CD8 T-cell responses responsible for cancer immunotherapy. It enhances the activation of anti-cancer T cell responses by enhanced APC maturation and antigen cross-presentation. The various vaccines that are recently used as cancer immunotherapeutic agents have been discussed in the following section [18].

6.5.3 Nanocarriers Potentiate Immunomodulation Through Multivalent Antigens and/or Adjuvants

Multiple copies of antigens and adjuvant molecules are permitted to occupy multiple sites of nanocarriers that increase the efficacy of immunomodulation in cancer therapy. The cytokine levels are elevated thereby reducing the tumor volume.

6.5.4 Self-Adjuvanted Nanocarriers

Immunoadjuvant is an additional characteristic of the NPs along with serving as a carrier for cancer nanovaccines. The best example includes chitosan NPs that promote cellular and humoral immunity in addition to a balanced Th1/Th2 response [19].

6.6 Nanovaccine Strategies in Cancer

Immunooncology is gaining popularity in the treatment of cancer with the conceptual use of nanotechnology. Nanovaccine-based immunotherapy has now shown a breakthrough in the treatment options for cancer that traditionally include only chemotherapy and radiotherapy. The following section discusses the significant nanovaccines used in cancer.

6.6.1 STING Agonist-Based Nanovaccines

STING is a signaling molecule that triggers the expression of type I interferons (IFNs) and pro-inflammatory cytokines. The activation of STING is brought about by leucocytes like CD11b+ and B cells. Innate and adaptive immune responses, therefore, play a role in cancer immunotherapy. Cyclic dinucleotides (CDNs) that are STING agonists activate its signaling pathway and have been used as part of vaccine for its therapeutic effect [20].

6.6.2 Neoantigen Nanovaccines

Somatic mutations in tumor cells form tumor neoantigens and their immunization has the capacity to overcome immune tolerance mechanisms and reduce autoimmunity. Cancer cells genomic sequencing help in the identification of these mutations and the development of neoantigen neovaccines [21, 22].

6.6.3 mRNA-Based Nanovaccines

The use of mRNA-based vaccines need prior antigen ingestion by antigen-presenting cells and escape from post-ingestion by endolysosomes for effective delivery and therapeutic effect in cancer. Liposomes-based mRNA nanovaccines are effective against spleen and dendritic cells [23].

6.6.4 aAPCs

These are artificial synthetic antigen presenting cells (APCs) that have an antigenic peptide and co-stimulatory molecules. The advantages of aAPCs include defined composition, uniform signal representation and large scale easy vaccine production. These vaccines cause T cell activation in cancer immunotherapy [5].

6.6.5 Nanovaccines for Combination Therapy

Nanovaccines with immunostimulatory cytokines or check point inhibitors have been successful in combination therapy owing to the heterogeneity of cancer. For example, tumor models *in vitro* have experimented the use of

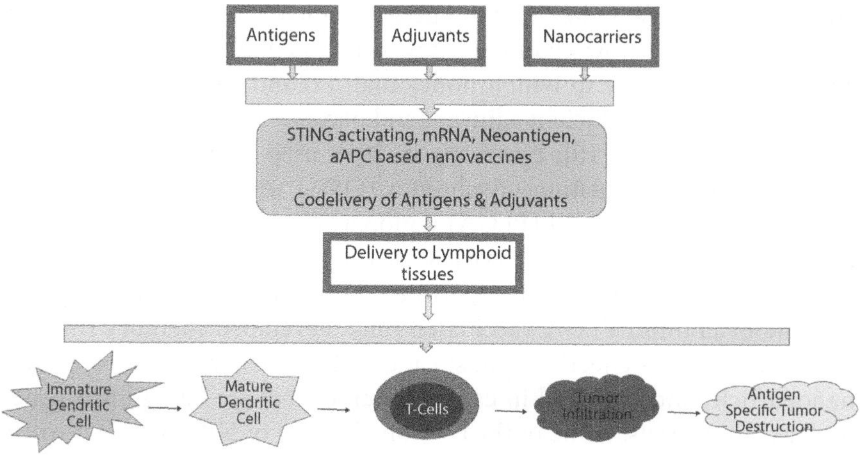

Figure 6.3 Mechanism of action of nanovaccines.

albumin-binding vaccines with immune checkpoint inhibitors and interleukin 2 and have found it to be efficient against treatment of cancer [17]. The mechanism of action of nanovaccines has been summarized in Figure 6.3.

6.7 Preclinical and Clinical Trials of Applications of Nanoimaging and Nanovaccinology in Cancer

The efficacy of any new drug is tested under preclinical and clinical phases of trials before it is practiced clinically. The preclinical phase includes pharmacological, toxicological, pharmacokinetic, and chemical analyses. The clinical trials are performed in 4 phases in which the 4th phase includes administration of the vaccine in the approved dose and way of administration [24, 25]. Various studies have been carried out as preclinical and clinical trials, which are applied to cancer imaging and treatment.

Zhu *et al.*, in 2017, have attempted an *in vitro* examination of self-assembled intertwining DNA-RNA nanocapsules (iDR-NCs) on cell lines for its efficacy as cancer immunotherapeutic agent. It was found that iDR-NC/neoantigen nanovaccines have 8-fold more frequent neoantigen-specific peripheral CD8+ T cells than cytosine–guanine oligodeoxynucleotides (CpG), induce T cell memory, and significantly inhibit the progression of neoantigen-specific colorectal tumors. It was inferred that iDR-NC have synergistic effect in immunotherapy along with DNA/RNA/peptide nanocarriers [16]. Zhu *et al.* have developed albumin/AlbiVax nanocomplexes and have experimented *in vivo* to check its efficiency in immunotherapy. PET imaging and flow cytometry have suggested 100- fold higher CpG and antigens delivery to lymph nodes than Freund's adjuvant. Albumin/AlbiVax is found an efficient adjuvant and plays a role in combination cancer immunotherapy [15]. Liu *et al.*, in 2019 used an innovative vaccine produced by encapsulating Ovalbumin (OVA) with $MPG^{\Delta NLS}$ into poly (lactide-co-glycolide) acid (PLGA) nanoparticles. This facilitated antigen cross penetration to cause cytotoxic CD8+ T-cell responses [26]. Liu *et al.*, in 2018 through their *in vivo* experiments have shown that hydroxychloroquine-ovalbumin-PLGA vaccinated mice developed memory immune responses that was effective against cancer [27]. There are many approved nanoparticles incorporated in cancer vaccines that are being investigated under clinical trials. Some of the lysosomal group of NPs include doxorubicin HCl liposome against Kaposi's sarcoma, ovarian cancer, and multiple myeloma and liposomal irinotecan for pancreatic cancer. Among the polymer NPs, leuprolide acetate is effectively used for prostate cancer. Protein NPs, such as albumin-bound paclitaxel, have shown increased delivery to pancreatic and breast cancer tissues [28].

6.8 Recent Developments in the Trials of Nanovaccinology in Cancer

The aim of the recent trials of nanovaccinology in cancer is to develop a novel immunotherapeutic agent that induces strong infiltration of immune cells into the tumor microenvironment thereby inhibiting tumor growth [13]. There are monoclonal antibodies that function as immune checkpoint inhibitors (ICIs) inhibiting the activity of cytotoxic T-lymphocyte antigen-4 (CTLA-4) or programmed cell death protein 1 (PD-1), expressed by T cells [2]. Studies have demonstrated that melanoma, renal cell, and colorectal carcinomas can be treated with the combined use of anti PD-1 mAb nivolumab, and 1-methyl-DL-tryptophan (1-MT), an immune modulating drug. The use of pembrolizumab is also widespread as an anti PD-1 agent in cancer therapy [29]. Similarly, nivolumab has been studied and found to be highly effective against melanoma and non-small cell lung carcinoma (NSCLC) [30–32]. ICIs were recently found to be successful in the treatment of cases of genetic mutations. Another study by Xu *et al.* in 2020 have experimented the benefit of cationic fluoropolymer on two subcutaneous tumour models and an orthotopic breast cancer tumour. Combining NPs with fluoropolymers and ovalbumin, activate the Toll-like receptor

4 (TLR4) signalling pathway resulting in effective antigen cross-presentation. This personalized cancer vaccine has been proved to be efficient in preventing post-operative cancer recurrence and metastasis [33].

6.9 Perspectives and Future Directions

The future of nanoimaging and nanovaccinology remains promising with new trials being carried out on various nanoparticles and delivery systems [19]. However, few challenges have surfaced during the development of nanovaccines. They have to be safe and non-toxic and the effect of new NPs on biological tissues should be predictable. The characteristics of NPs such as composition, size, shape, surface coatings, and their charge have to be well investigated. The drug release and biodistribution of these materials have to be examined. The vaccines should be assessed for favourable risk-benefit ratio and regulatory approval. *In vitro* assays have to be conducted to measure the biological activity and toxicity of vaccines used for cancer. It has been found that toxicity tests lack standard protocols that result in failure of the vaccine in late stages of the testing [6].

6.10 Conclusions

Nanovaccines and nanoimaging in cancer diagnostics and therapeutics are gaining lot of popularity in the medical field. Anti-cancer vaccines mainly target the immune system and trigger the lymphoid organs to release lymphocytes that have the capacity to combat the tumor cells. Newer vaccines are on the trials at the *in vitro* and *in vivo* levels by a team of investigators of various specialities who address pharmaceutical engineering principles, nanotechnology, and immuno-oncology. Many challenges face vaccine development in oncology research, it takes no longer for their application from bench to bed side. The future in this field is challenging to provide new processes to control T-cell development in immune-mediated diseases.

References

1. Siddique, S. and Chow, J.C., Application of nanomaterials in biomedical imaging and cancer therapy. *Nanomaterials*, 10, 9, 1700, 2020 Sep.

2. Krekorian, M., Fruhwirth, G.O., Srinivas, M., Figdor, C.G., Heskamp, S., Witney, T.H., Aarntzen, E.H., Imaging of T-cells and their responses during anti-cancer immunotherapy. *Theranostics*, 9, 25, 7924, 2019.
3. Toy, R., Bauer, L., Hoimes, C., Ghaghada, K.B., Karathanasis, E., Targeted nanotechnology for cancer imaging. *Adv. Drug Delivery Rev.*, 76, 79–97, 2014 Sep 30.
4. Jin, C., Wang, K., Oppong-Gyebi, A., Hu, J., Application of nanotechnology in cancer diagnosis and therapy-a mini-review. *Int. J. Med. Sci.*, 17, 18, 2964, 2020.
5. Zhang, Y., Lin, S., Wang, X.Y., Zhu, G., Nanovaccines for cancer immunotherapy. *Wiley Interdiscip. Rev.: Nanomed. Nanobiotechnol.*, 11, 5, e1559, 2019 Sep.
6. Liu, C.H. and Grodzinski, P., Nanotechnology for Cancer Imaging: Advances, Challenges, and Clinical Opportunities. *Radiol.: Imaging Cancer*, 3, 3, e200052, 2021.
7. Chapman, S., Dobrovolskaia, M., Farahani, K., Goodwin, A., Joshi, A., Lee, H., Meade, T., Pomper, M., Ptak, K., Rao, J., Singh, R., Nanoparticles for cancer imaging: The good, the bad, and the promise. *Nano Today*, 8, 5, 454–60, 2013 Oct 1.
8. Choi, H.S. and Frangioni, J.V., Nanoparticles for biomedical imaging: fundamentals of clinical translation. *Mol. Imag.*, 9, 6, 7290–2010, 2010 Nov 1.
9. Anselmo, A.C. and Mitragotri, S., Nanoparticles in the clinic. *Bioeng. Transl. Med.*, 1, 1, 10–29, 2016 Mar.
10. Jabir, N.R., Tabrez, S., Ashraf, G.M., Shakil, S., Damanhouri, G.A., Kamal, M.A., Nanotechnology-based approaches in anticancer research. *Int. J. Nanomed.*, 7, 4391, 2012.
11. Shi, J., Kantoff, P.W., Wooster, R., Farokhzad, O.C., Cancer nanomedicine: progress, challenges and opportunities. *Nat. Rev. Cancer*, 17, 1, 20–37, 2017 Jan.
12. Agarwal, M., Role of Nanovaccine in Immunotherapy. *J. Cell Sci. Ther.*, 1, S8, 1, 2015 Jan.
13. Grodzinski, P., Kircher, M., Goldberg, M., Gabizon, A., Integrating nanotechnology into cancer care. *ACS Nano,* 13, 7, 7370–7376, 2019.
14. Teixeira, V.M., Silva, A.C., Lopes, C.M., The role of nanotechnology in cancer treatment and diagnosis. 224–232, 2010.
15. Zhu, G., Lynn, G.M., Jacobson, O., Chen, K., Liu, Y., Zhang, H., Ma, Y., Zhang, F., Tian, R., Ni, Q., Cheng, S., Albumin/vaccine nanocomplexes that assemble *in vivo* for combination cancer immunotherapy. *Nat. Commun.*, 8, 1, 1–5, 2017 Dec 5.
16. Zhu, G., Mei, L., Vishwasrao, H.D., Jacobson, O., Wang, Z., Liu, Y., Yung, B.C., Fu, X., Jin, A., Niu, G., Wang, Q., Intertwining DNA-RNA nanocapsules loaded with tumor neoantigens as synergistic nanovaccines for cancer immunotherapy. *Nat. Commun.*, 8, 1, 1–3, 2017 Nov 14.

17. Zhu, G., Zhang, F., Ni, Q., Niu, G., Chen, X., Efficient nanovaccine delivery in cancer immunotherapy. *ACS Nano*, 11, 3, 2387–92, 2017 Mar 28.
18. Durgeau, A., Virk, Y., Corgnac, S., Mami-Chouaib, F., Recent advances in targeting CD8 T-cell immunity for more effective cancer immunotherapy. *Front. Immunol.*, 9, 14, 2018 Jan 22.
19. Shim, S. and Yoo, H.S., The application of mucoadhesive chitosan nanoparticles in nasal drug delivery. *Mar. Drugs*, 18, 12, 605, 2020 Dec.
20. Barber, G.N., Sting: infection, inflammation and cancer. *Nat. Rev. Immunol.*, 15, 12, 760–70, 2015 Dec.
21. Peng, M., Mo, Y., Wang, Y., Wu, P., Zhang, Y., Xiong, F., Guo, C., Wu, X., Li, Y., Li, X., Li, G., Neoantigen vaccine: an emerging tumor immunotherapy. *Mol. Cancer*, 18, 1, 1–4, 2019 Dec.
22. Si, P., Razmi, N., Nur, O., Solanki, S., Pandey, C.M., Gupta, R.K., Malhotra, B.D., Willander, M., de la Zerda, A., Gold nanomaterials for optical biosensing and bioimaging. *Nanoscale Adv.*, 3, 10, 2679–2698, 2021.
23. Si, P., Razmi, N., Nur, O., Solanki, S., Pandey, C.M., Gupta, R.K., Malhotra, B.D., Willander, M., de la Zerda, A., Gold nanomaterials for optical biosensing and bioimaging. *Nanoscale Adv.*, 3, 10, 2679–98, 2021.
24. Mackiewicz, J. and Mackiewicz, A., Design of clinical trials for therapeutic cancer vaccines development. *Eur. J. Pharmacol.*, 625, 1-3, 84–9, 2009 Dec 25.
25. Riggio, C., Pagni, E., Raffa, V., Cuschieri, A., Nano-oncology: clinical application for cancer therapy and future perspectives. *J. Nanomater.*, 2011, 1–10, 2011 Jan 1.
26. Liu, X., Liu, J., Liu, D., Han, Y., Xu, H., Liu, L., Leng, X., Kong, D., A cell-penetrating peptide-assisted nanovaccine promotes antigen cross-presentation and anti-tumor immune response. *Biomater. Sci.*, 7, 12, 5516–27, 2019.
27. Liu, J., Liu, X., Han, Y., Zhang, J., Liu, D., Ma, G., Li, C., Liu, L., Kong, D., Nanovaccine incorporated with hydroxychloroquine enhances antigen cross-presentation and promotes antitumor immune responses. *ACS Appl. Mater. Interfaces*, 10, 37, 30983–93, 2018 Aug 23.
28. Ventola, C.L., Progress in nanomedicine: approved and investigational nanodrugs. *Pharm. Ther.*, 42, 12, 742, 2017 Dec.
29. Riley, R.S., June, C.H., Langer, R., Mitchell, M.J., Delivery technologies for cancer immunotherapy. *Nat. Rev. Drug Discovery*, 18, 3, 175–96, 2019 Mar.
30. Postow, M.A., Chesney, J., Pavlick, A.C., Robert, C., Grossmann, K., McDermott, D., Linette, G.P., Meyer, N., Giguere, J.K., Agarwala, S.S., Shaheen, M., Nivolumab and ipilimumab versus ipilimumab in untreated melanoma. *N. Engl. J. Med.*, 372, 21, 2006–17, 2015 May 21.
31. Gettinger, S., Rizvi, N.A., Chow, L.Q., Borghaei, H., Brahmer, J., Ready, N., Gerber, D.E., Shepherd, F.A., Antonia, S., Goldman, J.W., Juergens, R.A., Nivolumab monotherapy for first-line treatment of advanced non–small-cell lung cancer. *J. Clin. Oncol.*, 34, 25, 2980, 2016 Sep 1.
32. Motzer, R.J., Tannir, N.M., McDermott, D.F., Frontera, O.A., Melichar, B., Choueiri, T.K., Plimack, E.R., Barthélémy, P., Porta, C., George, S., Powles, T.,

Nivolumab plus ipilimumab versus sunitinib in advanced renal-cell carcinoma. *N. Engl. J. Med.*, 2018 Mar 21.

33. Xu, J., Lv, J., Zhuang, Q., Yang, Z., Cao, Z., Xu, L., Pei, P., Wang, C., Wu, H., Dong, Z., Chao, Y., A general strategy towards personalized nanovaccines based on fluoropolymers for post-surgical cancer immunotherapy. *Nat. Nanotechnol.*, 15, 12, 1043–52, 2020 Dec.

7

Biomedical and Electronic Tune-Ups of 2C4NA Nanocrystalline Sample

Maalmarugan J.[1], Egbert Selwin Rose A.[2], Anbarasan P.[3], Poorani R.[4], Aarthi N.[5], Ganesan H.[6], Senthil Kannan K.[7]* and Flora G.[8]

[1]*Department of EEE, Sri Ranganathar Institute of Engineering and Technology, Athipalayam, Coimbatore, TN, India*

[2]*Department of Botany, St. Joseph's College – Autonomous, Tiruchirappalli, TN, India*

[3]*Department of EEE, St. Joseph's College of Engineering and Technology, Chennai, TN, India*

[4]*Department of Pharmacy Practice, Sri Ramakrishna Institute of Paramedical Sciences-College of Pharmacy, Coimbatore, TN, India*

[5]*Department of Zoology, PSGR Krishnammal College for Women, Coimbatore, TN, India*

[6]*Department of Mechanical Engineering, Sri Ranganathar Institute of Engineering and Technology, Athipalayam, Coimbatore, TN, India*

[7]*Department of R&D/Physics, Edayathangudy G.S. Pillay Arts and Science College (Autonomous – Affiliated to Bharathidasan University – Tiruchirappalli), Nagapattinam, Tamil Nadu, India*

[8]*Department of Botany, St. Mary's College (Autonomous), Thoothukudi, TN, India*

Abstract

2-chloro-4-nitroaniline (2C4NA) crystalline sample is grown by a solution growth method; it is milled to nanoform of 46 nm. The computational effect of the molecular arrangement of 2C4NA is shown with the ORTEP diagram and unit cell, and the nanotubular form, di-peptide linkage, super cell lattice are portrayed in a well manner for 2C4NA crystals. The interactions for the finger print effect of 2C4NA are well portrayed. The 2C4NA have superior extent for anti-diabetic as a result of the aniline existence and have augments in inhibition as the value of the concentration enhances and the IC-50 value as 37.9 for macro and in nanoform, it is 30.3. Also, the AD-nm variations have good efficiency, whereas the dimension of

**Corresponding author*: mscgoldmedalist@yahoo.in

Kaushik Pal (ed.) Nanovaccinology as Targeted Therapeutics, (131–144) © 2022 Scrivener Publishing LLC

the test decreases from 266 to 46 nm. The 2C4NA crystals are used in filter applications also as the data are represented and concluded with the inferences and reported with the utilities for electronic and pharma utilities and good FL data in nanoscaling and is used in anti-cancer and anti-inflammatory proviso and in tribology too.

Keywords: 2C4NA, FL, bio-use, electronic, theoretical

7.1 Introduction

The natural kind of large-scale crystal of 2C4NA is solitary full-grown by traditional evaporation manner and appropriately transferred to scaling of nm by milling. The natural sparklers have glowing depicted uses in electronic-mechano-bio disciplines and in expertise, here, the 2C4NA both scaling are acknowledged to continue for the nanotube assembly, ellipsoidal design, acidic outline of system, peptide contribution of 2C4NA, optimized force field—usefulness, VanderWaal's impact of the crystal, bio/pharma characterizations, and described [1–8].

This happens since the regular feeble intermolecular relations and since of the fragile cooperation that might happen among atomic degree of independence. In the cutting edge times, subatomic precious stones have ended up being the topic of amazing speculative investigations [9–16]. Generally, this has focused roughly mounting a thoughtful physical science of these plans in the appeal to lash it up for specialized purposes, like the average instance of subatomic hardware, despite current fulfillment presentation attempts to try to appreciate the climate of implicate carter in these constructions [17–23]. A field of district of consistently amazing development is that of super-atomic science. This enchanting district is based ahead the use of individual atoms managing to propose intentional subatomic precious stones that might be utilized for an assortment of specialized purposes [24–32].

The key in at the back this demeanor is that the gem construction and stuffing laid out by a game plan of atoms is set up to an incredible breadth by the intermolecular interfaces, for example, hydrogen bonds and van der Waals dealings. Atomic precious stones of natural particles are also propelling from the hereditary and biochemical insight [33–37]. A liberal amount of the hydrogen bond is irreplaceable to sort out various vital natural practices and particles. Atomic precious stones proffer an imitation where to understand the climate of the hydrogen bond in biochemical coordination in extra factor. The natural material [38–40] has great quality [41–43] and improved applications [44], particularly in electronic, mechanical, and bio than different materials [45]; 2C4NA precious stones are of better degree in electronic, primary, bio viable on account of essence of aniline [46, 47] and is of better tribological scope [47–52].

7.2 Computational, Tribological, Fluorescence, and Influx Study

The computational diagrams with super lattice of higher volume and peptide linkage and nanotubular as well as weak interactions with ORTEP for structural as well as unit cell based on these material and Hirshfeld interaction with finger printed full effect with fluorescence effect well portrayed from Figures 7.1 to 7.10. The tribological value is 16% more than the uncoated and 6% more than macro-coated stress values. Fluorescence data are 379 nm and corresponding 3.2739 eV for the blue emission FL from 2C4NA specimen of nanoscale. Influx value of 5.9572 microns of 2C4NA

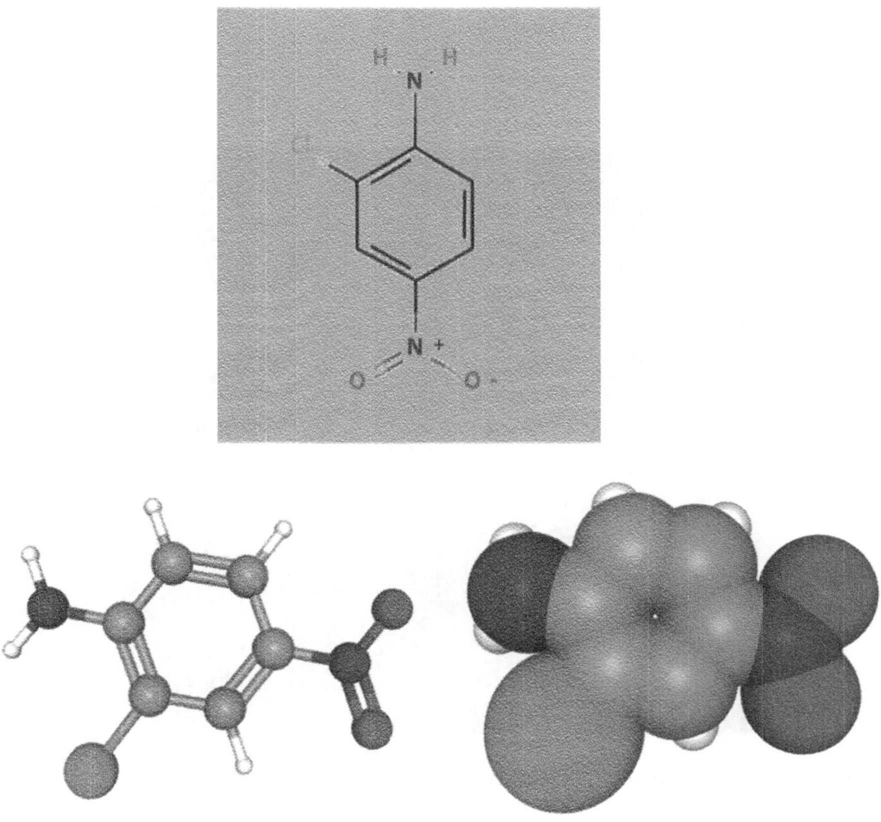

Figure 7.1 Molecule and ball, space filling of 2C4NA crystal [50–52].

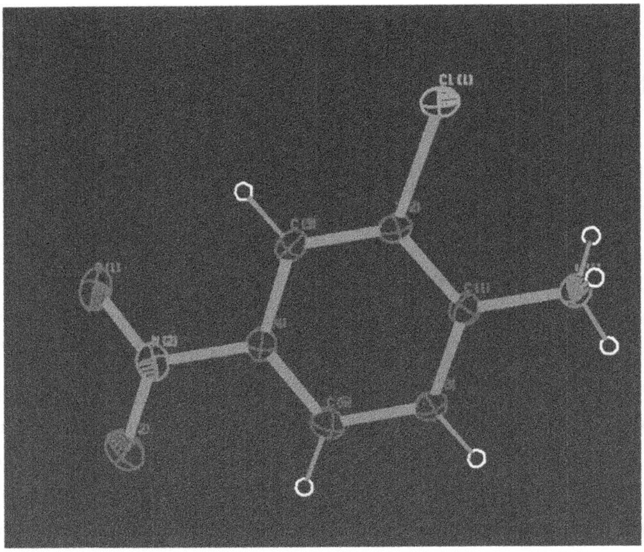

Figure 7.2 ORTEP of 2C4NA crystal [50–52].

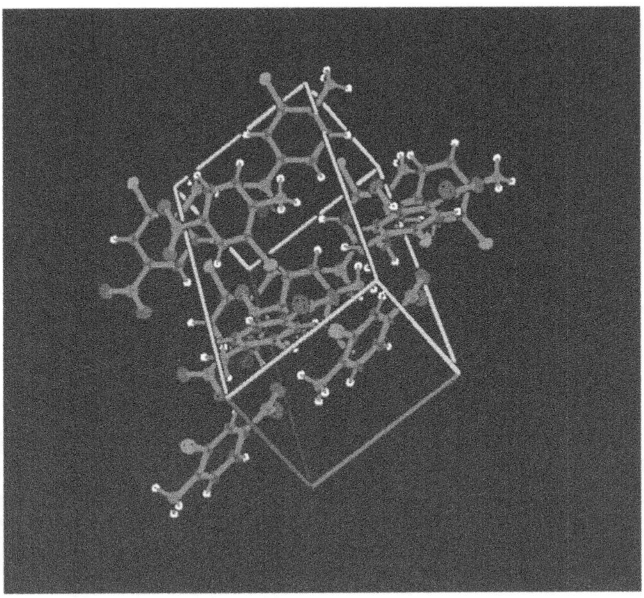

Figure 7.3 ORTEP—unit cell of 2C4NA crystal [50–52].

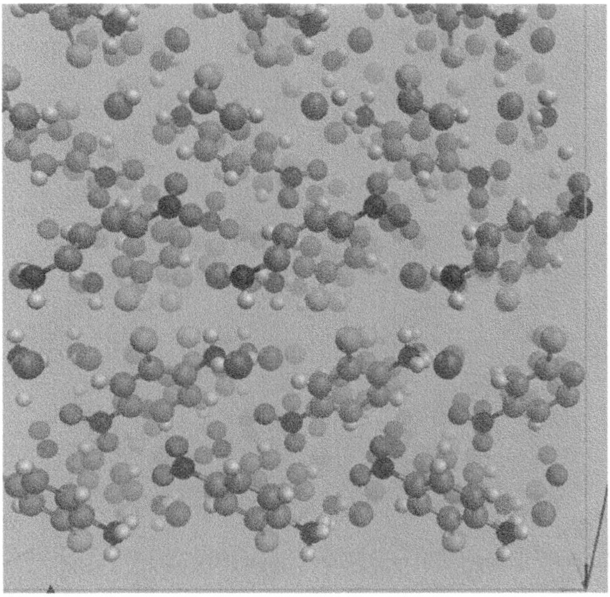

Figure 7.4 3 × 3 × 3 Super cell lattice of 2C4NA crystal [50–52].

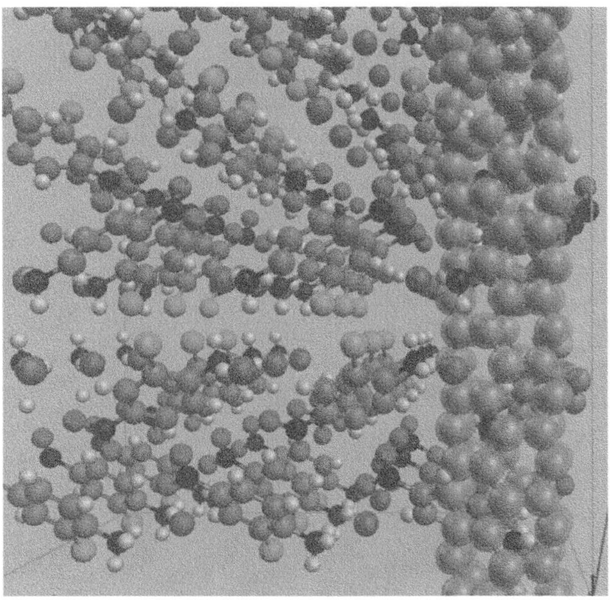

Figure 7.5 20 nm nanotubular of 2C4NA crystal [50–52].

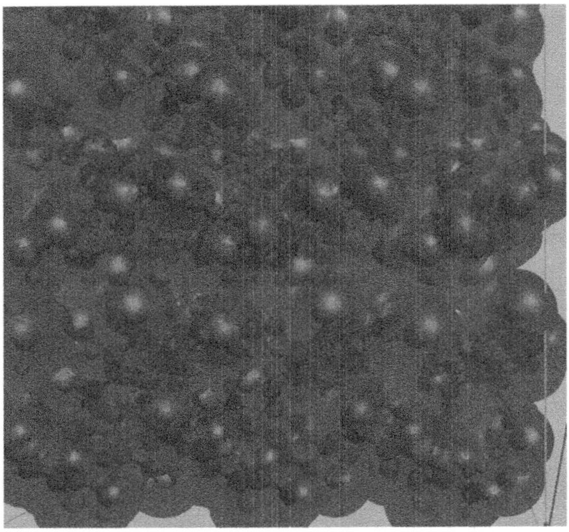

Figure 7.6 Vanderwall's medium of 2C4NA crystal [50–52].

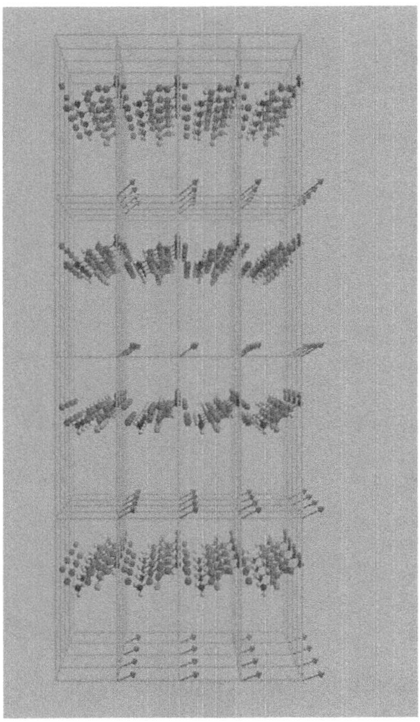

Figure 7.7 Miller's indices 4 × 4 × 4 unit cell 4 × 4 × 4 of 2C4NA crystal [50–52].

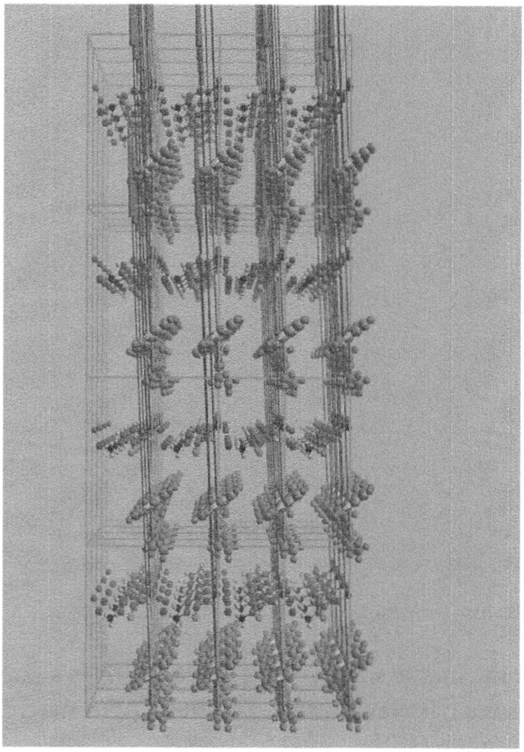

Figure 7.8 Miller's indices dipeptide linked of 2C4NA crystal [50–52].

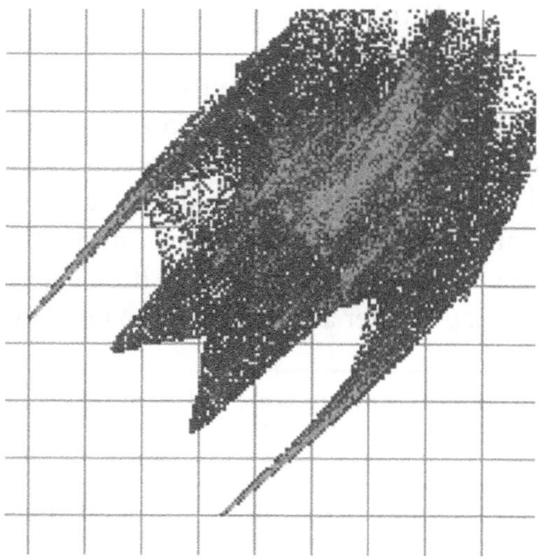

Figure 7.9 Hirshfield finger printed effect of 2C4NA crystal [50–52].

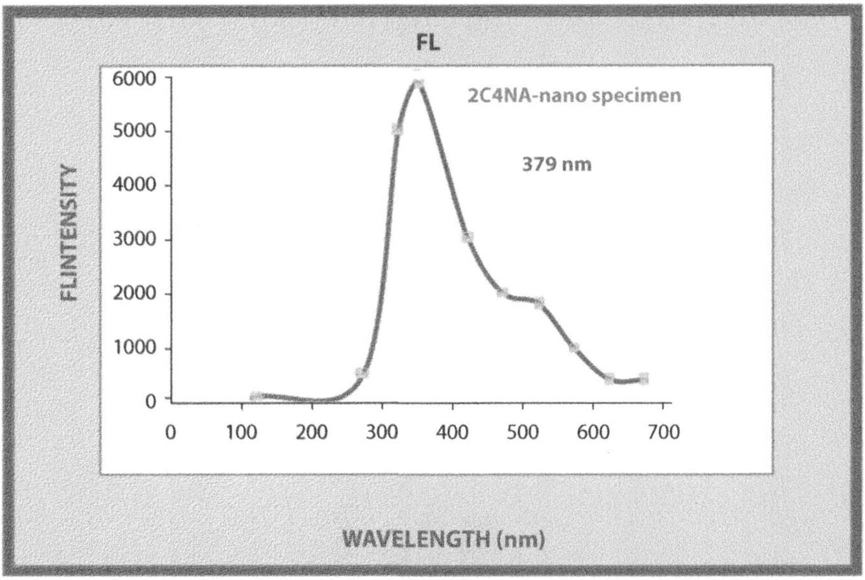

Figure 7.10 FL 379 nm—nanoscaled 2C4NA crystal.

represents that the macro influx refers that 2C4NA is a good NLO crystal, 5.9243 microns is a nanolevel influx. So, the 2C4NA macro and nanocrystals are utilized in filters.

7.3 Antidiabetic (AD) Study, Anticancer Study, and Anti-Inflammatory Study

The anti-diabetic (AD) studies for the grown 2C4NA crystals were carried out. The IC 50 values are 37.9 and 30.3 correspondingly for the AD of 2C4NA crystals, and the inflammatory data reveal that nano is preferred as per data for DPPH, FRAP, and total oxidant value. MTT attempt is a colorimetric examine used for the purpose on diminution to formazancrys KCs. The given test compounds 2C4NA show IC50 concentrations against HeLa cells at 161.67µg/ml after a treatment of 24 hours of incubation.

Samples	**% of DPPH for macro scale**	**% of DPPH for nanoscale**
2C4NA	35.43	36.25
Samples	**% of FRAP for macro scale**	**% of FRAP for nanoscale**
2C4NA	19.6	19.9

Samples	Total anti oxidant for macro scale	Total anti oxidant for nanoscale
2C4NA	43.3	45.1

7.4 Conclusion

The 2C4NA crystals are well grown and are analyzed for antidiabetic, anticancer, and anti-inflammatory cases and measured the mechanotribological and electronic influx and dipeptide linkage; super cell lattice are portrayed. The interactions for the finger print effect of 2C4NA are well portrayed. The 2C4NA includes high-quality possibility for antidiabetic by the aniline existence IC-50 value as 37.9 for macro, and in nanoform, it is 30.3. Also, the AD-nm variations will have good efficiency for sample size decrease from 266 to 46 nm. The 2C4NA crystals are used in filter applications also as the data are represented and concluded with the inferences and reported with the utilities for electronic and pharma utilities and good FL data in nanoscaling

References

1. Kalaipoonguzhali, V., SenthilKannan, K., Thirumoorthi, C., Chinnadurai, M., Jayanalina, T., Comparison of adsorption energy, ionization potential and electron affinity of CuS-ACT and CuS-Nit nanostructures monowire for nano device fabrication by computational approach. *Mater. Today: Proc.*, 33, 7, 2759–2760, 2020.
2. Gunasekaran, S. *et al.*, Structural studies on picolinium maleate crystal by density functional methods. *Indian J. Phys.*, 87, 12, 1189–1197, 2013.
3. Senthilkannan, K. *et al.*, Anti diabetic (AD) studies of bis-glycine hydro bromide (45 nm) nano crystals. *Mater. Today: Proc.*, 33, 7, 3201–3202, 2020.
4. Senthilkannan, K. *et al.*, Anti-diabetic activites of ZnO doped with Ce (5 at %) nano particles (NPs). *Mater. Today: Proc.*, 33, 7, 3056–3057, 2020.
5. Senthilkannan, K. *et al.*, Fluorescence, filter,nano tribological studies of 12-(4-Chlorophenyl)-9,9-Dimethyl-9,10-Dihydro-8H-Benzo[A]Xanthen-11(12H)-One-(CPDDHBXH) macro and nano crystals. *Mater. Today: Proc.*, 33, 7, 4163–4166, 2020.
6. Senthilkannan, K., Venkatachalam, K., Jothibas, M., Computational and experimental studies of acetoacetanilide crystals. *AIP Conf. Proc.*, 2270, 040014, 1–4, 2020.

7. Senthilkannan, K. and Venkatachalam K., Rajamani, A., Computational analysis of LPNPTH anisotropies for dementia for Alzheimer's syndrome by DFT and molecular harboring. *AIP Conf. Proc.*, 2270, 040008, 1–5, 2020.
8. Senthilkannan, K., Velu, S., Kalaipoonguzhali, V., Chinnadurai, M., Kannan, S., Electronic transport, HOMO–LUMO and computational studies of CuS monowire for nano device fabrication by DFT approach. *Mater. Today: Proc.*, 33, 7, 2746–2749, 2020.
9. Senthilkannan, K. and Gunasekaran, S., Spectroscopic studies and other novel studies of 4 bromo 4' chloro benzylidene aniline (BCBA) Crystal- A non linear optical material. *Int. J. Chemtech Res.*, 5, 6, 3051–3058, 2013.
10. Senthilkannan, K., Gayathri Devi, S., Nagarajan, P., Flora, G., Rajakumaravelu, R., Anti diabetic (AD) studies of picolinium maleate nano crystals. *Mater. Today: Proc.*, 33, 3, 3005–3007, 2020.
11. Senthilkannan, K., Ramamurthi, K., Bhakya, K., Velu, S., Kolanjinathan, M., Rajakumaravelu, R., Hardness, photoconductivity, anti-diabetic studies of L-Alaninium Fumarate (LAF) crystals. *AIP Conf. Proc.*, 2270, 100010, 1–4, 2020.
12. Senthilkannan, K., Baskaran, P., Seenivasan, R., Settu, P., Tribological, filter, FTIR and fluorescence studies of L-Alaninium tartrate (LAT) macro and nano crystals. *Mater. Today: Proc.*, 33, 7, 4148–4150, 2020.
13. Senthilkannan, K., Khan, K., Jaffar, A., Ponnusamy, V.K., Govindan, N.M., Effect of anti microbial and fluorescence on L-Alaninium maleate (LAM) macro and nano crystals. *Mater. Today: Proc.*, 33, 7, 2779–2781, 2020.
14. Senthilkannan, K., Ganesh, G., Abdul Jaffer Ali, H., Krishnaveni Ramamurthi, R., Khan, K., Anti diabetic (AD) activities of L-valinium picrate (LVP) macro and nano crystals. *Mater. Today: Proc.*, 33, 7, 2738–2740, 2020.
15. Senthilkannan, K., Bhakya, K., Iyanar, M., Growth and Influx, AC and DC conductivity studies of L-Alaninium Fumarate (LAF) Crystals. *AIP Conf. Proc.*, 2270, 100009, 1–4, 2020.
16. Senthilkannan, K., Growth, fluorescence and theoretical studies of B2CPCD crystals – Comparative analysis in macro and nano scaled crystals. *Mater. Today: Proc.*, 33, 7, 4368–4371, 2020.
17. Senthilkannan, K. *et al.*, Anti-diabetic (AD) activities of ZnO doped with Ce (7 at%) nano particles (NP). *Mater. Today: Proc.*, 33, 7, 3053–3055, 2020.
18. Senthilkannan, K. *et al.*, Tribological, filter studies of 3-Bromo-2-Hydroxy benzoic acid (BHBA) macro and nano crystals. *Mater. Today: Proc.*, 33, 7, 4145–4147, 2020.
19. Senthilkannan, K. *et al.*, Electronic transport, Homo-Lumo and computational studies of CuS-ACT monowire for nano device fabrication by software approach. *Mater. Today: Proc.*, 33, 7, 2756–2758, 2020.
20. Senthilkannan, K. *et al.*, Anti microbial and fluorescence activities of L-valinium picrate (LVP) macro and nano crystals. *Mater. Today: Proc.*, 33, 7, 2776–2778, 2020.

21. Senthilkumar, R. *et al.*, Anti-diabetic (AD) and hardness profile of 12-(4-Chlorophenyl)-9,9-Dimethyl-9,10-Dihydro-8H-benzo[a]xanthen-11(12H)-one–(CPDDHBXH) – Comparative analysis of macro and nano crystals. *Mater. Today: Proc.*, 33, 7, 4167–4170, 2020.
22. Sathishkumar, R. *et al.*, Synthesis, growth and characterization of 2,5 – Dimethyl-N-(3-phenylprop-2-en-1-ylidene) Aniline (2,5 DPPA) single crystal: A new second order nonlinear optical material for Photonic and optoelectronic applications, *Optik,* 226, 2, 1–11, 2020.
23. Patel, R.P. *et al.*, Growth and XRD, elemental, mechanical, dielectric, optical and photoconductivity, and surface morphological characterizations of 2-[4-(Trifluoromethyl) phenyl]-1H-benzimidazole (TFMPHB) crystals for electronic, mechanical applications. *Braz. J. Phys.*, 51, 3, 339–350, 2021.
24. Aarthi, R. *et al.*, Molecular structure-associated pharmacodynamic investigation on benzoyl peroxide using spectroscopic and quantum computational tools. *J. Taibah Univ. Sci.*, 12, 1, 104–122, 2018.
25. Saravanan, P. *et al.*, Biofriendly and competent domestic microwave assisted method for the synthesis of ZnO nanoparticles from the extract of Azadirachta indica leaves. *Mater. Today: Proc.*, 33, 7, 3160–3163, 2020.
26. Saravanan, P. *et al.*, A perspective approach towards appreciable size and cost-effective solar cell fabrication by synthesizing ZnO nanoparticles from Azadirachta indica leaves extract using domestic microwave oven. *J. Mater. Sci.: Mater. Electron.*, 31, 5, 4301–4309, 2020.
27. Saravanan, P. *et al.*, Dielectric and magnetic properties of Allium cepa and Raphanus sativus extracts biogenic ZnO nanoparticles. *J. Mater. Sci.: Mater. Electron.*, 32, 1, 1–14, 2021.
28. Periyathambi, P. *et al.*, Fluorescence and filter characterizations of NaBr-added L-alanine (LANB) – A comparative analysis in macro and nano scaled crystals. *Mater. Today: Proc.*, 33, 3766–3769, 2020.
29. Baskaran, P. *et al.*, Anti-diabetic activities of ZnO doped with Ce (3 at %) nano particles. *Mater. Today: Proc.*, 33, 7, 3051–3052, 2020.
30. Baskaran, P. *et al.*, Anti-diabetic studies of barium paranitro phenolate macro and nano crystals. *Mater. Today: Proc.*, 33, 7, 3058–3060, 2020.
31. Kolanjinathan, M., Senthilkannan, K., Paramasivam, S., Baskaran, P., Iyanar, M., Anti-diabetic studies of 4-(4-chlorophenyl)-7,7-dimethyl-7,8-dihydro-4H-1-benzopyran-2,5(3H,6H)-dione – (CPDMDHHBPHHD) nano crystals. *Mater. Today: Proc.*, 33, 7, 2750–2752, 2020.
32. Kolanjinathan, M. *et al.*, Dielectric, fluorescence, filter, nano tribological and photoconductivity studies of 4-(4-chlorophenyl)-7,7-dimethyl-7,8-dihydro-4H-1-benzopyran-2,5(3H,6H)-dione (CPDMDHHBPHHD) macro and nano crystals. *J. Mater. Sci.: Mater. Electron.*, 27, 4, 16907–16917, 2020.
33. Kolanjinathan, M., Hariharasuthan, R., Sivaramakrishnan, V. *et al.*, XRD, CHNSO, fluorescence, filter-influx, NLO, photoconductivity, hardness and helical spring-fabricated device stress analysis of 2′-chloro-4-methoxy-3-nitrobenzil (CMNB) crystal of different scalings for opto-electronic filter

and band gap engineering utilities. *J. Mater Sci: Mater. Electron.*, 32, 10049–10057, 2021.

34. Jothibas, M. *et al.*, Structural, optical and photo catatic activity of Ag doped ZnO nano particles obtained by sol-gel method. *AIP Conf. Proc.*, 2162, 1, 020151, 1–7, 2019.
35. Selvaraj, L. *et al.*, AS Anti-diabetic (AD) studies of Bis Glycine Hydro Bromide – BGHB macro crystals milled to nano scale of 219 nm as the preliminary fine particles. *Mater. Today: Proc.*, 33, 7, 3763–3765, 2020.
36. Kishore, N. *et al.*, CO and HCHO adsorption on FeO monowire devices: a DFT study. *Appl. Phys. A*, 123, 11, 706; 1–7, 2017, https://doi.org/10.1007/s00339-017-1330-6.
37. Senthilkannan, K., Gunasekaran, S., Gowtham, J., Wagish, R., UV, SEM, powder XRD studies of acetoacetanilide (AAC) Crystal. *Int. J. Chemtech Res.*, 6, 5, 3187–3190, 2014.
38. Kumar, K. *et al.*, Growth of diethyl 3,3′-[(2,4-dichlorophenyl) methylidene] bis(1H-indole-2-carboxylate)-(D32DMBC) organic NLO single crystal and its optical, thermal, mechanical, dielectric and computational studies. *J. Mater. Sci.: Mater. Electron.*, 31, 23, 1–8, 2020, https://doi.org/10.1007/s10854-020-04594-y.
39. SenthilKannan, K., Venkatachalam, K., Bhakya, K., Sharmidha, B., Kalaivani, M., Gayathri Devi, S., Senthilkannan, K., Growth and characterization of picolinium maleate (PM) crystals. *AIP Conf. Proc.*, 2270, 10014, 1–4, 2020, https://doi.org/10.1063/5.0019341.
40. SenthilKannan, K., Thamarikannan, P., Kalaipoonguzhali, V., Venkatachalam, K., Kannan, S., Baskar, A., Fluorescence, computational enactments of dimethyl N,N′-[(ethyne-1, 2-di-yl)Bis-(1,4- phenyl-ene carbon-yl)]bis-(l-alaninate) crystals. *AIP Conf. Proc.*, 2270, 100008, 1–4, 2020, https://doi.org/10.1063/5.0019334.
41. SenthilKannan, K., Thamaraikannan, P., Kalaipoonguzhali, V., Venkatachalam, K., Kannan, S., Ranadevan, R., Senthilkannan, K., Computational, I.R., Raman studies by DFT program and antidiabetic delineation by harboring of acetoacetanilide crystals. *AIP Conf. Proc.*, 2270, 10013, 1–4, 2020, https://doi.org/10.1063/5.0019339.
42. Flora, G. *et al.*, Anti-diabetic (AD) and crystal stiffness characterizations of NaBr-added L-alanine (LANB) – A comparative analysis in macro and nano scale crystals. *Mater. Today: Proc.*, 33, 7, 3937–3941, 2020.
43. Flora, G. *et al.*, Anti diabetic (AD), stiffness and hardness studies of 2-[4-(Trifluoromethyl) phenyl]-1H-benzimidazole crystals - (TFMPHB) macro and nano crystal. *Mater. Today: Proc.*, 33, 4233–4236, 2020.
44. Flora, G. *et al.*, Anti-inflammatory (AI) and crystalline hardness characterisations of 4-(4-chlorophenyl)-7,7-dimethyl-7,8-dihydro-4h-1-benzopyran-2,5(3h,6h)-dione-(CPDMDHHBPHHD) – comparative analysis of macro and nano scales crystals. *Mater. Today: Proc.*, 33, 3578–3582, 2020.

45. Ganesan, S., Gurunathan, R., Pasupuleti, R.R. *et al.*, Green synthesis of V_2O_5/ZnO nanocomposite materials for efficient photocatalytic and anti-bacterial applications. *Appl. Nanosci.*, 2021, https://doi.org/10.1007/s13204-021-01923-3.
46. Ganesan, H., SenthilKannan, K., Christy, S. *et al.*, Synthesis, growth, XRD, NLO, CHNSO, computational-structural, dielectric, photoconductivity, hardness and biostudies of diethyl 2-amino-5-{4-[bis (4-methyl phenyl) amino] benzamido} thiophene-3,4-dicarboxylate (DABMPABTD) macro-, nano crystals for device fabrication, pharma, electronic uses. *J. Mater. Sci.: Mater. Electron.*, 32, 15498–15508, 2021.
47. Maalmarugan, J., Yokeswaran, V., Divya, R. *et al.*, Synthesis, growth, XRD, NLO, CHNSO, structure by theoretical approach, dielectric, absorbance, photoconductivity and bio studies of 4-(4-Acetyl-5-Methyl-1H-1, 2, 3-Triazol-1-yl) Benzonitrile crystals for optical, opto-electronic, and photonics utilities. *J. Mater. Sci.: Mater. Electron.*, 32, 13850–13858, 2021, https://doi.org/10.1007/s10854-021-05960-0.
48. Rajkumar, M., Maalmarugan, J., Flora, G. *et al.*, Growth, characterizations, and the structural elucidation of diethyl-2-(3-oxoiso-1,3-dihydrobenzofuran-1-ylidene)malonate crystalline specimen for dielectric and electronic filters, thermal, optical, mechanical, and biomedical applications using conventional experimental and theoretical practices. *J. Mater. Sci.: Mater. Electron.*, 32, 22822–22839, 2021, https://doi.org/10.1007/s10854-021-06761-1.
49. SenthilKannan, K., Flora, G., Gunasekaran, S., Ali, H.A.J., Vimalan, M., Balasubramanian, S., Extraction of silver nanoparticles (Ag-NPs) by green synthesis from aqueous extract of seaweeds and their consequences on HeLa cell Line and Their utility on soil by spectroscopic tools, in: *Nanotechnology for Advances in Medical Microbiology*. Environmental and microbial biotechnology, Springer, Singapore, 2021, https://doi.org/10.1007/978-981-15-9916-3_5.
50. Momma, K. and Izumi, F., VESTA 3 for three-dimensional visualization of crystal, volumetric and morphology data. *J. Appl. Crystallogr.*, 44, 1272–1276, 2011.
51. Spackman, P.R., Turner, M.J., McKinnon, J.J., Wolff, S.K., Grimwood, D.J., Jayatilaka, D., Spackman, M.A., Crystal Explorer: A program for Hirshfeld surface analysis, visualization and quantitative analysis of molecular crystals. *J. Appl. Cryst.*, 54, 3, 2021, https://doi.org/10.1107/S1600576721002910.
52. Pek, A.J.S., Single – crystal structure validation with the program PLATON. *J. Appl. Cryst.*, 36, 7–11, 2003.

8

Biological, Electronic-Filter, Influx and Theoretical Practicalities of 2-Chloro-6-Nitroaniline (2C6NA) Crystals for Biomedical and Microelectronics Tasks

Maria Sumathi B.[1], Maalmarugan J.[2], Ganesan H.[3], Saravanan P.[4], Patel R.P.[5], Sheeba M.[6], Flora G.[1] and Senthil Kannan K.[7]*

[1]Department of Botany, St. Mary's College (Autonomous), Thoothukudi, TN, India
[2]Department of EEE, Sri Ranganathar Institute of Engineering and Technology, Athipalayam, Coimbatore, TN, India
[3]Department of Mechanical Engineering, Sri Ranganathar Institute of Engineering and Technology, Athipalayam, Coimbatore, TN, India
[4]P.G & Research Department of Physics, Arignar Anna Govt. Arts College, Cheyyar, India
[5]Department of Pure and Applied Physics, Guru Ghasidas Vishwavidyala, Bilaspur, Chhattisgarh, India
[6]Department of Zoology, PSGR Krishnammal College for Women, Coimbatore, TN, India
[7]Department of R&D/Physics, Edayathangudy G.S Pillay Arts and Science College (Autonomous – Affiliated to Bharathidasan University – Tiruchirappalli), Nagapattinam, Tamil Nadu, India

Abstract

The effect and impact of biomedical, electronic, and computational analysis are more on 2C6NA crystals and are based on aniline by means of the anticancer, antibacterial, antifungal, the structural effectiveness by computational and influx of 3.4679 microns influx data. The efficacy is by HeLa cell lines; for the cervical cancer and the *E. coli, B. subtilis, K. pneumoniae, A. niger,* and *A. terreus* and *A. flavus.* DPPH, FRAP, and antidiabetic utility of the 2C6NA nanocrystalline specimen are portrayed with conversion of milling with 43-nm scaling and the

**Corresponding author*: mscgoldmedalist@yahoo.in

Kaushik Pal (ed.) Nanovaccinology as Targeted Therapeutics, (145–156) © 2022 Scrivener Publishing LLC

structure effectiveness by means of software and optoelectronic filter utility is also discussed. The crystal is grown by evaporation method and properly milled to nm scalings. Aniline plays a major impact for bioactivity and in influx datum. The leading value of filter is applied to electronic functions and other NLO use, as well as biocompatibility of the titled crystal sample and is reported for these studies as a novel work and in the future can be preceded for harboring process.

Keywords: Biomedical, electronic, computational, influx, 2C6NA

8.1 Introduction

The utility of the crystalline materials is vast and focuses and emphasizes for new type of enhanced uses [1–5]. Organic nonlinear optical (NLO) materials are drawing marvelous conformity of contemplation appropriate to their relatable associations in optical arrangements, distinguished laser-upheld picture approach, communiques, data accumulation, higher mean-power NLO [6–13] transparent matters for optically definite amplifier interface and SHG accurate throughout the UV ethereal expanses [14–18]. Normalized organocrystals can have exceptionally unexpected nonlinear susceptibilities separated to inorganic variety of semitransparent sample [19–22]. Resourceful natural composite in formed amusement sketches, essential to exceedingly proficient incriminate transfer paths of accomplishment, has been influentially scrutinized. Organic materials are well compensated than the counterparts and nano [23–25] is preferred than macro [26–29], based on the utilities [30–34] and effectiveness of their crystalline data [35–39] and their major functions in computational [40–43], electronic [43–45], and biouses [46–52].

8.2 Computational and Influx

Figures 8.1 to 8.3 show the molecular arrangement, structure, and the space-filled effect for confirmation of the sample that is grown, as well as identifying the atomic scheme. The O-N=O and H-N-H and Cl bonds are narrated by software and ball bond nature by means of software using Java script coding by the networking people as the big data analysis part of the sample using crystal data, and for interactive frail method, the space-filled model is used. The influx 3.4679 microns for the filter relevances and opto electronic too for the sample for macro and 3.9767 microns for nano level to identify the betterment.

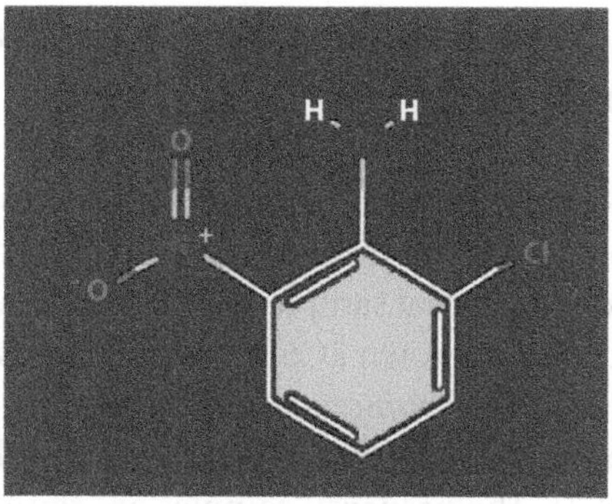

Figure 8.1 Molecular structural of 2C6NA crystals [50–52].

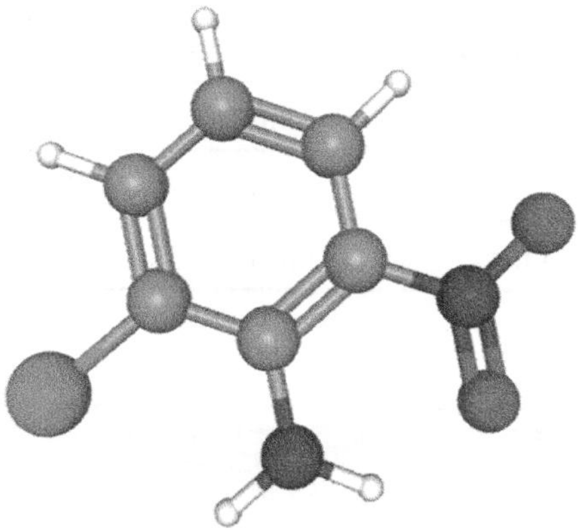

Figure 8.2 Ball and stick of 2C6NA crystals [50–52].

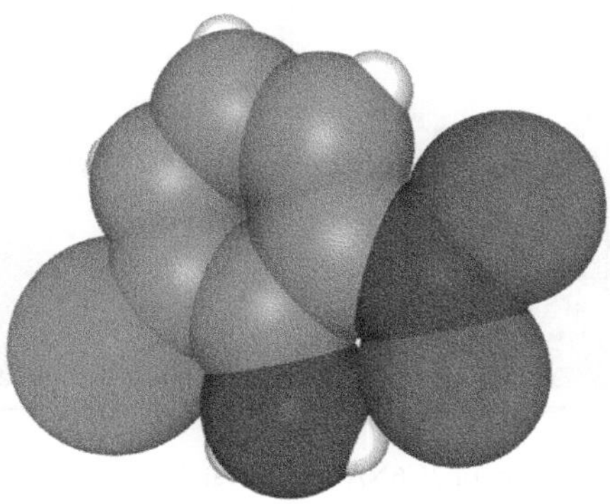

Figure 8.3 Space filled of 2C6NA crystals [50–52].

8.3 Antibacterial, Antifungal, Antidiabetic, DPPH, FRAP, Anticancer

The antibacterial action by region of reticence end results shows that the full-grown material reveals the motion as in Table 8.1 and Figure 8.4, the results perceptibly divulged that samples confirmed enhanced antibacterial commotion. The activity of grown 2C6NA nanocrystals is excellent against *E. coli, B. subtilis,* and *K. pneumoniae.* The viable antifungal medication fluconazoles was exercised as habitual. 2C6NA showed extensive antifungal activity (Table 8.2). The prepared samples are found to have the superior antifungal motion. 2C6NA crystals showed excellent activity against

Table 8.1 Antibacterial effect of 2C6NA nanocrystals.

Microorganisms used	50µL (2C6NA)	100 µL (2C6NA)	Disc (CAZ 10mcg)	$D.H_2O$
B.subtilis	2 mm	3mm	6mm	Nil
E.coli	3 mm	5mm	Nil	Nil
K. pneumoniae	3 mm	4mm	10mm	Nil

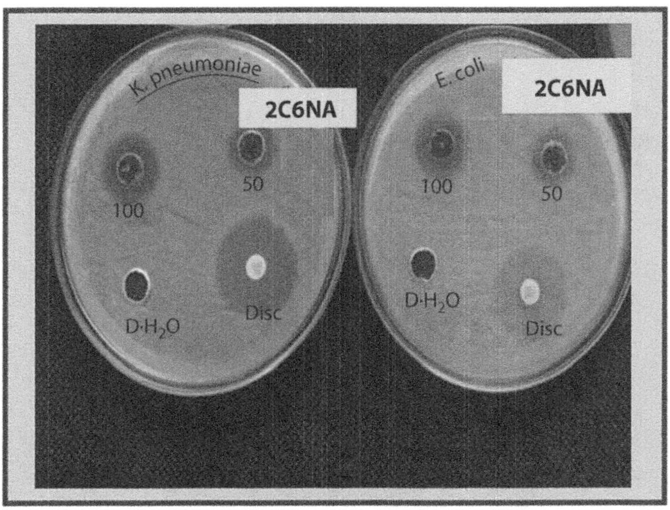

Figure 8.4 Atibacterial activity of 2C6NA nanocrystals.

A. niger and *A. terreus* and showed moderate activity against *A. flavus*. Table 8.3 presents the anti-diabetic and the anti-oxidant data. The antidiabetic study was performed by means of an alpha-glucosidase reserve assay, whereas acarbose was used as the standard drug. The alpha amylase and alpha glucosidase reticence of the sample in assessment with acarbose is shown in Table 8.3. DPPH radical was estimated, 1 mL of ligands solution in DMSO was added to 1 mL of DPPH radical solution in methanol. The *in vitro* cell growth inhibitory activity in opposition to the human cancer cell lines. 100 μL of the investigation trials (5(25, 50, 100, 200, and 400 μg/ml)) were as in Tables 8.4 and 8.5 added to the wells, and the cells were further incubated for another 2 days at a range of around 37°C to 38°C in an environment of CO_2.

Table 8.2 Fungal approach of 2C6NA nanocrystals.

Microorganisms used	50 μL (2C6NA)	100 μL (2C6NA)	Standard
A. niger	4 mm	7 mm	Nil
A. flavus	5 mm	6 mm	Nil
A. terreus	6 mm	7 mm	Nil

Table 8.3 Antioxidant and antidiabetic data of 2C6NA nanocrystals.

Samples	% of DPPH
2C6NA	69.12
Samples	**Mg/g of FRAP**
2C6NA	26.92
Sample	**Alpha -amylase**
2C6NA	52.12
Sample	**Alpha - glucosidase**
2C6NA	50.20

Table 8.4 Details of samples received for the study.

Sl. no.	Sample name/code	Concentrations	Cell lines
1	2C6NA	5 (25, 50, 100, 200, and 400 μg/ml)	HeLa

Table 8.5 Concentrations used for the study.

Sl. no	Test compounds	Cell line	Concentration treated to cells
1	Untreated	Hela	No treatment
2	Standard (doxorubicin)	Hela	15uM
3	Blank	-	Only Media without cells
4	2C6NA	He La	5(25,50,100,200 & 400ug/ ml)

8.4 Conclusion

The impact of biomedical, electronic, and computational analyses is more on 2C6NA crystals and are based on aniline by means of the anticancer, antibacterial, antifungal, the structural effectiveness by computational, and influx of 3.4679 microns influx data. The efficacy is by HeLa cell lines (Figure 8.5); for the cervical cancer and the *E. coli, B. subtilis K. pneumoniae. A. niger, terreus,* and *A. flavus.* DPPH, FRAP, and antidiabetic utility of the 2C6NA nanocrystalline specimen are portrayed with the conversion of milling with 43 nm scaling, and the structure effectiveness by means of software and optoelectronic filter utility is also discussed. The crystal is grown by evaporation method and milled to nm scalings. Aniline plays

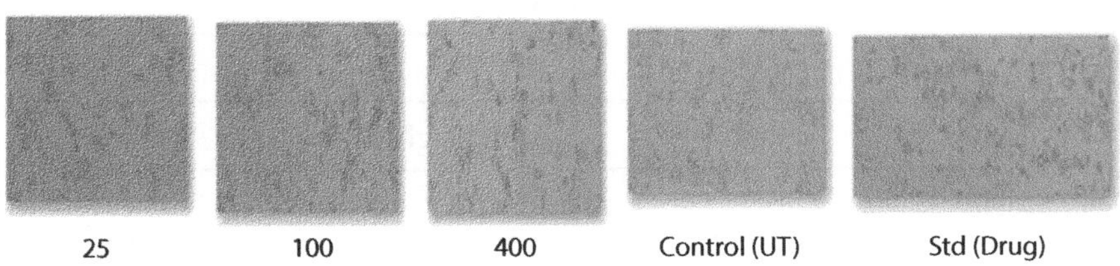

Figure 8.5 HeLa cell of 26CNA of 25, 100, 400 microg/ml.

a major impact for bioactivity and in influx. The prime value of filter is applied to electronic functions and other NLO use, as well as biocompatibility of the sample, and in the future, harboring bio use can be enabled for industrial use of microelectronic sector and in anticancer drugs as a major or derivative use and in big data analytics in software.

References

1. Kalaipoonguzhali.V., SenthilKannan. K., Thirumoorthi.C., Chinnadurai.M, Jayanalina.T., Comparison of adsorption energy, ionization potential and electron affinity of CuS-ACT and CuS-Nit nanostructures monowire for nano device fabrication by computational approach, Mater. Today: Proc. 33 (7), 2759-2760, 2020
2. Sethu Gunasekaran *et al.*, Structural studies on picolinium maleate crystal by density functional methods, Indian J. Phys. 87(12), 1189–1197, 2013.
3. Senthilkannan.K, *et al.*, Anti diabetic (AD) studies of bis-glycine hydro bromide (45 nm) nano crystals, Mater. Today: Proc. 33(7), 3201-3202,2020.
4. Senthilkannan.K *et al.*, Anti-diabetic activites of ZnO doped with Ce (5 at %) nano particles (NPs), Mater. Today: Proc. 33(7), 3056-3057, (2020).
5. Senthilkannan.K *et al.*, Fluorescence, filter,nano tribological studies of 12-(4-Chlorophenyl)-9,9-Dimethyl-9,10-Dihydro-8H-Benzo[A]Xanthen-11(12H)-One-(CPDDHBXH) macro and nano crystals, Mater. Today: Proc. 33(7), 4163-4166, 2020.
6. Senthilkannan . K., Venkatachalam K, M. Jothibas, Computational and experimental studies of acetoacetanilide crystals, AIP Conf Proc. 2270 (2270):040014;1-4, 2020.
7. Senthilkannan . K., Venkatachalam K, Ashokkumar Rajamani, Computational analysis of LPNPTH anisotropies for dementia for Alzheimer's syndrome by DFT and molecular harboring, AIP Conf Proc. 2270(2270), 040008;1-5, 2020.
8. Senthilkannan . K., Sivaramakrishnan Velu., Kalaipoonguzhali.V., Chinnadurai.M., Kannan.S., Electronic transport, HOMO–LUMO and computational studies of CuS monowire for nano device fabrication by DFT approach, Mater. Today: Proc. 33(7), 2746-2749, 2020.
9. Senthilkannan . K., Gunasekaran.S, Spectroscopic studies and other novel studies of 4 bromo 4' chloro benzylidene aniline (BCBA) Crystal- A non linear optical material, Int. J. Chemtech Res. 5(6), 3051-3058,2013.
10. Senthilkannan . K., Gayathri Devi.S, Prithiviraj Nagarajan, Flora.G, Ranadevan Rajakumaravelu, Anti diabetic (AD) studies of picolinium maleate nano crystals, Mater. Today: Proc. 33(3), 3005-3007, 2020.
11. Senthilkannan . K., Krishnaveni Ramamurthi., Bhakya.K., Sivaramakrishnan Velu, Kolanjinathan.M., Ranadevan Rajakumaravelu, Hardness,

Photoconductivity, Anti-diabetic Studies of L -AlaniniumFumarate (LAF) Crystals, AIP Conf Proc. 2270:100010;1-4, 2020.
12. Senthilkannan . K., P. Baskaran, Renuka Seenivasan, P. Settu, Tribological, Filter, FTIR and fluorescence studies of L-Alaninium tartrate (LAT) Macro and nano crystals, Mater. Today: Proc. 33(7), 4148-4150,2020.
13. Senthilkannan . K., Kaleemullah Khan., Abdul Jaffar., Vinoth Kumar Ponnusamy., Natana Murugaraj Govindan., Effect of anti microbial and fluorescence on L-Alaninium maleate (LAM) macro and nano crystals, Mater. Today: Proc. 33(7), 2779-2781, 2020.
14. Senthilkannan.K.,Ganesh.G.,AbdulJafferAli.H.,KrishnaveniRamamurthi.R, Kaleemullah Khan, Anti diabetic (AD) activities of L-valinium picrate (LVP) macro and nano crystals, Mater. Today: Proc. 33(7), 2738-2740, 2020.
15. Senthilkannan. K., Bhakya.K, Iyanar.M, Growth and Influx, AC and DC Conductivity Studies of L-AlaniniumFumarate (LAF) Crystals, AIP Conf Proc. 2270:100009;1-4, 2020.
16. Senthilkannan . K, Growth, fluorescence and theoretical studies of B2CPCD crystals – Comparative analysis in macro and nano scaled crystals, Mater. Today: Proc., 33(7), 4368-4371, 2020.
17. Senthilkannan . K, *et al.*, Anti-diabetic (AD) activities of ZnO doped with Ce (7 at%) nano particles (NP), Mater. Today: Proc. 33(7), 3053-3055, 2020.
18. Senthilkannan . K *et al.*, Tribological, filter studies of 3-Bromo-2-Hydroxy benzoic acid (BHBA) macro and nano crystals, Mater. Today: Proc. 33(7), 4145-4147,2020.
19. Senthilkannan . K *et al.*, Electronic transport, Homo-Lumo and computational studies of CuS-ACT monowire for nano device fabrication by software approach, Mater. Today: Proc. 33(7), 2756-2758, 2020.
20. Senthilkannan . K *et al.*, Anti microbial and fluorescence activities of L-valinium picrate (LVP) macro and nano crystals, Mater. Today: Proc. 33(7), 2776-2778 (2020).
21. Senthilkumar.R *et al.*, Anti-diabetic (AD) and hardness profile of 12-(4-Chlorophenyl)-9,9- Dimethyl-9,10-Dihydro-8H-benzo[a]xanthen-11(12H)-one –(CPDDHBXH) – Comparative analysis of macro and nano crystals, Mater. Today: Proc. 33(7), 4167-4170, 2020.
22. Sathishkumar.R *et al.*, Synthesis, Growth and Characterization of 2,5 – Dimethyl-N-(3-phenylprop-2-en-1-ylidene) Aniline (2,5 DPPA) Single Crystal: A New Second Order Nonlinear Optical Material for Photonic and Optoelectronic Applications, Optik, 226(2), 1-11, 2020.
23. Patel.R.P *et al.*, Growth and XRD, Elemental, Mechanical, Dielectric, Optical and Photoconductivity, and Surface Morphological Characterizations of 2-[4-(Trifluoromethyl) phenyl]-1H-benzimidazole (TFMPHB) Crystals for Electronic, Mechanical Applications, *Braz. J. Phys.*, 51(3), 339-350, 2021.
24. Aarthi.R *et al.*, Molecular structure- associated pharmacodynamic investigation on benzoyl peroxide using spectroscopic and quantum computational tools, J. Taibah Univ. Sci. 12(1), 104-122,2018.

25. Saravanan.P, *et al.*, Biofriendly and competent domestic microwave assisted method for the synthesis of ZnO nanoparticles from the extract of Azadirachta indica leaves, Mater. Today: Proc. 33(7), 3160-3163, 2020.
26. Saravanan.P, *et al.*, A perspective approach towards appreciable size and cost-effective solar cell fabrication by synthesizing ZnO nanoparticles from Azadirachta indica leaves extract using domestic microwave oven, J. Mater. Sci.: Mater. Electron.31(5),4301–4309, 2020.
27. Saravanan.P *et al.*, Dielectric and magnetic properties of Allium cepa and Raphanus sativus extracts biogenic ZnO nanoparticles, J. Mater. Sci.: Mater. Electron. 32(1), 1-14, 2021.
28. Periyathambi.P *et al.*, Fluorescence and filter characterizations of NaBr-added L-alanine (LANB) – A comparative analysis in macro and nano scaled crystals, Mater. Today: Proc. 33, 3766-3769, 2020.
29. Baskaran.P, *et al.*, Anti-diabetic activities of ZnO doped with Ce (3 at %) nano particles, Mater. Today: Proc. 33(7), 3051-3052, 2020.
30. Baskaran.P *et al.*, Anti-diabetic studies of barium paranitro phenolate macro and nano crystals, Mater. Today: Proc. 33(7), 3058-3060, 2020.
31. Kolanjinathan.M, Senthilkannan.K., Sivagurunathan Paramasivam, Baskaran.P, Iyanar.M, Anti-diabetic studies of 4-(4-chlorophenyl)-7,7-di-methyl-7,8-dihydro-4H-1-benzopyran-2,5(3H,6H)-dione – (CPDMDHHBPHHD) nano crystals, Mater. Today: Proc. 33(7), 2750-2752, 2020.
32. Kolanjinathan.M *et al.*, Dielectric, fluorescence, filter, nano tribological and photoconductivity studies of 4-(4-chlorophenyl)-7,7-dimethyl-7,8-di-hydro-4H-1-benzopyran-2,5(3H,6H)-dione (CPDMDHHBPHHD) macro and nano crystals, J. Mater. Sci.: Mater. Electron. 27(4), 16907–16917, 2020.
33. Kolanjinathan, M., Hariharasuthan, R., Sivaramakrishnan, V. *et al.* XRD, CHNSO, fluorescence, filter-influx, NLO, photoconductivity, hardness and helical spring-fabricated device stress analysis of 2′-chloro-4-methoxy-3-ni-trobenzil (CMNB) crystal of different scalings for opto-electronic filter and band gap engineering utilities. J Mater Sci: Mater Electron **32,** 10049–10057, 2021.
34. Jothibas.M *et al.*, Structural, optical and photo catatic activity of Ag doped ZnO nano particles obtained by sol-gel method, AIP Conf Proc. 2162(1):020151, 1-7,2019.
35. Logeshwari Selvaraj *et al.*, AS Anti-diabetic (AD) studies of Bis Glycine Hydro Bromide – BGHB macro crystals milled to nano scale of 219 nm as the preliminary fine particles, Mater. Today: Proc. 33(7), 3763-3765, 2020.
36. Kishore.N *et al.*, CO and HCHO adsorption on FeO monowire devices: a DFT study, Applied Physics A 123(11), 706; 1-7 (2017), https://doi.org/10.1007/s00339-017-1330-6.
37. Senthilkannan.K, Gunasekaran.S , Gowtham.J, Retwik Wagish, UV, SEM, Powder XRD Studies of Acetoacetanilide (AAC) Crystal, Int. J. Chemtech Res. 6(5), 3187-3190, 2014.

38. Kumar.K *et al.*, Growth of diethyl 3,3′-[(2,4-dichlorophenyl) methylidene] bis(1H-indole-2-carboxylate)-(D32DMBC) organic NLO single crystal and its optical, thermal, mechanical, dielectric and computational studies, J. Mater. Sci.: Mater. Electron. 31(23):1-8, (2020) https://doi.org/10.1007/s10854-020-04594-y.
39. SenthilKannan.K, Venkatachalam.K, Bhakya.K, Sharmidha.B, Kalaivani.M, Gayathri Devi.S, Senthilkannan.K, Growth and Characterization of Picolinium Maleate (PM) Crystals, AIP Conf Proc. 2270:10014;1-4 (2020) https://doi.org/10.1063/5.0019341
40. SenthilKannan.K, Thamarikannan.P, Kalaipoonguzhali.V, Venkatachalam K, Kannan.S, Baskar.A, Fluorescence, computational enactments of dimethyl N,N′-[(ethyne-1, 2-di-yl)Bis-(1,4- phenyl-ene carbon-yl)]bis-(l-al-aninate) crystals, AIP Conf Proc.,2270:100008;1-4, (2020) https://doi.org/10.1063/5.0019334
41. SenthilKannan.K,Thamaraikannan.P,Kalaipoonguzhali.V,Venkatachalam.K, Kannan.S, Ranadevan.R, Senthilkannan.K, Computational IR, Raman studies by DFT program and antidiabetic delineation by harboring of ace-toacetanilide crystals, AIP Conf Proc., 2270:10013;1-4 (2020) https://doi.org/10.1063/5.0019339
42. Flora.G *et al.*, Anti-diabetic (AD) and crystal stiffness characterizations of NaBr-added L-alanine (LANB) – A comparative analysis in macro and nano scale crystals, Mater. Today: Proc. 33(7), 3937-3941, (2020).
43. Flora.G *et al.*, Anti diabetic (AD), stiffness and hardness studies of 2-[4-(Trifluoromethyl) phenyl]-1H-benzimidazole crystals - (TFMPHB) macro and nano crystal, Mater. Today: Proc., 33, 4233-4236, 2020.
44. Flora.G *et al.*, Anti-inflammatory (AI) and crystalline hardness character-isations of 4-(4-chlorophenyl)-7,7-dimethyl-7,8-dihydro-4h-1-benzopy-ran-2,5(3h,6h)-dione-(CPDMDHHBPHHD) – comparative analysis of macro and nano scales crystals, Mater. Today: Proc. 33, 3578-3582, 2020.
45. Ganesan,S., Gurunathan,R., Pasupuleti, R.R. *et al.* Green synthesis of V_2O_5/ZnO nanocomposite materials for efficient photocatalytic and anti-bacterial applications. Appl Nanosci (2021). https://doi.org/10.1007/s13204-021-01923-3.
46. Ganesan, H., SenthilKannan, K., Christy, S. *et al.* Synthesis, growth, XRD, NLO, CHNSO, computational-structural, dielectric, photoconductivity, hardness and biostudies of diethyl 2-amino-5-{4-[bis (4-methyl phenyl) amino] benzamido} thiophene-3,4-dicarboxylate (DABMPABTD) macro-, nano crystals for device fabrication, pharma, electronic uses. J Mater Sci: Mater Electron 32, 15498–15508, 2021.
47. Maalmarugan, J., Yokeswaran, V., Divya, R. *et al.* Synthesis, growth, XRD, NLO, CHNSO, structure by theoretical approach, dielectric, absorbance, photoconductivity and bio studies of 4-(4-Acetyl-5-Methyl-1H-1, 2, 3-Triazol-1-yl) Benzonitrile crystals for optical, opto-electronic, and

photonics utilities. J Mater Sci: Mater Electron 32, 13850–13858 (2021), https://doi.org/10.1007/s10854-021-05960-0.
48. Rajkumar, M., Maalmarugan, J., Flora, G. *et al.* Growth, characterizations, and the structural elucidation of diethyl-2-(3-oxoiso-1,3-dihydrobenzofuran-1-ylidene)malonate crystalline specimen for dielectric and electronic filters, thermal, optical, mechanical, and biomedical applications using conventional experimental and theoretical practices. J Mater Sci: Mater Electron, 32, 22822–22839, 2021, https://doi.org/10.1007/s10854-021-06761-1
49. SenthilKannan K., Flora G., Gunasekaran S., Ali H.A.J., Vimalan M., Balasubramanian S. (2021) Extraction of Silver Nanoparticles (Ag-NPs) by Green Synthesis from Aqueous Extract of Seaweeds and Their Consequences on HeLa Cell Line and Their Utility on Soil by Spectroscopic Tools. Nanotechnology for Advances in Medical Microbiology. Environmental and Microbial Biotechnology. Springer, Singapore. https://doi.org/10.1007/978-981-15-9916-3_5
50. K. Momma and F. Izumi, "VESTA 3 for three-dimensional visualization of crystal, volumetric and morphology data," J. Appl. Crystallogr., 44, 1272-1276 (2011).
51. Spackman, P. R., Turner, M. J., McKinnon, J. J., Wolff, S. K., Grimwood, D. J., Jayatilaka, D. & Spackman, M. A. Crystal Explorer: a program for Hirshfeld surface analysis, visualization and quantitative analysis of molecular crystals (2021). J. Appl. Cryst. 54, 3, 2021 https://doi.org/10.1107/S1600576721002910
52. A.J.SPek, J.Appl.Cryst.2003, 36, 7-11. Single – crystal structure validation with the program PLATON

9

Antidiabetic, Anti-Oxidant, Computational, Filter, and Tribological Characterizations of Bis Glycine Lithium Bromide Monohydrate Nano (32 nm) Scaled Crystals

Dayana Lobo F.[1], Senthil Kannan K.[2*], Mathivanan V.[3], Jacintha Tamil Malar A.[1], Christy S.[4], Flora G.[1], Ganesan H.[5] and Maalmarugan J.[6]

[1]*Department of Botany, St.Mary's College - Autonomous, Thoothukudi, Tamilnadu, India*
[2]*Department of R&D/Physics, Edayathangudy G.S Pillay Arts and Science College (Autonomous - Affiliated to Bharathidasan University - Tiruchirappalli, Nagapattinam, Tamilnadu, India*
[3]*Department of Physics, Shri Sapthagiri Institute of Technology, Ocheri, Ranipet, Tamilnadu, India*
[4]*Department of Information Technology, Saveetha School of Engineering, Saveetha Institute of Medical and Technical Sciences, Saveetha University, Chennai, TN-India*
[5]*Department of Mechanical Engineering, Sri Ranganathar Institute of Engineering and Technology, Athipalayam, Coimbatore, TN, India*
[6]*Department of EEE, Sri Ranganathar Institute of Engineering and Technology, Athipalayam, Coimbatore, TN, India*

Abstract
Crystals are generally intended for multipurpose applications and effectiveness in almost all the day to day activities, as well as areas, primarily in electronics and biology. The aim is that the current exploration is paying attention on Bis Glycine Lithium Bromide Monohydrate (BGLBMH nanocrystals), its production and the variety of studies, characterizations. BGLBMH are grown in regulated way by a solution growing process, and nano crystal change is mainly by milled

**Corresponding author*: mscgoldmedalist@yahoo.in

Kaushik Pal (ed.) Nanovaccinology as Targeted Therapeutics, (157–168) © 2022 Scrivener Publishing LLC

methodology to 32 nm. The Single XRD, PXRD investigation, filter, tribology, anti-diabetic, and antioxidant (AD and AO) studies are performed for nano BGLBMH. The single crystal XRD study exposes the lattice parameters of the BGLBMH with a, b, c in Å as 7.5397, 17.4174, 8.2727, and β as 118.14° as the crystalline system is of monoclinic with the space group of $P2_1/c$. The nanoscaled crystalline samples are properly and well analyzed for fluorescence activity. The 395-nm wavelength of nanoscaling of 32 nm with band gap value of 3.139 eV is identified and is a perfect match with earlier work. The nanosketch out of BGLBMH nano-crystals are of 32 nm likewise for the end schema of final grilling by milled effect. The thermal ellipsoidal plot by promolecular effect by software is analyzed. The BGLBMH have the proper utilities in electro, mechano, and bio/pharma utilities based on the influx for filters, tribological data, and AD/AO data.

***Keywords*:** Fluorescence, influx, nano, tribology

9.1 Introduction

Crystalline specimen are of gracious and circumstantial utility with regard to their way of studies and achieving goals and have tremendous major specific functionalities by the chemical compositions [1–8] and the chains of catena present in the crystalline sample [9–13] and also the presence of solute/solvent in the model for further processing [14–18] and the composites of glycine have in recent times paying attention, appeal owing to their possible relevances in the field of ferro-electricity [19–24], dielectrics nature of properties [25–29] and nonlinear optical—SHG/THG/HHG properties [29–33]. Nonlinear optical materials—NLOs [33–37]—are extremely significant for the existing and present case of researchers due to its consequence for bring into being the second, as well as the type of third harmonic generations [38–43]. Single crystalline X-ray diffracted beam structural investigation reveals that the glycine lithium bromide taken the shape in the crystalline zone as the monoclinic type of system, with the crystalline spacegroup as the $P2_1/c$. Fluorescence, filter use influx, tribological, AD and AO work for BGLBMH macro and nanoscalings of the crystalline specimen are studied and reported [43–52].

9.2 Experimental

9.2.1 Synthesis

Bis-glycine lithiumbromide (BGLB) crystalline chemical salt was synthesized by dissolving glycine and lithiumbromide in proper stoichiometric proportion in the double distilled refined water to get the titled block of specimen, the ambience of the temperature of the schematic crystal growth setup and arrangement was properly kept at a constant and consistent bath of temperature of 52-53°C, and the BGLBMH crystals are yielded out. The salt was expelled out by progressive recrystallizations and purified product is obtained.

9.3 Results and Discussions

9.3.1 Single Crystalline XRD (SXRD) Study and Powder XRD (PXRD) Studies

The single crystalline XRD (SXRD) study as well as the Powder XRD (PXRD) for crystals of the BGLBMH are properly represented by the proper data of SXRD as mentioned in Table 9.1, and the PXRD indexed data pattern in Figure 9.1 with the versatile planes of proper and referred reflections was regulated by using the product AUTOX93 and greatly in the effect of matched with PXRD indexed pattern and milled ones as in Table 9.2.

Table 9.1 Data of SXRD of BGLBMH crystals.

System	Data
a in Å	7.5397
b in Å	17.4174
c in Å	8.2727
Crystal size – macro scale	13 x 7 x 5 mm^3
Crystal size—nanoscale	32 nm
space group	$P2_1/c$
System	monoclinic
β	118.14°

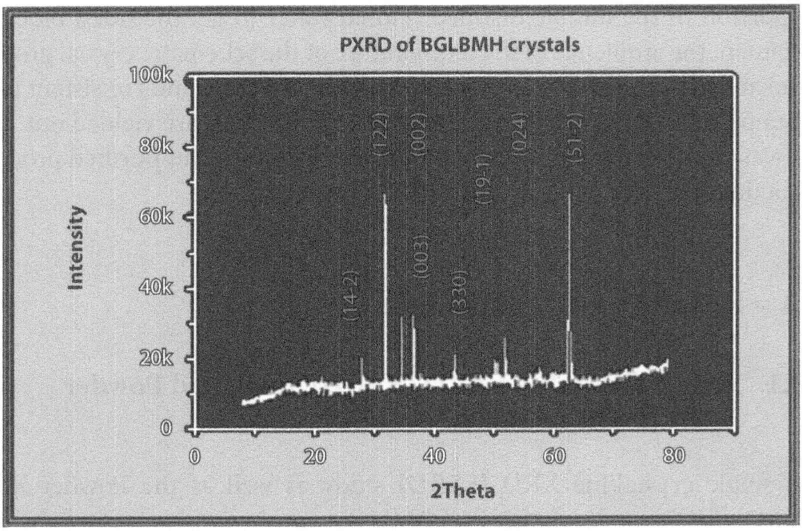

Figure 9.1 PXRD of BGLBMH crystals.

Table 9.2 Milling of BGLBMH crystals for nanoscaling.

Sample	Crystal size
BGLBMH nanocrystals after milling	**32 nm**

9.3.2 Fluorescence (FL) Study for 32-nm Scale

The effectiveness of the FL data of the sample is properly analyzed for 32-nm scaling and obtained the 395-nm emission cum emanated value of the FL wavelength of BGLBMH crystals with the band gap of 3.139 eV and is a higher energy value than the 34-nm scale of titled specimen, and the proper refranged data are obtained for the 32-nm scale of the present specimen for FL outfit. The FL spectrum is portrayed in Figure 9.2 as given below.

9.3.3 Antidiabetic (AD) Study and Influx Study

The antidiabetic (AD) studies for the BGLBMH crystals are properly measured for the two enzymatic representation of alpha-amylase (AA), as well as alpha-glucosidase (AG), and the IC-50 data for macroscales and nanoscales are 35.4 and 29.3 for the AA and 37.1 and 30.2 for the AG-AD of BGLBMH crystals of 32 nm, and in IC-50 proviso, its diminutived

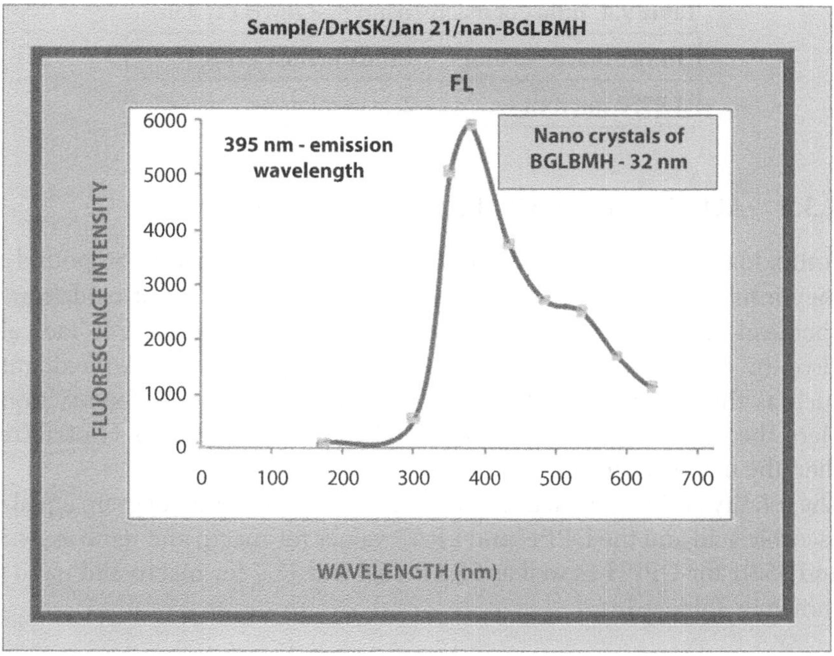

Figure 9.2 FL of nano BGLBMH crystals.

assessment from macroscaling to nanoscaling, which is suitable for AD, is shown in Table 9.3. The AD work of BGLBMH is particularly due to the presence of glycine and not due to the effect of bromine and lithium especially when scale is nanoscale by the chemical structure and shape and size parameters and the physical properties. Influx value of the extent of 1.9750 microns of macro leveled BGLBMH portrays that the BGLBMH is very good and a proper client for NLO property and 2.4316 microns is a nanolevel influx of the entitled specimen. So the BGLBMH are mainly used in filter type of proviso purposes too as shown in the statistics presented in Table 9.4.

Table 9.3 AD of macro, nano BGLBMH crystals.

Type of AD	IC-50 - macro BGLBMH	IC-50 – nano BGLBMH
Alpha-amylase	35.4	29.3
Alpha-glucosidase	37.1	30.2

Table 9.4 Influx of macro, nano BGLBMH crystals.

Influx macro scaling	Influx nanoscaling
1.9750 microns	2.4316 microns

9.3.4 AO-DPPH, FRAP of Antioxidant Activity

Antioxidants are a type of chemical substance or chemical compound as they inhibit the process and the proceedings of the state of oxidation, a chemical-based normalized reaction to produce a type of free radicals, also, the chain reactions that may harm/damage the cells. Antioxidants, such as thiol/ascorbic acid, are the best kind of inhibitors for reactions. Here the case DPPH and FRAP of BGLBMH nanoscalings is preferred than the macroscalings.

The totality antioxidant action is expressed as the quantity of gram equal of ascorbic acid and the DPPH and FRAP values for macro and nano as 34.34 and 35.01 for DPPH as well as FRAP 16.4 and 17.7 for macro and nano as shown in Table 9.5.

9.3.5 Tribology—Load Capacity by the Compressive Strength Model of the Polymeric Bearings, Software-Based Thermal Ellipsoidal Plot

The diameter of the shaft is 20 mm; length of bearing, 20 mm; E, 1.799 Gpa; dR as radial data, 0.2 mm; wall thickness, 1.5 mm and maxi pressure as 9 MPa for nanoscaling coated data and final yield of load capacity as 6.417 hecta Newtons and stiffness of 85.6 MN/m, and for macro scaled coating data, the same input except the 1.5 mm of wall thickness replaced as 2.0 mm, final yield of load capacity as 7.352 hecta Newtons and stiffness 73.5 MN/m. The mechano tribology parameters of BGLBMH coating shows that nano is preferred for the work than bulk.

Table 9.5 AO of macro, nano BGLBMH crystals.

Samples	% of DPPH for macro scale	% of DPPH for nanoscale
BGLBMH	34.34	35.01
Samples	**% of FRAP for macroscale**	**% of FRAP for nanoscale**
BGLBMH	16.4	17.7

The software program for the thermal ellipsoidal of 50% effectiveness of the sample with promolecular generation with the interactions are specified for curvedness effect represents the atomic close relativeness by software and intended for low or high profile, and as per Figure 9.3, it is a high-profile curved effect by software and Figure 9.4 as shape index profile for the titled material.

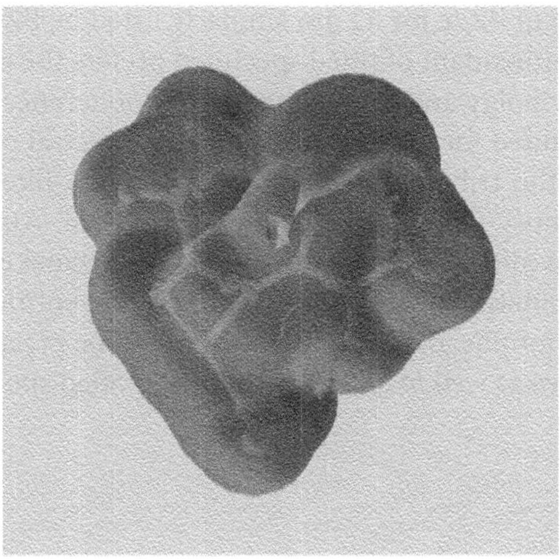

Figure 9.3 Software based thermal ellipsoidal plot-promolecular generation system – curvedness interactions [50–52].

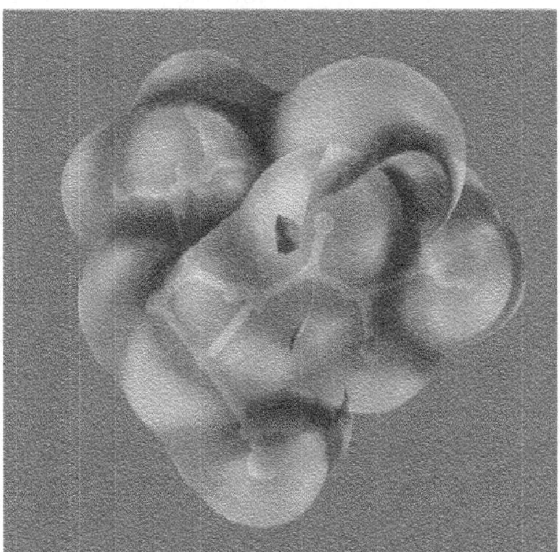

Figure 9.4 Software based thermal ellipsoidal plot-promolecular generation system – shaped index interactions [50–52].

9.4 Conclusion

Crystalline materials impact more intense spectral utility especially of nanoscale than micro or macro ones and the BGLBMH crystals of versatile scaling are mainly placed and used in arrangement by proper stratagem of macro and nanolevel by processing technique of slow leveled evaporation, as well as apposite milling. BGLBMH are of the framework as monoclinic with space group of $P2_1/c$ for 32 nm similarly listed by PXRD and antidiabetic as well as antioxidant of titled specimen prefers the nano than macro and influx and tribolgy and FL data reveal the preference of a nanoscaled one and is well suited for mechano, electronics, spectral physics, and biology to identify the tribological stiffness, electronic filter conglomeratic value, FL to identify flaws, bio as AD and AO data. Also, the software-based curvedness and shape index by means of thermal ellipsoidal plot is mentioned computationally for the structure of the entitled sample and is better candidate for pharma use and in future can be preceded for the harboring and *in-vivo* as well *in-silico* forms for the titled specimen.

References

1. Kalaipoonguzhali, V., SenthilKannan, K., Thirumoorthi, C., Chinnadurai, M., Jayanalina, T., Comparison of adsorption energy, ionization potential and electron affinity of CuS-ACT and CuS-Nit nanostructures monowire for nano device fabrication by computational approach. *Mater. Today: Proc.*, 33, 7, 2759–2760, 2020.
2. Gunasekaran, S. *et al.*, Structural studies on picolinium maleate crystal by density functional methods. *Indian J. Phys.*, 87, 12, 1189–1197, 2013.
3. Senthilkannan, K. *et al.*, Anti diabetic (AD) studies of bis-glycine hydro bromide (45 nm) nano crystals. *Mater. Today: Proc.*, 33, 7, 3201–3202, 2020.
4. Senthilkannan, K. *et al.*, Anti-diabetic activites of ZnO doped with Ce (5 at %) nano particles (NPs). *Mater. Today: Proc.*, 33, 7, 3056–3057, 2020.
5. Senthilkannan, K. *et al.*, Fluorescence, filter,nano tribological studies of 12-(4-Chlorophenyl)-9,9-Dimethyl-9,10-Dihydro-8H-Benzo[A]Xanthen-11(12H)-One-(CPDDHBXH) macro and nano crystals. *Mater. Today: Proc.*, 33, 7, 4163–4166, 2020.
6. Senthilkannan, K., Venkatachalam, K., Jothibas, M., Computational and experimental studies of acetoacetanilide crystals. *AIP Conf Proc.*, 2270, 2270, 1–4, 2020.
7. Senthilkannan ., K., Venkatachalam, K., Rajamani, A., Computational analysis of LPNPTH anisotropies for dementia for Alzheimer's syndrome by DFT and molecular harboring. *AIP Conf Proc*, vol. 2270, pp. 1–5, 2020.

8. Senthilkannan, K., Sivaramakrishnan, V., Kalaipoonguzhali, V., Chinnadurai, M., Kannan, S., Electronic transport, HOMO–LUMO and computational studies of CuS monowire for nano device fabrication by DFT approach. *Mater. Today: Proc.*, 33, 7, 2746–2749, 2020.
9. Senthilkannan, K. and Gunasekaran, S., Spectroscopic studies and other novel studies of 4 bromo 4' chloro benzylidene aniline (BCBA) Crystal- A non linear optical material. *Int. J. Chemtech Res.*, 5, 6, 3051–3058, 2013.
10. Senthilkannan, K., Gayathri Devi, S., Nagarajan, P., Flora, G., Rajakumaravelu, R., Anti diabetic (AD) studies of picolinium maleate nano crystals. *Mater. Today: Proc.*, 33, 3, 3005–3007, 2020.
11. Senthilkannan, K., Ramamurthi., K., Bhakya, K., Velu, S., Kolanjinathan, M., Rajakumaravelu, R., Hardness, Photoconductivity, Anti-diabetic Studies of L-AlaniniumFumarate (LAF) Crystals. *AIP Conf Proc*, vol. 2270:100010, pp. 1–4, 2020.
12. Senthilkanna, K., Baskaran, P., Seenivasan, R., Settu, P., Tribological, Filter, FTIR and fluorescence studies of L-Alaninium tartrate (LAT) Macro and nano crystals. *Mater. Today: Proc.*, 33, 7, 4148–4150, 2020.
13. Senthilkannan, K., Kaleemullah, K., Abdul, J., Vinoth Kumar, P., Natana Murugaraj, G., Effect of anti microbial and fluorescence on L-Alaninium maleate (LAM) macro and nano crystals. *Mater. Today: Proc.*, 33, 7, 2779–2781, 2020.
14. Senthilkannan, K., Ganesh, G., Abdul Jaffer, A.H., Krishnaveni Ramamurthi, R., Khan, K., Anti diabetic (AD) activities of L-valinium picrate (LVP) macro and nano crystals. *Mater. Today: Proc.*, 33, 7, 2738–2740, 2020.
15. Senthilkannan, K., Bhakya, K., Iyanar, M., Growth and Influx, AC and DC Conductivity Studies of L-AlaniniumFumarate (LAF) Crystals. *AIP Conf Proc.*, 2270:100009, 1–4, 2020.
16. Senthilkannan, K., Growth, fluorescence and theoretical studies of B2CPCD crystals – Comparative analysis in macro and nano scaled crystals. *Mater. Today: Proc.*, 33, 7, 4368–4371, 2020.
17. Senthilkannan, K. *et al.*, Anti-diabetic (AD) activities of ZnO doped with Ce (7 at%) nano particles (NP). *Mater. Today: Proc.*, 33, 7, 3053–3055, 2020.
18. Senthilkannan, K. *et al.*, Tribological, filter studies of 3-Bromo-2-Hydroxy benzoic acid (BHBA) macro and nano crystals. *Mater. Today: Proc.*, 33, 7, 4145–4147, 2020.
19. Senthilkannan, K. *et al.*, Electronic transport, Homo-Lumo and computational studies of CuS-ACT monowire for nano device fabrication by software approach. *Mater. Today: Proc.*, 33, 7, 2756–2758, 2020.
20. Senthilkannan, K. *et al.*, Anti microbial and fluorescence activities of L-valinium picrate (LVP) macro and nano crystals. *Mater. Today: Proc.*, 33, 7, 2776–2778, 2020.
21. Senthilkumar, R. *et al.*, Anti-diabetic (AD) and hardness profile of 12-(4-Chlorophenyl)-9,9-Dimethyl-9,10-Dihydro-8H-benzo[a]xanthen-

11(12H)-one –(CPDDHBXH) – Comparative analysis of macro and nano crystals. *Mater. Today: Proc.*, 33, 7, 4167–4170, 2020.
22. Sathishkumar, R. *et al.*, Synthesis, Growth and Characterization of 2,5 – Dimethyl-N-(3-phenylprop-2-en-1-ylidene) Aniline (2,5 DPPA) Single Crystal, in: *A New Second Order Nonlinear Optical Material for Photonic and Optoelectronic Applications*, vol. 226, pp. 1–11, 2020.
23. Patel, R.P. *et al.*, Growth and XRD, Elemental, Mechanical, Dielectric, Optical and Photoconductivity, and Surface Morphological Characterizations of 2-[4-(Trifluoromethyl) phenyl]-1H-benzimidazole (TFMPHB) Crystals for Electronic, Mechanical Applications. *Braz. J. Phys.*, 51, 3, 339–350, 2021.
24. Aarthi, R. *et al.*, Molecular structure- associated pharmacodynamic investigation on benzoyl peroxide using spectroscopic and quantum computational tools. *J. Taibah Univ. Sci.*, 12, 1, 104–122, 2018.
25. Saravanan, P. *et al.*, Biofriendly and competent domestic microwave assisted method for the synthesis of ZnO nanoparticles from the extract of Azadirachta indica leaves. *Mater. Today: Proc.*, 33, 7, 3160–3163, 2020.
26. Saravanan, P. *et al.*, A perspective approach towards appreciable size and cost-effective solar cell fabrication by synthesizing ZnO nanoparticles from Azadirachta indica leaves extract using domestic microwave oven. *J. Mater. Sci.: Mater. Electron*, 31, 5, 4301–4309, 2020.
27. Saravanan, P. *et al.*, Dielectric and magnetic properties of Allium cepa and Raphanus sativus extracts biogenic ZnO nanoparticles. *J. Mater. Sci.: Mater. Electron*, 32, 1, 1–14, 2021.
28. Periyathambi, P. *et al.*, Fluorescence and filter characterizations of NaBr-added L-alanine (LANB) – A comparative analysis in macro and nano scaled crystals. *Mater. Today: Proc.*, 33, 3766–3769, 2020.
29. Baskaran, P. *et al.*, Anti-diabetic activities of ZnO doped with Ce (3 at %) nano particles. *Mater. Today: Proc.*, 33, 7, 3051–3052, 2020.
30. Baskaran, P. *et al.*, Anti-diabetic studies of barium paranitro phenolate macro and nano crystals. *Mater. Today: Proc.*, 33, 7, 3058–3060, 2020.
31. Kolanjinathan, M., Senthilkannan, K., Paramasivam, S., Baskaran, P., Iyanar, M., Anti-diabetic studies of 4-(4-chlorophenyl)-7,7-dimethyl-7,8-dihydro-4H-1-benzopyran-2,5(3H,6H)-dione – (CPDMDHHBPHHD) nano crystals. *Mater. Today: Proc.*, 33, 2750–2752, 7, 2020.
32. Kolanjinathan, M. *et al.*, Dielectric, fluorescence, filter, nano tribological and photoconductivity studies of 4-(4-chlorophenyl)-7,7-dimethyl-7,8-dihydro-4H-1-benzopyran-2,5(3H,6H)-dione(CPDMDHHBPHHD) macro and nano crystals. *J. Mater. Sci.: Mater. Electron.*, 27, 4, 16907–16917, 2020.
33. Kolanjinathan, M., Hariharasuthan, R., Sivaramakrishnan, V. *et al.*, XRD, CHNSO, fluorescence, filter-influx, NLO, photoconductivity, hardness and helical spring-fabricated device stress analysis of 2′-chloro-4-methoxy-3-nitrobenzil (CMNB) crystal of different scalings for opto-electronic filter and band gap engineering utilities. *J. Mater Sci: Mater Electron*, 32, 10049–10057, 2021.

34. Jothibas, M. *et al.*, Structural, optical and photo catatic activity of Ag doped ZnO nano particles obtained by sol-gel method. *AIP Conf Proc*, vol. 2162, pp. 1–7, 2019.
35. Selvaraj, L. *et al.*, AS Anti-diabetic (AD) studies of Bis Glycine Hydro Bromide – BGHB macro crystals milled to nano scale of 219 nm as the preliminary fine particles. *Mater. Today: Proc.*, 33, 7, 3763–3765, 2020.
36. Kishore, N. *et al.*, CO and HCHO adsorption on FeO monowire devices: a DFT study. *Appl. Phys. A*, 123, 11, 1–7, 2017, https://doi.org/10.1007/s00339-017-1330-6.
37. Senthilkannan, K., Gunasekaran, S., Gowtham, J., Wagish, R., UV, SEM, Powder XRD Studies of Acetoacetanilide (AAC) Crystal. *Int. J. Chemtech Res.*, 6, 5, 3187–3190, 2014.
38. Kumar, K. *et al.*, Growth of diethyl 3,3′-[(2,4-dichlorophenyl) methylidene] bis(1H-indole-2-carboxylate)-(D32DMBC) organic NLO single crystal and its optical, thermal, mechanical, dielectric and computational studies. *J. Mater. Sci.: Mater. Electron.*, 31, 23, 1–8, 2020, https://doi.org/10.1007/s10854-020-04594-y.
39. SenthilKannan, K., Venkatachalam, K., Bhakya, K., Sharmidha, B., Kalaivani, M., Gayathri Devi, S., Senthilkannan, K., Growth and Characterization of Picolinium Maleate (PM) Crystals. *AIP Conf Proc.*, 2270:10014, 1–4, 2020, https://doi.org/10.1063/5.0019341.
40. SenthilKannan, K., Thamarikannan, P., Kalaipoonguzhali, V., Venkatachalam, K., Kannan, S., Baskar, A., Fluorescence, computational enactments of dimethyl N,N′-[(ethyne-1, 2-di-yl)Bis-(1,4- phenyl-ene carbon-yl)]bis-(l-alaninate) crystals. *AIP Conf Proc*, vol. 2270:100008, pp. 1–4, 2020, https://doi.org/10.1063/5.0019334.
41. SenthilKannan, K., Thamaraikannan, P., Kalaipoonguzhali, V., Venkatachalam, K., Kannan, S., Ranadevan, R., Senthilkannan, K., Computational IR, Raman studies by DFT program and antidiabetic delineation by harboring of aceto-acetanilide crystals. *AIP Conf Proc*, vol. 2270:10013, pp. 1–4, 2020, https://doi.org/10.1063/5.0019339.
42. Flora, G. *et al.*, Anti-diabetic (AD) and crystal stiffness characterizations of NaBr-added L-alanine (LANB) – A comparative analysis in macro and nano scale crystals. *Mater. Today: Proc.*, 33, 7, 3937–3941, 2020.
43. Flora, G. *et al.*, Anti diabetic (AD), stiffness and hardness studies of 2-[4-(Trifluoromethyl) phenyl]-1H-benzimidazole crystals - (TFMPHB) macro and nano crystal. *Mater. Today: Proc.*, 33, 4233–4236, 2020.
44. Flora, G. *et al.*, Anti-inflammatory (AI) and crystalline hardness characterisations of 4-(4-chlorophenyl)-7,7-dimethyl-7,8-dihydro-4h-1-benzopyran-2,5(3h,6h)-dione-(CPDMDHHBPHHD) – comparative analysis of macro and nano scales crystals. *Mater. Today: Proc.*, 33, 3578–3582, 2020.
45. Ganesan, S., Gurunathan, R., Pasupuleti, R.R. *et al.*, Green synthesis of V_2O_5/ZnO nanocomposite materials for efficient photocatalytic and

anti-bacterial applications. *Appl. Nanosci*, 2021, https://doi.org/10.1007/s13204-021-01923-3.

46. Ganesan, H., SenthilKannan, K., Christy, S. *et al.*, Synthesis, growth, XRD, NLO, CHNSO, computational-structural, dielectric, photoconductivity, hardness and biostudies of diethyl 2-amino-5-{4-[bis (4-methyl phenyl) amino] benzamido} thiophene-3,4-dicarboxylate (DABMPABTD) macro-, nano crystals for device fabrication, pharma, electronic uses. *J. Mater Sci: Mater Electron*, 32, 15498–15508, 2021.
47. Maalmarugan, J., Yokeswaran, V., Divya, R. *et al.*, Synthesis, growth, XRD, NLO, CHNSO, structure by theoretical approach, dielectric, absorbance, photoconductivity and bio studies of 4-(4-Acetyl-5-Methyl-1H-1, 2, 3-Triazol-1-yl) Benzonitrile crystals for optical, opto-electronic, and photonics utilities. *J. Mater Sci: Mater Electron*, 32, 13850–13858, 2021, https://doi.org/10.1007/s10854-021-05960-0.
48. Rajkumar, M., Maalmarugan, J., Flora, G. *et al.*, Growth, characterizations, and the structural elucidation of diethyl-2-(3-oxoiso-1,3-dihydrobenzofuran-1-ylidene)malonate crystalline specimen for dielectric and electronic filters, thermal, optical, mechanical, and biomedical applications using conventional experimental and theoretical practices. *J. Mater Sci: Mater Electron*, 32, 22822–22839, 2021, https://doi.org/10.1007/s10854-021-06761-1.
49. SenthilKannan, K., Flora, G., Gunasekaran, S., Ali, H.A.J., Vimalan, M., Balasubramanian, S., Extraction of Silver Nanoparticles (Ag-NPs) by Green Synthesis from Aqueous Extract of Seaweeds and Their Consequences on HeLa Cell Line and Their Utility on Soil by Spectroscopic Tools, in: *Nanotechnology for Advances in Medical Microbiology. Environmental and Microbial Biotechnology*, Springer, Singapore, 2021, https://doi.org/10.1007/978-981-15-9916-3_5.
50. Momma, K. and Izumi, F., VESTA 3 for three-dimensional visualization of crystal, volumetric and morphology data. *J. Appl. Crystallogr.*, 44, 1272–1276, 2011.
51. Spackman, P.R., Turner, M.J., McKinnon, J.J., Wolff, S.K., Grimwood, D.J., Jayatilaka, D., Spackman, M.A., Crystal Explorer: a program for Hirshfeld surface analysis, visualization and quantitative analysis of molecular crystals, *J. Appl. Cryst.*, 54, 3, 20212021, https://doi.org/10.1107/S1600576721002910.
52. Pek, A.J.S., Single – crystal structure validation with the program PLATON. *J. Appl. Cryst.*, 36, 7–11, 2003.

10

Device Utility, Energy, and Bioutility of N2MNM4MBH Macro, Nano Models

Pauline Jenifer S.[1], Flora G.[1], Zozimus Divya Lobo C.[2], Charles A.[3], Senthil Kannan K.[4]*, Anbuvel D.[5], Prajith V.[6] and Jemma Hermelin Jesy Diaz[7]

[1]*Department of Botany, St. Mary's College (Autonomous), Thoothukudi, TN, India*
[2]*Department of Chemistry, St. Mary's College (Autonomous), Thoothukudi, Tamil Nadu, India*
[3]*Department of Chemistry, Thirumali Engineering College, Kilambi, Kanchipuram, TN, India*
[4]*Department of R&D/Physics, Edayathangudy G.S Pillay Arts and Science College (Autonomous – Affiliated to Bharathidasan University – Tiruchirappalli), Nagapattinam, Tamil Nadu, India*
[5]*Department of Chemistry, Vivekananda College, Kanyakumari, TN, India*
[6]*Sri Ramakrishna Institute of Paramedical Sciences, Coimbatore TN, India*
[7]*Department of Zoology, St.Mary's College (Autonomous), Thoothukudi, TN, India*

Abstract

The organic crystalline N¢-[(2-Methoxynaphthalen-1-yl) methyl-idene]-4-methyl-benzo hydrazide (N2MNM4MBH) materials are enhanced for better applications in mechanofield, electronic zones, and bio uses mainly here mentioned for diabetic and COX legendary data. N2MNM4MBH are of orthorhombic in nature; with space group of $Pna2_1$. The COX construction is better scrutinized for harboring data; the unit cell by ORTEP, as well as 4 × 4 × 4 super lattice and 16-nm nanodevices fabricated tool by computational way; energized tool bar and energy interactions by Hirshfeld are well portrayed. The antidiabetic calculation, as well as efficacy of the entitled crystalline specimen of macroleveled and nanoleveled data for alpha amylase and alpha glucosidase, is well exposed as the best tool by nano over the macro. The bio use is by naphthalene for cleaned effect and by benzo hydrazide for the enhanced and enabled use in diabetic, microbial, cancer, and so on. Thus, the entitled crystal is focused for XRD, COX, diabetic, device invention, super lattice structure, and so on.

**Corresponding author*: mscgoldmedalist@yahoo.in

Kaushik Pal (ed.) Nanovaccinology as Targeted Therapeutics, (169–182) © 2022 Scrivener Publishing LLC

Keywords: COX, diabetic, lattice, nanotubular, interactions

10.1 Introduction

Organic materials are the predominant ones for the applications in all fields than their counterparts. Cyclooxygenase (COX), better branded as prostaglandin-endoperoxide-synthase (PTGS), is an enzyme with the purpose of being accountable and meant for the construction of prostanoids [1–3]. The harboring is effectively [4–7] studied, and the device utility [8–11] is also promptly enabled [13–16] and the diabetic enhancement [17–21] is also well reported for macroline, as well as nanoline [22–28]. The benzohydrazide is the typical organic type of material having discerning proficient pharmaceutical exercises [23–27]. The organic crystals are having well-exposed uses in electro-mechano-bio and in techno, here, the N2MNM4MBH are branded to progress for the nanotube assembly, ellipsoidal design, acidic sketches of complex, peptide contribution of N2MNM4MBH, optimized force field—usefulness, VanderWaal's propel of the crystal, antidiabetic, antifungal, and anti-inflammatory characterizations is reported [28–33]. Molecular crystals put frontward an affluent level of corporeal incident conspicuously assorted commencement the optoelectronic and obligatory way demonstrated by conventional obdurate, such as covalent/ionic nature of crystals [34–37]. This happened moderately since the usually feeble intermolecular ways, and fairly since the fragile interface that valor transpires among molecular degree of sovereignty [38–42]. In contemporary occasions, molecular crystals have revolved elsewhere to be the matter of authoritative imaginary and trial survey. To a large amount, this has interior roughly increasing a caring of the schemes to fasten it up for practical rationales, such as the emblematic crate of molecular electronics, in addition to this conclusion, at dispense recitation attempts are undertaken to figure out the surroundings of implicate mover in these configurations [43–45]. An enabled field of section of unvaryingly controlling association is that of supramolecular chemistry. This engrossing zone is based further on the consumption of being the molecules in a position to standardize the attempt to recommend persistent molecular crystals that may be exercised for a range of procedural intentions. The input in at the nurture this position is that the crystal configuration and stuffing summarized by an understanding of the molecules is well set up to an immense extent by the intermolecular boundaries, such as weak bond deals [46–52].

10.2 Synthesis and XRD

To the proper methanol chemical solution, the solution of 5-bromosalicylaldehyde and 4-nitrobenzohydrazide with drops of acetic acid was slowly and perfectly added. The assortment was refluxed for about an hour and then evaporated to room temperature. The white crystalline solid was accumulated by filtration. The XRD data portray that the system is orthorhombic, space group is $Pna2_1$, a = 26.739Å, b = 4.894Å, c = 12.733Å, V = 1666.25Å^3, Mo Kα radiation with $\lambda = 0.71073$ Å.

10.3 Influx

The nano influx as well as the thin film influx is 4.7997 and 4.0304 microns, respectively, for the optoelectronic filter utility of the N2MNM4MBH crystal for the betterment and predominancy lead to NLO studies to predict the photonic, as well as optoelectronic applications. Nano is preferred than the thin film influx for the usage.

10.4 Computational

Figures 10.1 to 10.8 specify the unit-cell by ORTEP; 4 × 4 × 4 super lattice; 16 nm tubular device data; energy interactions from Figure 10.4 and Table 10.1; ribbon structure, COX ribbon structure; COX bonded title crystal and the ball structure of harboring process tells the interactions and Table 10.1 tells the colored effect of specimen based on versatile energies.

10.4.1 Antidiabetic Study

The antidiabetic effect of both scalings for AA and AG are portrayed, and nano is preferred than macro. For AA, it is 52.14 and 50.16, and for AG, it is 56.12 and 53.13 for macro and nano, and AA is well preferred than AG, as shown in Table 10.2 and Figure 10.9 and is due to the existence of benzo hydrazide in the entitled crystal.

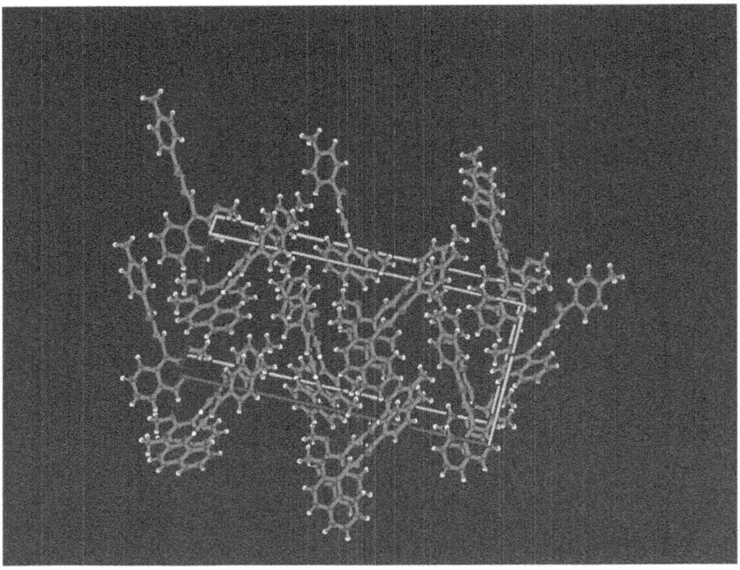

Figure 10.1 Unit cell by ORTEP [50–52].

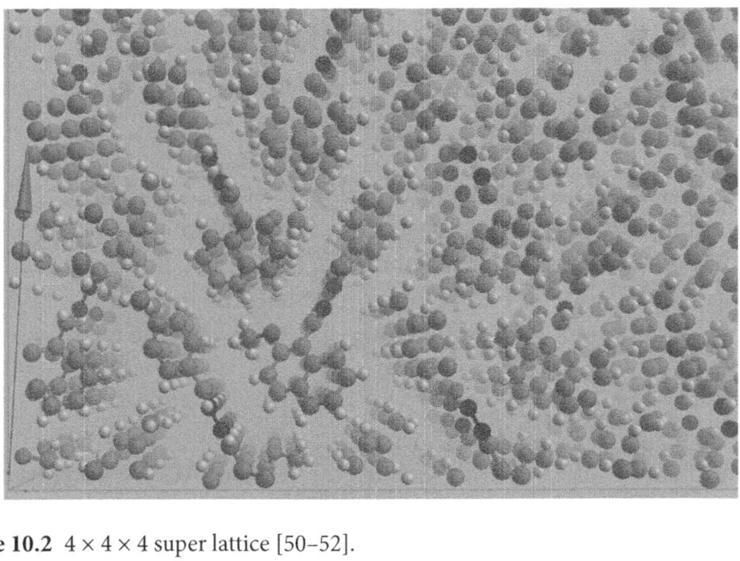

Figure 10.2 4 × 4 × 4 super lattice [50–52].

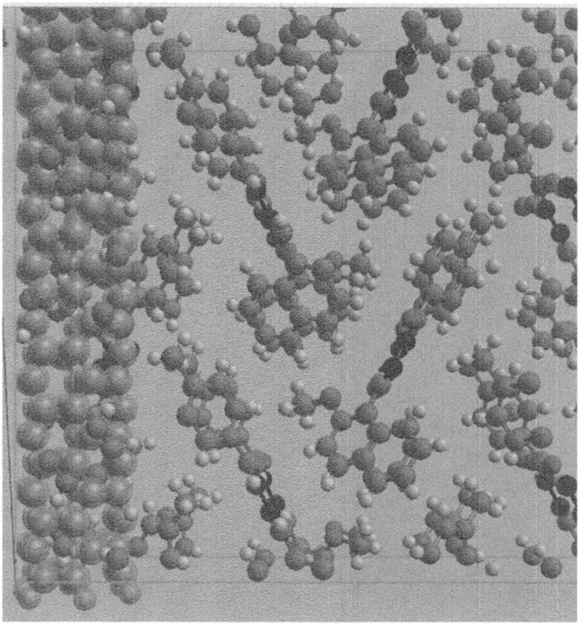

Figure 10.3 16 nm nano tubular effect on N2MNM4MBH [50–52].

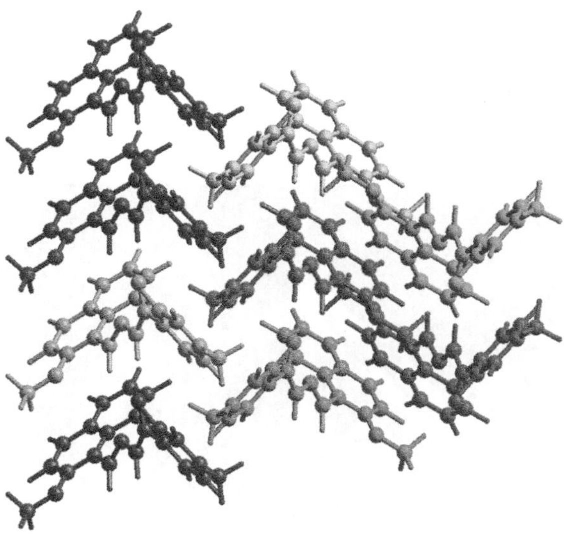

Figure 10.4 Energized titled crystal with colored effect by software [50–52].

Table 10.1 Energy densities of crystals of N2MNM4MBH.

Crystal Atoms Surface Energies

four energy components, scaled appropriately (see the scale factor table below)

	N	Symop	R	Electron Density	E_ele	E_pol	E_dis	E_rep	E_tot
	2	-x, -y, z+1/2	9.32	HF/3-21G	-3.6	-2.5	-25.5	8.4	-21.5
	2	x, y, z	4.89	HF/3-21G	-45.5	-23.1	-74.4	59.0	-80.6
	2	-x+1/2, y+1/2, z +1/2	10.21	HF/3-21G	-5.1	-1.9	-23.3	9.4	-19.9
	2	x, y, z	13.64	HF/3-21G	-1.0	-0.3	-8.6	2.5	-6.9
	2	-x, -y, z+1/2	8.69	HF/3-21G	-19.5	-7.5	-29.1	13.6	-39.9
	2	-x+1/2, y+1/2, z +1/2	12.34	HF/3-21G	-1.5	-0.5	-2.0	0.0	-3.6
	2	-x+1/2, y+1/2, z +1/2	10.21	HF/3-21G	4.2	-0.9	-8.3	1.4	-2.6
	2	x, y, z	12.74	HF/3-21G	-3.6	-1.0	-11.0	4.4	-10.6

Scale factors for benchmarked energy models
See Mackenzie et al. IUCrJ (2017)

Energy Model	k_ele	k_pol	k_disp	k_rep
CE-HF ... HF/3-21G electron densities	1.019	0.651	0.901	0.811
CE-B3LYP ... B3LYP/6-31G(d,p) electron densities	1.057	0.740	0.871	0.618

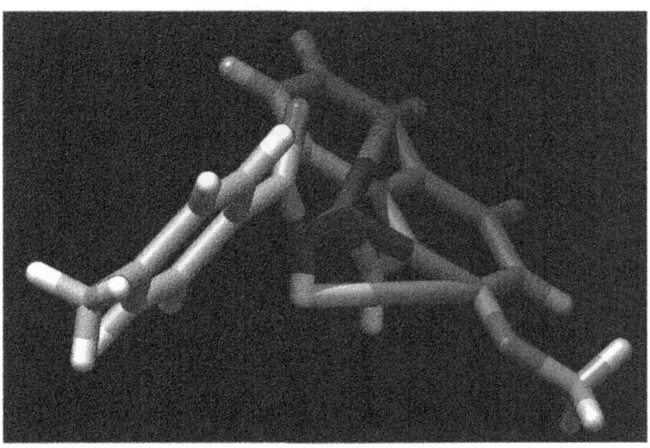

Figure 10.5 Ribbon structure of N2MNM4MBH crystals [50–52].

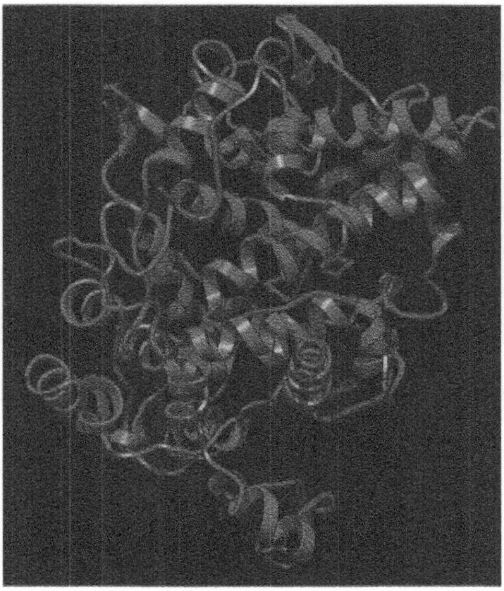

Figure 10.6 COX structure [50–52].

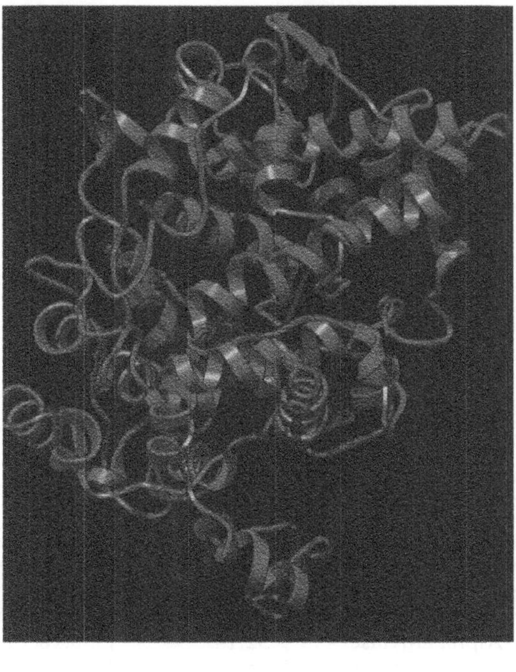

Figure 10.7 COX ribbon structure bonded with molecule of N2MNM4MBH crystals [50–52].

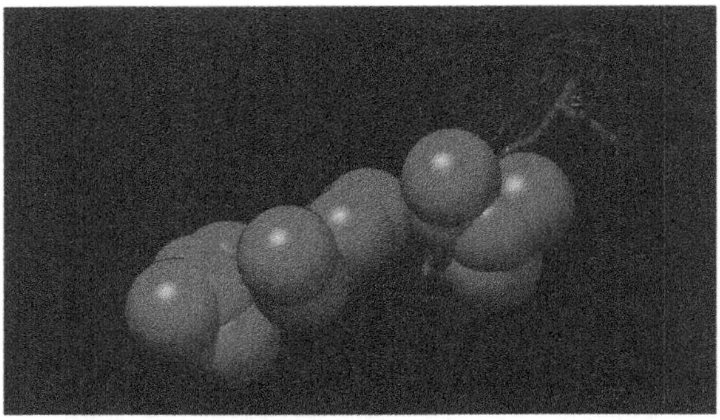

Figure 10.8 Cyclooxygenase with ball orientation with crystal [50–52].

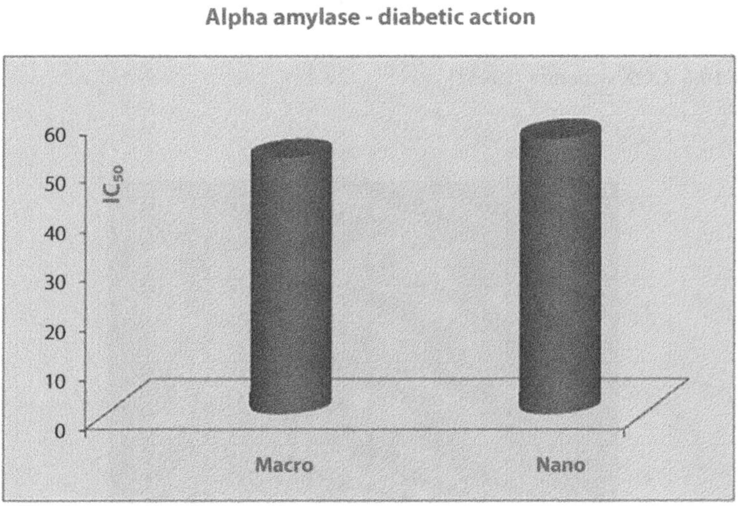

Figure 10.9 AA of diabetic representation of titled crystal of both scalings.

Table 10.2 Antidiabetic effects of both scales.

S. no.	Macro	Nano
AA-Alpha amylase	52.14	50.16
AG-Alpha glucosidase	56.12	53.13

10.5 Conclusion

The organic crystalline N′-[(2-Methoxynaphthalen-1-yl) methyl-idene]-4-methyl-benzo hydrazide (N2MNM4MBH) materials are well grown and are of orthorhombic in nature, with a space group of $Pna2_1$. The COX construction is better scrutinized for harboring data; the unit cell by ORTEP as well as 4 × 4 × 4 super lattice and 16-nm nanodevices fabricated tool by computational way; energized tool bar and energy interactions by Hirshfeld are well portrayed; The antidiabetic calculation, as well as efficacy of the entitled crystalline specimen of macro and nano leveled data for alpha amylase and alpha glucosidase, is well exposed as the best tool by nano over the macro. The bio use is by benzo hydrazide for the enhanced and enabled use in diabetic. The bio use by naphthalene for cleaned effect and by benzo hydrazide for the enhanced and enabled use in diabetic, microbial, cancer, and so on. Thus, the entitled crystal focused on XRD, COX, diabetic, device invention super lattice structure, and so on.

References

1. Kalaipoonguzhali, V., SenthilKannan, K., Thirumoorthi, C., Chinnadurai, M., Jayanalina, T., Comparison of adsorption energy, ionization potential and electron affinity of CuS-ACT and CuS-Nit nanostructures monowire for nano device fabrication by computational approach. *Mater. Today: Proc.*, 33, 7, 2759–2760, 2020.
2. Gunasekaran, S. *et al.*, Structural studies on picolinium maleate crystal by density functional methods. *Indian J. Phys.*, 87, 12, 1189–1197, 2013.
3. Senthilkannan, K. *et al.*, Anti diabetic (AD) studies of bis-glycine hydro bromide (45 nm) nano crystals. *Mater. Today: Proc.*, 33, 7, 3201–3202, 2020.
4. Senthilkannan, K. *et al.*, Anti-diabetic activites of ZnO doped with Ce (5 at %) nano particles (NPs). *Mater. Today: Proc*, vol. 33, pp. 3056–3057, 2020.
5. Senthilkannan, K. *et al.*, Fluorescence, filter,nano tribological studies of 12-(4-Chlorophenyl)-9,9-Dimethyl-9,10-Dihydro-8H-Benzo[A]Xanthen-11(12H)-One-(CPDDHBXH) macro and nano crystals. *Mater. Today: Proc.*, 33, 7, 4163–4166, 2020.
6. Senthilkannan, K., Venkatachalam, K., and Jothibas, M., Computational and experimental studies of acetoacetanilide crystals. *AIP Conf Proc*, vol. 2270, pp. 1–4, 2020.
7. Senthilkannan., K., Venkatachalam, K., Rajamani, A., Computational analysis of LPNPTH anisotropies for dementia for Alzheimer's syndrome by DFT and molecular harboring. *AIP Conf Proc*, vol. 2270, pp. 1–5, 2020.

8. Senthilkannan, K., Sivaramakrishnan, V., Kalaipoonguzhali, V., Chinnadurai, M., Kannan, S., Electronic transport, HOMO–LUMO and computational studies of CuS monowire for nano device fabrication by DFT approach. *Mater. Today: Proc.*, 33, 7, 2746–2749, 2020.
9. Senthilkannan, K. and Gunasekaran, S., Spectroscopic studies and other novel studies of 4 bromo 4' chloro benzylidene aniline (BCBA) Crystal- A non linear optical material. *Int. J. Chemtech Res.*, 5, 6, 3051–3058, 2013.
10. Senthilkannan, K., Gayathri, D.S., Nagarajan, P., Flora, G., Rajakumaravelu, R., Anti diabetic (AD) studies of picolinium maleate nano crystals. *Mater. Today: Proc.*, 33, 3, 3005–3007, 2020.
11. Senthilkannan, K., Ramamurthi., K., Bhakya, K., Velu, S., Kolanjinathan, M., Rajakumaravelu, R., Hardness, Photoconductivity, Anti-diabetic Studies of L-AlaniniumFumarate (LAF) Crystals. *AIP Conf. Proc.*, 2270:100010, 1–4, 2020.
12. Senthilkannan, K., Baskaran, P., Seenivasan, R., Settu, P., Tribological, Filter, FTIR and fluorescence studies of L-Alaninium tartrate (LAT) Macro and nano crystals. *Mater. Today: Proc.*, 33, 7, 4148–4150, 2020.
13. Senthilkannan, K., Khan, K., Jaffar, A., Ponnusamy, V.K., Govindan, N.M., Effect of anti microbial and fluorescence on L-Alaninium maleate (LAM) macro and nano crystals. *Mater. Today: Proc.*, 33, 7, 2779–2781, 2020.
14. Senthilkannan., K., Ganesh, G., Abdul Jaffer Ali, H., Krishnaveni Ramamurthi, R., Khan, K., Anti diabetic (AD) activities of L-valinium picrate (LVP) macro and nano crystals. *Mater. Today: Proc.*, 33, 7, 2738–2740, 2020.
15. Senthilkannan., K., Bhakya, K., Iyanar, M., Growth and Influx, AC and DC Conductivity Studies of L-AlaniniumFumarate (LAF) Crystals. *AIP Conf Proc.*, 2270:100009, 1–4, 2020.
16. Senthilkannan, K., Growth, fluorescence and theoretical studies of B2CPCD crystals – Comparative analysis in macro and nano scaled crystals. *Mater. Today: Proc.*, 33, 7, 4368–4371, 2020.
17. Senthilkannan, K. *et al.*, Anti-diabetic (AD) activities of ZnO doped with Ce (7 at%) nano particles (NP). *Mater. Today: Proc.*, 33, 7, 3053–3055, 2020.
18. Senthilkannan., K. *et al.*, Tribological, filter studies of 3-Bromo-2-Hydroxy benzoic acid (BHBA) macro and nano crystals. *Mater. Today: Proc.*, 33, 7, 4145–4147, 2020.
19. Senthilkannan, K. *et al.*, Electronic transport, Homo-Lumo and computational studies of CuS-ACT monowire for nano device fabrication by software approach. *Mater. Today: Proc.*, 33, 7, 2756–2758, 2020.
20. Senthilkannan, K. *et al.*, Anti microbial and fluorescence activities of L-valinium picrate (LVP) macro and nano crystals. *Mater. Today: Proc.*, 33, 7, 2776–2778, 2020.
21. Senthilkumar, R. *et al.*, Anti-diabetic (AD) and hardness profile of 12-(4-Chlorophenyl)-9,9-Dimethyl-9,10-Dihydro-8H-benzo[a]xanthen-11(12H)-one –(CPDDHBXH) – Comparative analysis of macro and nano crystals. *Mater. Today: Proc.*, 33, 7, 4167–4170, 2020.

22. Sathishkumar, R. *et al.*, Synthesis, Growth and Characterization of 2,5 – Dimethyl-N-(3-phenylprop-2-en-1-ylidene) Aniline (2,5 DPPA) Single Crystal. *A New Second Order Nonlinear Optical Mater. Photonic Optoelectronic Appl.*, 226, 2, 1–11, 2020.
23. Patel, R.P. *et al.*, Growth and XRD, Elemental, Mechanical, Dielectric, Optical and Photoconductivity, and Surface Morphological Characterizations of 2-[4-(Trifluoromethyl) phenyl]-1H-benzimidazole (TFMPHB) Crystals for Electronic, Mechanical Applications. *Braz. J. Phys.*, 51, 3, 339–350, 2021.
24. Aarthi, R. *et al.*, Molecular structure- associated pharmacodynamic investigation on benzoyl peroxide using spectroscopic and quantum computational tools. *J. Taibah Univ. Sci.*, 12, 1, 104–122, 2018.
25. Saravanan, P. *et al.*, Biofriendly and competent domestic microwave assisted method for the synthesis of ZnO nanoparticles from the extract of Azadirachta indica leaves. *Mater. Today: Proc.*, 33, 7, 3160–3163, 2020.
26. Saravanan, P. *et al.*, A perspective approach towards appreciable size and cost-effective solar cell fabrication by synthesizing ZnO nanoparticles from Azadirachta indica leaves extract using domestic microwave oven. *J. Mater. Sci.: Mater. Electron.*, 31, 5, 4301–4309, 2020.
27. Saravanan, P. *et al.*, Dielectric and magnetic properties of Allium cepa and Raphanus sativus extracts biogenic ZnO nanoparticles. *J. Mater. Sci.: Mater. Electron.*, 32, 1, 1–14, 2021.
28. Periyathambi, P. *et al.*, Fluorescence and filter characterizations of NaBr-added L-alanine (LANB) – A comparative analysis in macro and nano scaled crystals. *Mater. Today: Proc.*, 33, 3766–3769, 2020.
29. Baskaran, P. *et al.*, Anti-diabetic activities of ZnO doped with Ce (3 at %) nano particles. *Mater. Today: Proc.*, 33, 7, 3051–3052, 2020.
30. Baskaran, P. *et al.*, Anti-diabetic studies of barium paranitro phenolate macro and nano crystals. *Mater. Today: Proc.*, 33, 7, 3058–3060, 2020.
31. Kolanjinathan, M., Senthilkannan, K., Paramasivam, S., Baskaran, P., Iyanar, M., Anti-diabetic studies of 4-(4-chlorophenyl)-7,7-dimethyl-7,8-dihydro-4H-1-benzopyran-2,5(3H,6H)-dione – (CPDMDHHBPHHD) nano crystals. *Mater. Today: Proc.*, 33, 7, 2750–2752, 2020.
32. Kolanjinathan, M. *et al.*, Dielectric, fluorescence, filter, nano tribological and photoconductivity studies of 4-(4-chlorophenyl)-7,7-dimethyl-7,8-dihydro-4H-1-benzopyran-2,5(3H,6H)-dione (CPDMDHHBPHHD) macro and nano crystals. *J. Mater. Sci.: Mater. Electron.*, 27, 4, 16907–16917, 2020.
33. Kolanjinathan, M., Hariharasuthan, R., Sivaramakrishnan, V. *et al.*, XRD, CHNSO, fluorescence, filter-influx, NLO, photoconductivity, hardness and helical spring-fabricated device stress analysis of 2′-chloro-4-methoxy-3-nitrobenzil (CMNB) crystal of different scalings for opto-electronic filter and band gap engineering utilities. *J. Mater Sci: Mater Electron*, 32, 10049–10057, 2021.

34. Jothibas, M. *et al.*, Structural, optical and photo catatic activity of Ag doped ZnO nano particles obtained by sol-gel method. *AIP Conf Proc*, vol. 2162, pp. 1–7, 2019.
35. Selvaraj, L. *et al.*, AS Anti-diabetic (AD) studies of Bis Glycine Hydro Bromide – BGHB macro crystals milled to nano scale of 219 nm as the preliminary fine particles. *Mater. Today: Proc.*, 33, 7, 3763–3765, 2020.
36. Kishore, N. *et al.*, CO and HCHO adsorption on FeO monowire devices: a DFT study. *Appl. Phys. A*, 123, 11, 1–7, 2017, https://doi.org/10.1007/s00339-017-1330-6.
37. Senthilkannan, K., Gunasekaran, S., Gowtham, J., Wagish, R., UV, SEM, Powder XRD Studies of Acetoacetanilide (AAC) Crystal. *Int. J. Chemtech Res.*, 6, 5, 3187–3190, 2014.
38. Kumar, K. *et al.*, Growth of diethyl 3,3′-[(2,4-dichlorophenyl) methylidene] bis(1H-indole-2-carboxylate)-(D32DMBC) organic NLO single crystal and its optical, thermal, mechanical, dielectric and computational studies. *J. Mater. Sci.: Mater. Electron.*, 31, 23, 1–8, 2020, https://doi.org/10.1007/s10854-020-04594-y.
39. SenthilKannan, K., Venkatachalam, K., Bhakya, K., Sharmidha, B., Kalaivani, M., Gayathri Devi, S., Senthilkannan, K., Growth and Characterization of Picolinium Maleate (PM) Crystals. *AIP Conf Proc*, vol. 2270:10014, pp. 1–4, 2020, https://doi.org/10.1063/5.0019341.
40. SenthilKannan, K., Thamarikannan, P., Kalaipoonguzhali, V., Venkatachalam, K., Kannan, S., Baskar, A., Fluorescence, computational enactments of dimethyl N,N′-[(ethyne-1, 2-di-yl)Bis-(1,4- phenyl-ene carbon-yl)]bis-(l-alaninate) crystals. *AIP Conf Proc*, vol. 2270:100008, pp. 1–4, 2020, https://doi.org/10.1063/5.0019334.
41. SenthilKannan, K., Thamaraikannan, P., Kalaipoonguzhali, V., Venkatachalam, K., Kannan, S., Ranadevan, R., Senthilkannan, K., Computational IR, Raman studies by DFT program and antidiabetic delineation by harboring of aceto-acetanilide crystals. *AIP Conf Proc*, vol. 2270:10013, pp. 1–4, 2020, https://doi.org/10.1063/5.0019339.
42. Flora, G. *et al.*, Anti-diabetic (AD) and crystal stiffness characterizations of NaBr-added L-alanine (LANB) – A comparative analysis in macro and nano scale crystals. *Mater. Today: Proc.*, 33, 7, 3937–3941, 2020.
43. Flora, G. *et al.*, Anti diabetic (AD), stiffness and hardness studies of 2-[4-(Trifluoromethyl) phenyl]-1H-benzimidazole crystals - (TFMPHB) macro and nano crystal. *Mater. Today: Proc.*, 33, 4233–4236, 2020.
44. Flora, G. *et al.*, Anti-inflammatory (AI) and crystalline hardness characterisations of 4-(4-chlorophenyl)-7,7-dimethyl-7,8-dihydro-4h-1-benzopyran-2,5(3h,6h)-dione-(CPDMDHHBPHHD) – comparative analysis of macro and nano scales crystals. *Mater. Today: Proc.*, 33, 3578–3582, 2020.
45. Ganesan, S., Gurunathan, R., Pasupuleti, R.R. *et al.*, Green synthesis of V_2O_5/ZnO nanocomposite materials for efficient photocatalytic and

anti-bacterial applications. *Appl. Nanosci.*, 2021, https://doi.org/10.1007/s13204-021-01923-3.

46. Ganesan, H., SenthilKannan, K., Christy, S. *et al.*, Synthesis, growth, XRD, NLO, CHNSO, computational-structural, dielectric, photoconductivity, hardness and biostudies of diethyl 2-amino-5-{4-[bis (4-methyl phenyl) amino] benzamido} thiophene-3,4-dicarboxylate (DABMPABTD) macro-, nano crystals for device fabrication, pharma, electronic uses. *J. Mater. Sci.: Mater. Electron.*, 32, 15498–15508, 2021.
47. Maalmarugan, J., Yokeswaran, V., Divya, R. *et al.*, Synthesis, growth, XRD, NLO, CHNSO, structure by theoretical approach, dielectric, absorbance, photoconductivity and bio studies of 4-(4-Acetyl-5-Methyl-1H-1, 2, 3-Triazol-1-yl) Benzonitrile crystals for optical, opto-electronic, and photonics utilities. *J. Mater Sci: Mater Electron*, 32, 13850–13858, 2021, https://doi.org/10.1007/s10854-021-05960-0.
48. Rajkumar, M., Maalmarugan, J., Flora, G. *et al.*, Growth, characterizations, and the structural elucidation of diethyl-2-(3-oxoiso-1,3-dihydrobenzofuran-1-ylidene)malonate crystalline specimen for dielectric and electronic filters, thermal, optical, mechanical, and biomedical applications using conventional experimental and theoretical practices. *J. Mater Sci: Mater Electron*, 32, 22822–22839, 2021, https://doi.org/10.1007/s10854-021-06761-1.
49. SenthilKannan, K., Flora, G., Gunasekaran, S., Ali, H.A.J., Vimalan, M., Balasubramanian, S., Extraction of Silver Nanoparticles (Ag-NPs) by Green Synthesis from Aqueous Extract of Seaweeds and Their Consequences on HeLa Cell Line and Their Utility on Soil by Spectroscopic Tools, in: *Nanotechnology for Advances in Medical Microbiology. Environmental and Microbial Biotechnology*, Springer, Singapore, 2021, https://doi.org/10.1007/978-981-15-9916-3_5.
50. Momma, K. and Izumi, F., VESTA 3 for three-dimensional visualization of crystal, volumetric and morphology data. *J. Appl. Crystallogr.*, 44, 1272–1276, 2011.
51. Spackman, P.R., Turner, M.J., McKinnon, J.J., Wolff, S.K., Grimwood, D.J., Jayatilaka, D., Spackman, M.A., Crystal Explorer: a program for Hirshfeld surface analysis, visualization and quantitative analysis of molecular crystals, *J. Appl. Cryst.*, 54, 3, 2021, https://doi.org/10.1107/S1600576721002910.
52. Pek, A.J.S., Single – crystal structure validation with the program PLATON. *J. Appl. Cryst.*, 36, 7–11, 2003.

11

Biocurative, Tribological, Electro-Functionalities of ZnO-MIZN Nanoparticles

Senthil Kannan K.[1*], Prabhjeet Kaur Dhillon[2], Jemma Hermelin Jesy Diaz[3], Padmavathi P.[4], Flora G.[5], Irudhya Sahaya Lancy S.[6], Jeeva Rani Thangam G.[7] and Sheeba M.[8]

[1]*Department of R&D/Physics, Edayathangudy G.S. Pillay Arts and Science College (Autonomous – Affiliated to Bharathidasan University – Tiruchirappalli), Nagapattinam, Tamil Nadu, India*
[2]*Department of Basic Sciences, Guru Nanak College, Sri Muktsar Sahib, Punjab, India*
[3]*Department of Zoology, St. Mary's College (Autonomous), Thoothukudi TN, India*
[4]*Department of Physics, St. Mary's College (Autonomous), Thoothukudi, TN, India*
[5]*Department of Botany, St. Mary's College (Autonomous), Thoothukudi, TN, India*
[6]*Department of Physics, Kamaraj College (Autonomous), Thoothukudi, TN, India*
[7]*Department of Physics, Pope's College (Autonomous), Thoothukudi, TN, India*
[8]*Department of Zoology, PSGR Krishnammal College for Women, Coimbatore, TN, India*

Abstract
Nano, as well as the functional materials, covers up the advancement and the swot up of new nano-materials and their congregation into multi-functional elucidation and enhanced structures, fabricating the novel devices for applications in the core techno-areas. ZnO nano particles (ZnO-NPs) are successfully grown as the product of green synthesis methodological from mango leaves (*Mangifera indica* as ZnO-MIZN) and verified the formation by powder XRD as the nano scaling with wurtzite-category structure, the crystallite size is nearly 18 nm and is a weak ferromagnetic modules which have oxygen vacancy sites, diamagnetic into paramagnetic transition is possible for the ZnO NPs and circular-helical, torque-tightened preloading tribological parameters were performed for mango-extorted ZnO NPs,

**Corresponding author*: mscgoldmedalist@yahoo.in

Kaushik Pal (ed.) Nanovaccinology as Targeted Therapeutics, (183–194) © 2022 Scrivener Publishing LLC

4.5796 microns for nano influx of titled NPs. With the well-diffusion technology, the bacterial cultures at 4°C represent the *Escherichia coli, Staphylococcus aureus*, and *Staphylococcus typhi* for 10, 20, and 30 microliters with the inhibitions zones in mm, respectively, for the organisms as 4,7 and 12; 12, 13 and 5; 0, 2, and 0. For the DMSO, nil data are obtained for all organisms and DISC with Cefazolin (CE) (0.030 mg) antibiotic disc was properly and perfect manner used as an element for positive control for nearly 1 day with 37°C with 6, 3, and 0 for corresponding organism, such as *E. coli, S. aureus*, and *S. typhi* and ZnO NPs are good scope and better tool for antidiabetics too.

Keywords: Influx, tribology, magnetic, antibacterial, antidiabetic

11.1 Introduction

Nanoparticles are in nm in diameter [1–6]. The properties of nanoparticles regularly vary particularly from those of greater particles of a similar substance [7–12]. Subsequently, the properties of that surface layer might overwhelm over those of the mass material.

Nanoparticles happen broadly in nature and are objects of study in numerous sciences, like science, physical science, geography, and science [13–17].

Being at the progress between mass materials and nuclear or atomic designs, they frequently display marvels that are not seen at one or the other scale. They are a significant part of environmental blemish, and key fixings in many industrialized items, like paints, plastics, metals, pottery, and attractive items [18–23].

However, nanoparticles demonstrate various disentanglement mechanics, which, along with their one of kind surface constructions, brings about mechanical properties that are not the same as the mass material [24–27].

Noncircular calculations of nano prisms lead to high successful cross-areas and more profound shades of the colloidal solutions [28–33].

Anisotropic nanoparticles show a particular retention conduct and stochastic molecule direction under unpolarized light, showing an unmistakable reverberation mode for each sensitive hub [34–40].

Nano materials are focused for multifunctional, multilevel uses than bulk by means of their size, shape, and behavior [41–49].

Here, ZnO NPs are portrayed which are having excellent influx, tribo-mechano, PXRD, magnetic as well as antibacterial utility and is the extorted one from mango leaves. Macro and nano materials are differed due to the characters [49].

11.2 Antibacterial Activity

The antibacterial action was properly and effectively performed with the well-diffusion methodology, and the bacterial cultures were reserved at 4°C after effective subcultured incubation of 1 day at 37°C in the ambience of the incubator. Mueller Hinton Agar (39 g/1000 ml, Himedia-Mumbai) was efficiently prepared and proper manner sterilized at the range of 121°C for 900 s.

Mueller Hinton agar plate were properly and perfectly preceded and prepared and after solidification 60 µl of *Staphylococcus aureus, Escherichia coli*, and *Staphylococcus typhi* were properly transferred and widened with sterilized cotton wad and dried for 120 to 180 s.

Cefazolin (CE, 0.030 mg) antibiotic disc was properly and perfect manner used as an element for positive control and all the plates were proper manner and finely incubated at 37°C for 1 day. The inhibition zones generated by the ZnO nanoparticles were finely and proper manner measured in mm following the period of incubation as in Figures 11.1 and 11.2 and in Table 11.1.

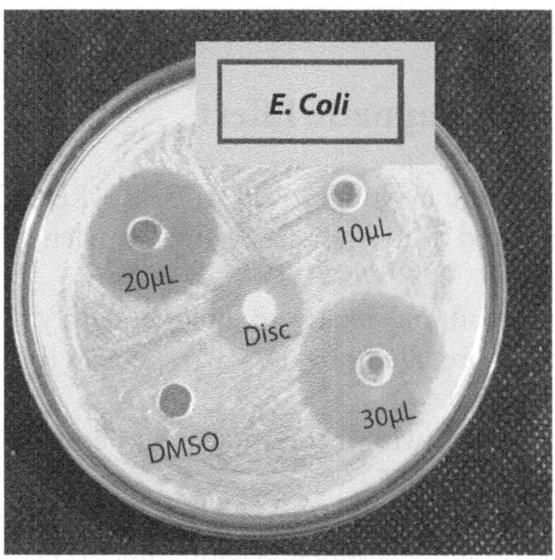

Figure 11.1 Bio activity of ZnO NPs—*E. coli*.

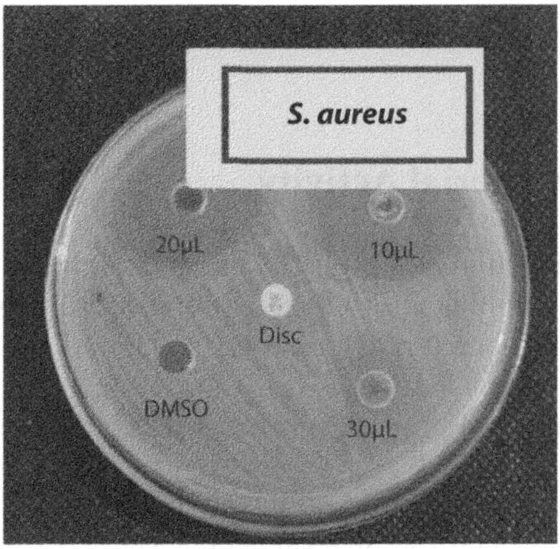

Figure 11.2 Bio activity of ZnO NPs—*S. aureus.*

Table 11.1 ZnO-MIZN—antibacterial activity.

Organisms	10µL	20µL	30µL	DMSO	DISC (CE30)
E. coli	4	7	12	nil	6
S. aureus	12	13	5	nil	3
S. typhi	nil	2	nil	nil	nil

11.3 XRD and Magnetic Effect

Figure 11.3 displays the evolution of POWDER XRD -PXRD patterns of biogenic ZnO prepared from zinc acetate, urea, ethylene glycol, and extract of *Mangifera indica.*

The peaks are broad and relatively intense, signifying the nano crystalline nature of the prepared powders, irrespective the concentration of *Mangifera indica extract.*

All peaks are indexed within the wurtzite-type of ZnO phase, in pact with JCPDS No. 01-080-0075.

The XRD patterns were refined using the whole profile fitting (WPF) program by Rietveld way and incorporated within the PDXL software by Figure 11.4 with refined XRD pattern of sample refinements as in Table 11.2.

It can be observed that all peaks are well fitted, i.e., the goodness of fit parameter is in the range of 1.4 to 1.6, a confirmation of ZnO single phase.

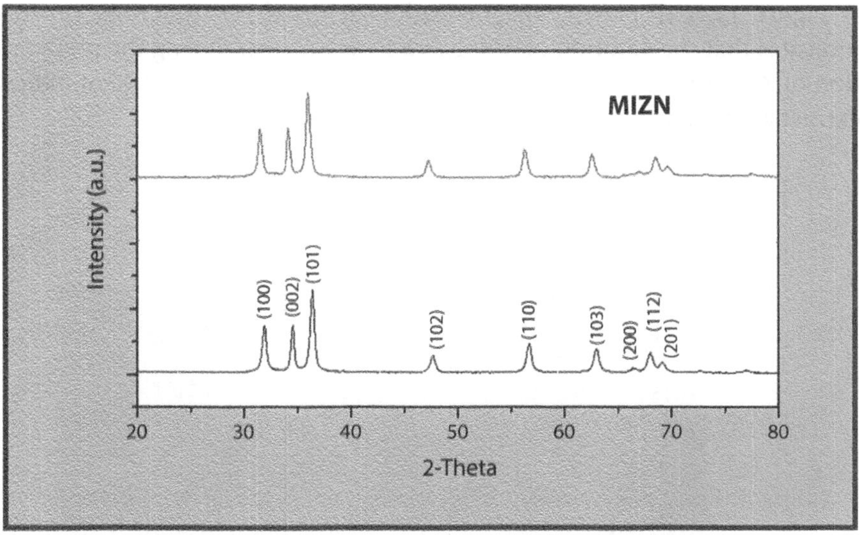

Figure 11.3 PXRD of MIZN NPs.

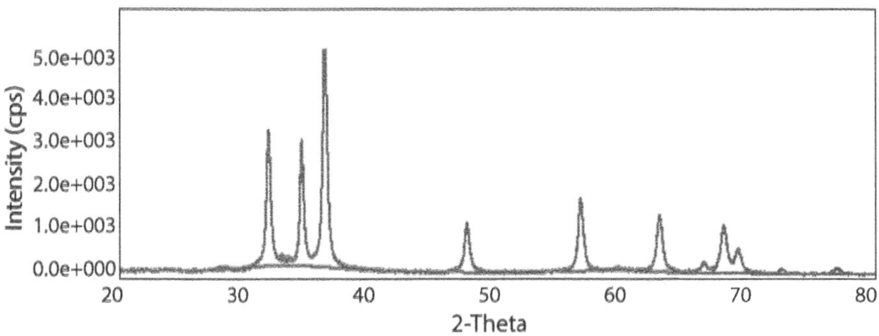

Figure 11.4 Evolution of XRD patterns of biogenic MIZN NPs.

Table 11.2 Phase composition, structural, and microstructural parameters as obtained by the Rietveld refinements of XRD patterns of biogenic ZnO nanopowders.

Sample	Crystallite size (nm)	Micro strain (%)
ZnO-MIZN	18.8	0.24

Figure 11.5, displaying magnetization-field (M-H) hysteresis curves, indicates that the addition of *Mangifera indica extract* during the preparation of ZnO induces magnetic transition: pure ZnO and *Mangifera indica* extract are paramagnetic as shown in Table 11.3.

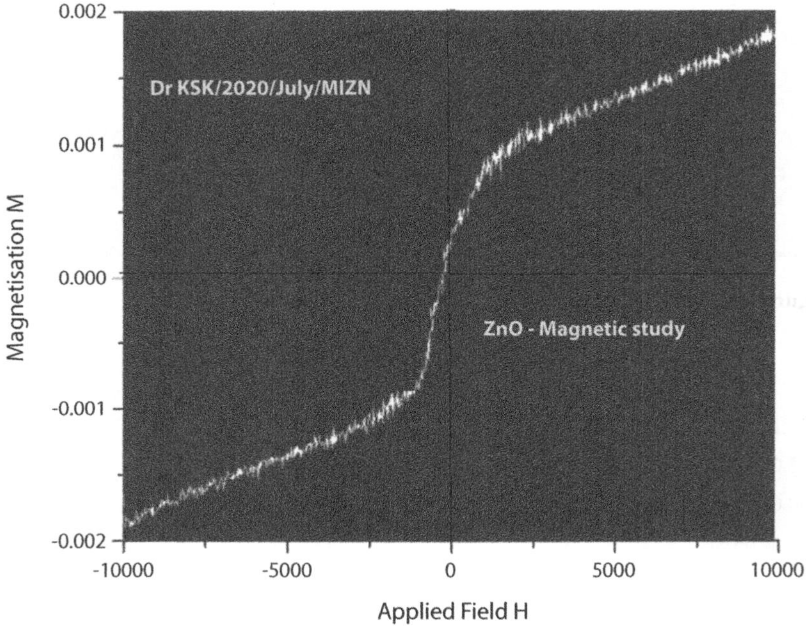

Figure 11.5 Magnetization-field hysteresis curves of biogenic MIZN-NPs.

Table 11.3 Magnetic properties of biogenic ZnO nano powders.

Sample	Behavior	Hc (Oe)	Mr (μemu/g)	M (memu/g)	Ms (memu/g)
ZnO-MIZN	F	43.1	55.3	-	0.796
	P+F	40.7	55.3	1.83	-

11.4 Tribological Data for Nano Sample Coatings of ZnO-MIZN

a) **Circular wire helical springs**
The frontier parameters represents the effective stress, deflective estimations, rigidity information of titled nano samples of ZnO-MIZN, and the impact in the gadgets of electronic industries and in mechano-elastic designs primarily of nano level tribology, which has better quality by deflection statistics and by string rigidity data.
The nano tribology gives data in which the radius is 0.01 mm and the coil radius is 0.07 mm, the shear value is 0.91 GPa, the string stiffness value is 0.016 kN/m, the shear stress value is 11.14 GPa, and the spring deflective coefficient or deflection value is 40 mm. Bulk as well as nano materials show this behavior [27–36]

b) **Torque tightened to bolt by nano-coated ZnO-MIZN samples for preloading**
Preload is a manufacturing appearance with numerous significance. In the universal logic, it refers to the interior appliance of tension to definite mechanical schemes and domains and zones. The ZnO-MIZN–coated sample with thread of grade 1 with thread friction as 0.15 and head facial coefficient of friction as 0.12 and identified as tensile stress zone of 0.120 inch^2 and stress is 19.9 kpsi and positive friction and negative friction of the thread as 97 and -58 lb.in and initial preload is 2353 lb and torque tightened total is 177 lb.in [37–43].
ZnO-MIZN is essential and best suited for mechano industries and other solidity zones where the coated springs and bolts are needed for tribological improvement than the normal bearings. For convenience, the scaling can be adjusted or modified to Newton scale by proper addition of factors to convert for universal utility [44–49].

11.5 Filter Utility

The filter utility and the influx for ZnO-MIZN are identified with the help of filter components and apparatus, and the 4.5796 microns for nano influx of ZnO-MIZN; it is the change over value cum variation in the zone when the filter use by longest wave is occurred and its esteem is generally in micron scale rarely nano scaling. It is identified to represent the filter effective value and also the NLO property if the sample is in bulk scale and the application in opto-electronics in nano scale. The variation in nano influx of ZnO series is due to size of the particle as it may vary from sample to sample. Here, the samples are chosen to best outfit based on filter nano influx as ZnO-MIZN is preferred over for the opto electronic filter value and the utility for the sample to pass through depends on purity and quality and by dimension and scaling in macro/nano.

11.6 Conclusion

Nano, as well as the functional materials cover up the advancement and the major research contribution over the globe, and the ZnO nano particles (ZnO-NPs) are successfully grown by green synthesis methodological way.

From the mango leaves (*Mangifera indica*), the ZnO NPs are extracted and verified the formation by powder XRD as the nano scaling with wurtzite-category structure, the crystallite size nearly 18 nm and weak ferromagnetic modules which are having oxygen vacancy sites, diamagnetic into paramagnetic transition is possible for the ZnO NPs.

Also circular-helical, torque tightened preloading tribological parameters were performed for mango extorted ZnO NPs, 4.5796 microns, for nano influx of titled NPs.

With the well-diffusion technology, bacterial cultures, such as *E. coli*, *S. aureus*, and *S. typhi* and ZnO NPs are good scope and better tool for antidiabetics too.

References

1. Kalaipoonguzhali, V., Senthilkannan, K., Thirumoorthi, C., Chinnadurai, M., Jayanalina, T., Comparison of adsorption energy, ionization potential and electron affinity of CuS-ACT and CuS-Nit nanostructures monowire for nano device fabrication by computational approach. *Mater. Today: Proc.*, 33, 7, 2759–2760, 2020.
2. Gunasekaran, S. *et al.*, Structural studies on picolinium maleate crystal by density functional methods. *Indian J. Phys.*, 87, 12, 1189–1197, 2013.
3. Senthilkannan, K. *et al.*, Anti diabetic (AD) studies of bis-glycine hydro bromide (45 nm) nano crystals. *Mater. Today: Proc.*, 33, 7, 3201–3202, 2020.

4. Senthilkannan, K. *et al.*, Anti-diabetic activites of ZnO doped with Ce (5 at %) nano particles (NPs). *Mater. Today: Proc.*, 33, 7, 3056–3057, 2020.
5. Senthilkannan, K. *et al.*, Fluorescence, filter,nano tribological studies of 12-(4-Chlorophenyl)-9,9-Dimethyl-9,10-Dihydro-8H-Benzo[A]Xanthen-11(12H)-One-(CPDDHBXH) macro and nano crystals. *Mater. Today: Proc.*, 33, 7, 4163–4166, 2020.
6. Senthilkannan, K., Venkatachalam, K., Jothibas, M., Computational and experimental studies of acetoacetanilide crystals. *AIP Conf. Proc.*, vol. 2270, pp. 040014, 1–4, 2020.
7. Senthilkannan, K., Venkatachalam, K., Rajamani, A., Computational analysis of LPNPTH anisotropies for dementia for Alzheimer's syndrome by DFT and molecular harboring. *AIP Conf. Proc.*, vol. 2270, pp. 040008, 1–5, 2020.
8. Senthilkannan, K., Sivaramakrishnan, V., Kalaipoonguzhali, V., Chinnadurai, M., Kannan, S., Electronic transport, HOMO–LUMO and computational studies of CuS monowire for nano device fabrication by DFT approach. *Mater. Today: Proc.*, 33, 7, 2746–2749, 2020.
9. Senthilkannan, K. and Gunasekaran, S., Spectroscopic studies and other novel studies of 4 bromo 4' chloro benzylidene aniline (BCBA) Crystal- A non linear optical material. *Int. J. Chemtech Res.*, 5, 6, 3051–3058, 2013.
10. Senthilkannan, K., Gayathri Devi, S., Nagarajan, P., Flora, G., Ranadevan, R., Anti diabetic (AD) studies of picolinium maleate nano crystals. *Mater. Today: Proc.*, 33, 3, 3005–3007, 2020.
11. Senthilkannan, K., Ramamurthi, K., Bhakya, K., Sivaramakrishnan, V., Kolanjinathan, M., Ranadevan, R., Hardness, Photoconductivity, Anti-diabetic Studies of L -AlaniniumFumarate (LAF) Crystals. *AIP Conf. Proc.*, vol. 2270, pp. 100010, 1–4, 2020.
12. Senthilkannan, K., Baskaran, P., Seenivasan, R., Settu, P., Tribological, Filter, FTIR and fluorescence studies of L-Alaninium tartrate (LAT) Macro and nano crystals. *Mater. Today: Proc.*, 33, 7, 4148–4150, 2020.
13. Senthilkannan, K., Kaleemullah, K., Abdul, J., Ponnusamy., V.K., Govindan, N.M., Effect of anti microbial and fluorescence on L-Alaninium maleate (LAM) macro and nano crystals. *Mater. Today: Proc.*, 33, 7, 2779–2781, 2020.
14. Senthilkannan, K., Ganesh, G., Abdul Jaffer Ali, H., Krishnaveni Ramamurthi, R., Kaleemullah, K., Anti diabetic (AD) activities of L-valinium picrate (LVP) macro and nano crystals. *Mater. Today: Proc.*, 33, 7, 2738–2740, 2020.
15. Senthilkannan, K., Bhakya, K., Iyanar, M., Growth and Influx, AC and DC Conductivity Studies of L-AlaniniumFumarate (LAF) Crystals. *AIP Conf. Proc.*, vol. 2270, pp. 100009, 1–4, 2020.
16. Senthilkannan, K., Growth, fluorescence and theoretical studies of B2CPCD crystals – Comparative analysis in macro and nano scaled crystals. *Mater. Today: Proc.*, 33, 7, 4368–4371, 2020.
17. Senthilkannan, K. *et al.*, Anti-diabetic (AD) activities of ZnO doped with Ce (7 at%) nano particles (NP). *Mater. Today: Proc.*, 33, 7, 3053–3055, 2020.

18. Senthilkannan, K. *et al.*, Tribological, filter studies of 3-Bromo-2-Hydroxy benzoic acid (BHBA) macro and nano crystals. *Mater. Today: Proc.*, 33, 7, 4145–4147, 2020.
19. Senthilkannan, K. *et al.*, Electronic transport, Homo-Lumo and computational studies of CuS-ACT monowire for nano device fabrication by software approach. *Mater. Today: Proc.*, 33, 7, 2756–2758, 2020.
20. Senthilkannan, K. *et al.*, Anti microbial and fluorescence activities of L-valinium picrate (LVP) macro and nano crystals. *Mater. Today: Proc.*, 33, 7, 2776–2778, 2020.
21. Senthilkumar, R. *et al.*, Anti-diabetic (AD) and hardness profile of 12-(4-Chlorophenyl)-9,9-Dimethyl-9,10-Dihydro-8H-benzo[a]xanthen-11(12H)-one -(CPDDHBXH) – Comparative analysis of macro and nano crystals. *Mater. Today: Proc.*, 33, 7, 4167–4170, 2020.
22. Sathishkumar, R. *et al.*, Synthesis, growth and characterization of 2,5-dimethyl-N-(3-phenylprop-2-en-1-ylidene) aniline (2,5 DPPA) single crystal: A new second order nonlinear optical material for photonic and optoelectronic applications. *Optik*, 226, 2, 1–11, 2020.
23. Patel, R.P. *et al.*, Growth and XRD, elemental, mechanical, dielectric, optical and photoconductivity, and surface morphological characterizations of 2-[4-(Trifluoromethyl) phenyl]-1H-benzimidazole (TFMPHB) Crystals for electronic, mechanical applications. *Braz. J. Phys.*, 51, 3, 339–350, 2021.
24. Aarthi, R. *et al.*, Molecular structure-associated pharmacodynamic investigation on benzoyl peroxide using spectroscopic and quantum computational tools. *J. Taibah Univ. Sci.*, 12, 1, 104–122, 2018.
25. Saravanan, P. *et al.*, Biofriendly and competent domestic microwave assisted method for the synthesis of ZnO nanoparticles from the extract of Azadirachta indica leaves. *Mater. Today: Proc.*, 33, 7, 3160–3163, 2020.
26. Saravanan, P. *et al.*, A perspective approach towards appreciable size and cost-effective solar cell fabrication by synthesizing ZnO nanoparticles from Azadirachta indica leaves extract using domestic microwave oven. *J. Mater. Sci. Mater. El.*, 31, 5, 4301–4309, 2020.
27. Saravanan, P. *et al.*, Dielectric and magnetic properties of Allium cepa and Raphanus sativus extracts biogenic ZnO nanoparticles. *J. Mater. Sci. Mater. El.*, 32, 1, 1–14, 2021.
28. Periyathambi, P. *et al.*, Fluorescence and filter characterizations of NaBr-added L-alanine (LANB) – A comparative analysis in macro and nano scaled crystals. *Mater. Today: Proc.*, 33, 3766–3769, 2020.
29. Baskaran, P. *et al.*, Anti-diabetic activities of ZnO doped with Ce (3 at %) nano particles. *Mater. Today: Proc.*, 33, 7, 3051–3052, 2020.
30. Baskaran, P. *et al.*, Anti-diabetic studies of barium paranitro phenolate macro and nano crystals. *Mater. Today: Proc.*, 33, 7, 3058–3060, 2020.
31. Kolanjinathan, M., Senthilkannan, K., Paramasivam, S., Baskaran, P., Iyanar, M., Anti-diabetic studies of 4-(4-chlorophenyl)-7,7-dimethyl-7,8-dihydro-

4H-1-benzopyran-2,5(3H,6H)-dione – (CPDMDHHBPHHD) nano crystals. *Mater. Today: Proc.*, 33, 7, 2750–2752, 2020.

32. Kolanjinathan, M. *et al.*, Dielectric, fluorescence, filter, nano tribological and photoconductivity studies of 4-(4-chlorophenyl)-7,7-dimethyl-7,8-dihydro-4H-1-benzopyran-2,5(3H,6H)-dione (CPDMDHHBPHHD) macro and nano crystals. *J. Mater. Sci. Mater. El.*, 27, 4, 16907–16917, 2020.
33. Kolanjinathan, M., Hariharasuthan, R., Sivaramakrishnan, V. *et al.*, XRD, CHNSO, fluorescence, filter-influx, NLO, photoconductivity, hardness and helical spring-fabricated device stress analysis of 2′-chloro-4-methoxy-3-nitrobenzil (CMNB) crystal of different scalings for opto-electronic filter and band gap engineering utilities. *J. Mater Sci. Mater El.*, 32, 10049–10057, 2021.
34. Jothibas, M. *et al.*, Structural, optical and photo catatic activity of Ag doped ZnO nano particles obtained by sol-gel method. *AIP Conf. Proc.*, vol. 2162, pp. 020151, 1–7, 2019.
35. Selvaraj, L. *et al.*, AS Anti-diabetic (AD) studies of Bis Glycine Hydro Bromide – BGHB macro crystals milled to nano scale of 219 nm as the preliminary fine particles. *Mater. Today: Proc.*, 33, 7, 3763–3765, 2020.
36. Kishore, N. *et al.*, CO and HCHO adsorption on FeO monowire devices: A DFT study. *Appl. Phys. A*, 123, 11, 706, 1–7, 2017. https://doi.org/10.1007/s00339-017-1330-6.
37. Senthilkannan, K., Gunasekaran, S., Wagish, J.G.R., UV, SEM, Powder XRD studies of Acetoacetanilide (AAC) Crystal. *Int. J. Chemtech Res.*, 6, 5, 3187–3190, 2014.
38. Kumar, K. *et al.*, Growth of diethyl 3,3′-[(2,4-dichlorophenyl) methylidene] bis(1H-indole-2-carboxylate)-(D32DMBC) organic NLO single crystal and its optical, thermal, mechanical, dielectric and computational studies. *J. Mater. Sci. Mater. El.*, 31, 23, 1–8, 2020. https://doi.org/10.1007/s10854-020-04594-y.
39. Senthilkannan, K., Venkatachalam, K., Bhakya, K., Sharmidha, B., Kalaivani, M., Gayathri Devi, S., Growth and characterization of picolinium maleate (PM) Crystals. *AIP Conf. Proc.*, vol. 2270, pp. 10014, 1–4, 2020, https://doi.org/10.1063/5.0019341.
40. Senthilkannan, K., Thamarikannan, P., Kalaipoonguzhali, V., Venkatachalam, K., Kannan, S., Baskar, A., Fluorescence, computational enactments of dimethyl N,N′-[(ethyne-1, 2-di-yl)Bis-(1,4- phenyl-ene carbon-yl)]bis-(l-alaninate) crystals. *AIP Conf. Proc.*, vol. 2270, pp. 100008, 1–4, 2020, https://doi.org/10.1063/5.0019334.
41. Senthilkannan, K., Thamaraikannan, P., Kalaipoonguzhali, V., Venkatachalam, K., Kannan, S., Ranadevan, R., Computational IR, Raman studies by DFT program and antidiabetic delineation by harboring of acetoacetanilide crystals. *AIP Conf. Proc.*, vol. 2270, pp. 10013, 1–4, 2020, https://doi.org/10.1063/5.0019339.

42. Flora, G. *et al.*, Anti-diabetic (AD) and crystal stiffness characterizations of NaBr-added L-alanine (LANB) – A comparative analysis in macro and nano scale crystals. *Mater. Today: Proc.*, 33, 7, 3937–3941, 2020.
43. Flora, G. *et al.*, Anti diabetic (AD), stiffness and hardness studies of 2-[4-(Trifluoromethyl) phenyl]-1H-benzimidazole crystals - (TFMPHB) macro and nano crystal. *Mater. Today: Proc.*, 33, 4233–4236, 2020.
44. Flora, G. *et al.*, Anti-inflammatory (AI) and crystalline hardness characterisations of 4-(4-chlorophenyl)-7,7-dimethyl-7,8-dihydro-4h-1-benzopyran-2,5(3h,6h)-dione-(CPDMDHHBPHHD) – comparative analysis of macro and nano scales crystals. *Mater. Today: Proc.*, 33, 3578–3582, 2020.
45. Ganesan, S., Gurunathan, R., Pasupuleti, R.R. *et al.*, Green synthesis of V2O5/ZnO nanocomposite materials for efficient photocatalytic and anti-bacterial applications. *Appl. Nanosci.*, 2021. https://doi.org/10.1007/s13204-021-01923-3.
46. Ganesan, H., Senthilkannan, K., Christy, S. *et al.*, Synthesis, growth, XRD, NLO, CHNSO, computational-structural, dielectric, photoconductivity, hardness and biostudies of diethyl 2-amino-5-{4-[bis (4-methyl phenyl) amino] benzamido} thiophene-3,4-dicarboxylate (DABMPABTD) macro-, nano crystals for device fabrication, pharma, electronic uses. *J. Mater. Sci. Mater. El.*, 32, 15498–15508, 2021.
47. Maalmarugan, J., Yokeswaran, V., Divya, R. *et al.*, Synthesis, growth, XRD, NLO, CHNSO, structure by theoretical approach, dielectric, absorbance, photoconductivity and bio studies of 4-(4-Acetyl-5-Methyl-1H-1, 2, 3-Triazol-1-yl) Benzonitrile crystals for optical, opto-electronic, and photonics utilities. *J. Mater. Sci. Mater. El.*, 32, 13850–13858, 2021. https://doi.org/10.1007/s10854-021-05960-0.
48. Rajkumar, M., Maalmarugan, J., Flora, G. *et al.*, Growth, characterizations, and the structural elucidation of diethyl-2-(3-oxoiso-1,3-dihydrobenzofuran-1-ylidene)malonate crystalline specimen for dielectric and electronic filters, thermal, optical, mechanical, and biomedical applications using conventional experimental and theoretical practices. *J. Mater. Sci. Mater. El.*, 32, 22822–22839, 2021. https://doi.org/10.1007/s10854-021-06761-1.
49. Senthilkannan, K., Flora, G., Gunasekaran, S., Ali, H.A.J., Vimalan, M., Balasubramanian, S., Extraction of silver nanoparticles (Ag-NPs) by green synthesis from aqueous extract of seaweeds and Their consequences on HeLa cell line and their utility on soil by spectroscopic tools, in: *Nanotechnology for Advances in Medical Microbiology. Environmental and Microbial Biotechnology*, Springer, Singapore, 2021, https://doi.org/10.1007/978-981-15-9916-3_5.

12

Nanotubular Device Effect, Super Cell Effectiveness, Hirshfeld Energy Analysis and Biomedicinal Efficacy of 2-Fluoro-5-Nitro-Aniline (2F5NA) Crystals

Flora G.[1], Munikumari A.[2] Sheeba M.[3], Jemma Hermelin Jesy Diaz[4], Senthil Kannan K.[5*], Ponrathy T.[6], Muthu Sheeba M.[6] and Joshua Steve Abishek B.[7]

[1]*Department of Botany, St. Mary's College – Autonomous, Thoothukudi, Tamil Nadu, India*
[2]*Department of Genetics and Genomics, Yogi Vemana University Kadapa, A.P., India*
[3]*Department of Zoology, PSGR Krishnammal College for Women, Coimbatore, Tamil Nadu, India*
[4]*Department of Zoology, St. Mary's College – Autonomous, Thoothukudi, Tamil Nadu, India*
[5]*Department of R&D/Physics, Edayathangudy G.S Pillay Arts and Science College (Autonomous – Affiliated to Bharathidasan University – Tiruchirappalli), Nagapattinam, Tamil Nadu, India*
[6]*Department of Botany, Kamaraj College, Thoothukudi, Tamil Nadu, India*
[7]*Department of Bioinformatics, SASTRA University, Thanjavur, Tamil Nadu, India*

Abstract

The effective mechanism for the growth of 2-fluoro-5-nitro-aniline (2F5NA) crystals is by the traditional cost-effective solution growth method; the crystalline sample is monoclinic with $P2_1/n$ space group; the XRD data reveal the crystal data of 2F5NA; the nanotubular, super cell, Hirshfeld analysis, and biomedical utility of 2F5NA crystalline samples are well portrayed using suitable softwares for the better outcome, super cell lattice, as well as the device with nanotube and with acidic, peptide link are well portrayed with the internal, external, shaping

**Corresponding author*: mscgoldmedalist@yahoo.in

Kaushik Pal (ed.) Nanovaccinology as Targeted Therapeutics, (195–212) © 2022 Scrivener Publishing LLC

indexing, curvedness effect, patching, and 3 × 3 × 3 order of the lattice are also discussed. The titled organic crystalline specimen is a well and effective utility in bio as antifungal and antidiabetic are properly delineated. The interaction energy by HF/B3LYP is given in the tabular representation for energy in kJ/mol; ORTEP of crystal for the molecular way and unit cell by ORTEP are presented for a proper and clear picture of the crystal confirmation. The novelty is mainly for bio medicinal use (antibacterial) and enhanced electronic sectors; the material is having nanotube device use mainly the predominant use of the sample.

Keywords: 2F5NA, ORTEP, Hirshfeld, super lattice, nanotube

12.1 Introduction

Macro and nano crystals are the excellent ones in utility based and in NLO; the predominance behavior is measured; here, 2F5NA are prepared by traditional evaporation method and grown in 30 plus days and are reported for the structural elucidation, nanotubes, interactions as well as bio uses, and their enhancement above the other counterparts. The materials is so chosen to be the dextro with Ala-Glu-Leu-Ser building with phi; psi each of 180° N and C data as NH_2 and COOH. Customary nonlinear optical (NLO) materials are drawing a huge understanding of thought fitting to their appropriate connections in optical frameworks [1–3]. In order, there are particular plans of purposes for beneficial, similarly as negligible cost, high-reaction, higher-mean-power NLO clear substances for optically characterized speaker connection and SHG common organo-crystals can have extraordinarily nonlinear susceptibilities separated to inorganic sort of clear model [1–7]. Imaginative regular compound particles with one or other sweet-smelling engineered materials scheme in framed strategies; crucial for unimaginably proficient charge relocate blueprints have been intensely analyzed [8–16]. These composites are obliged to come to fruition in the standard noncentrosymmetric division in assessment of purposes creation employments of quadratic optically nonlinear results [17–23]. Normal composites are shaped by powerless Van der Waal's and hydrogen bonds and get more genuine degree of delocalization [24–31]. In such a manner, amino acids are stirring regular class of materials for the force in NLO sort of uses. Essentially, amino acids characteristically secure nonlinear optical result since the time which incorporating a digressed carbon particle come to fruition in noncentrosymmetric class of room bundle.

Amino destructive in firm condition encases a deprotonated carboxylic destructive get-together and protonated amino grouping. The dipolar nature depicts uncommon physiocompound attributes in amino acids, which make them outrageous contenders for NLO contraptions [31–37]. The properties of 2F5NA have been as of now investigated by and large [38–43]. The current assessment has principle center essentially around the improvement of 2F5NA single precious stones and analyzes its nonlinear optical properties [44–52]. The created crystals are seen by an extent of systems, including X-pillar diffractometry (XRD) and so on.

12.2 XRD and Computational

The 2F5NA formula is $C_6H_5FN_2O_2$, space group as $P2_1/n$, crystal system is monoclinic; temperature (K) is 296; a, b, c (Å) as 12.1967, 3.7560, 14.4540; β (°) is 102.143. The consequence of molecular effectiveness, such as structure, unit-cell, 3D image, are well portrayed; the 3 × 3 × 3 model is also given for device building; the Hirshfeld interactions, the device of nano with peptides and acidic and 5 × 5 × 5 modal way is delineated for the crystalline specimen with ORTEP diagram and with interaction effectiveness and the Homo-Lumo and other densities with void space are portrayed for efficient spacing of 2F5NA from Figures 12.1 to 12.19 and from Table 12.1.

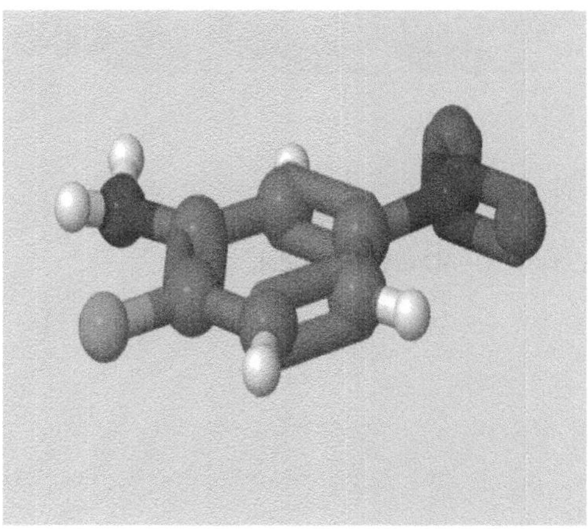

Figure 12.1 2F5NA crystals—molecular model.

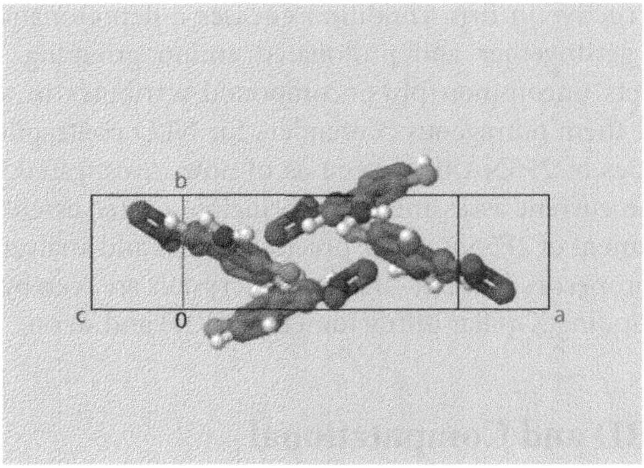

Figure 12.2 2F5NA crystals—unit cell [50–52].

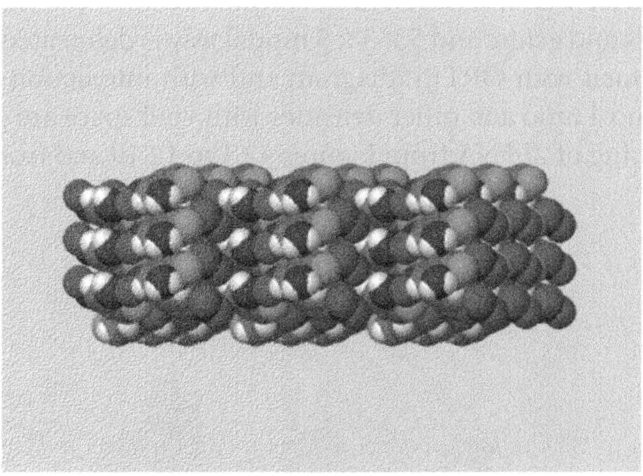

Figure 12.3 2F5NA crystals—3D crystal model.

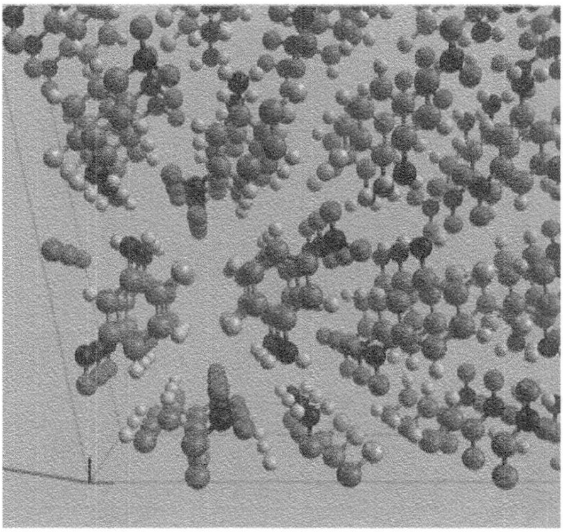

Figure 12.4 2F5NA crystals—3 × 3 × 3 model [50–52].

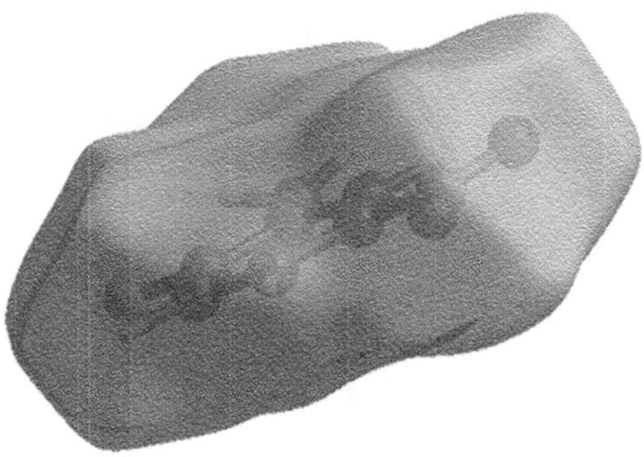

Figure 12.5 2F5NA crystals—HFA without surface effect.

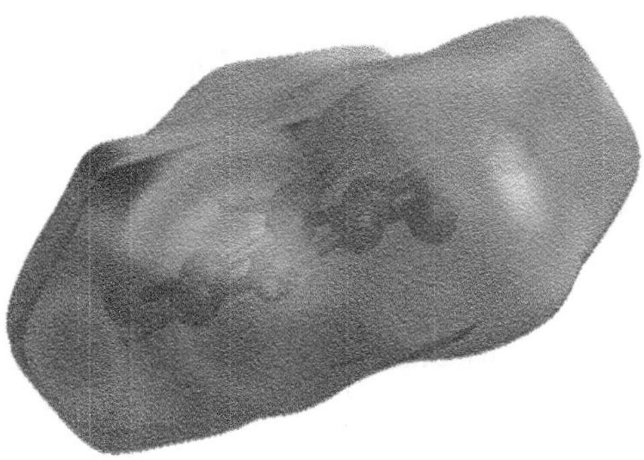

Figure 12.6 2F5NA crystals—HFA d_i effect [50–52].

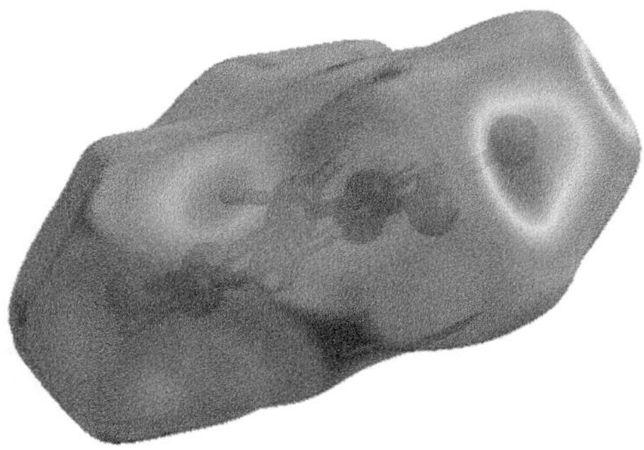

Figure 12.7 2F5NA crystals—HFA d_e effect.

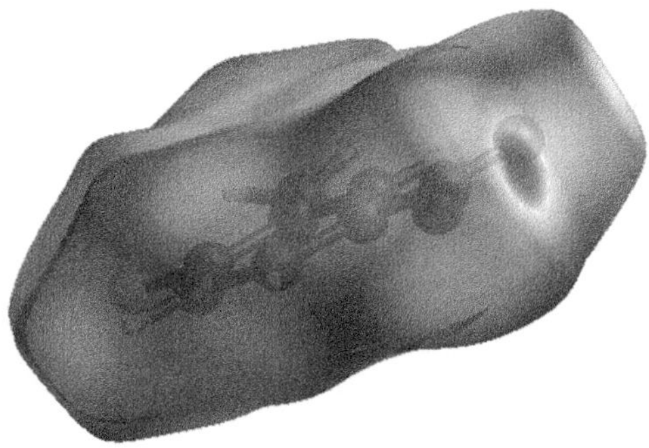

Figure 12.8 2F5NA crystals—HFA d_{norms} effect [50–52].

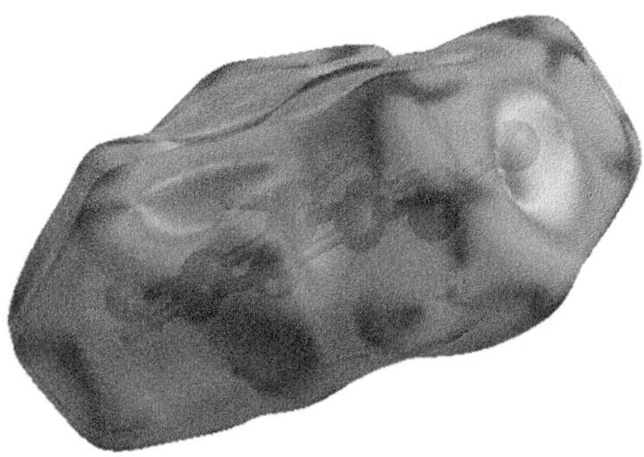

Figure 12.9 2F5NA crystals—shape index effect.

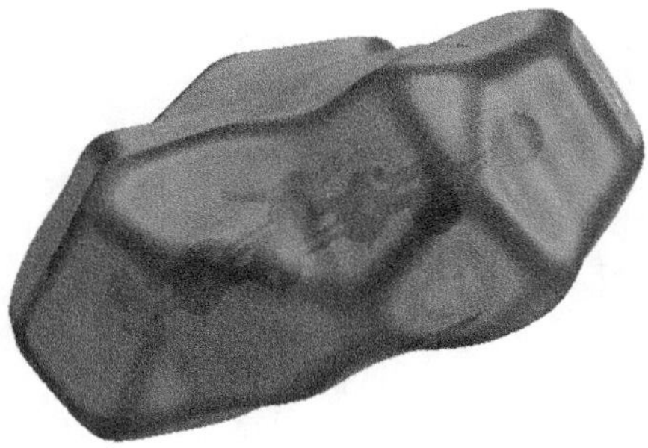

Figure 12.10 2F5NA crystals—HFA curvedness effect [50–52].

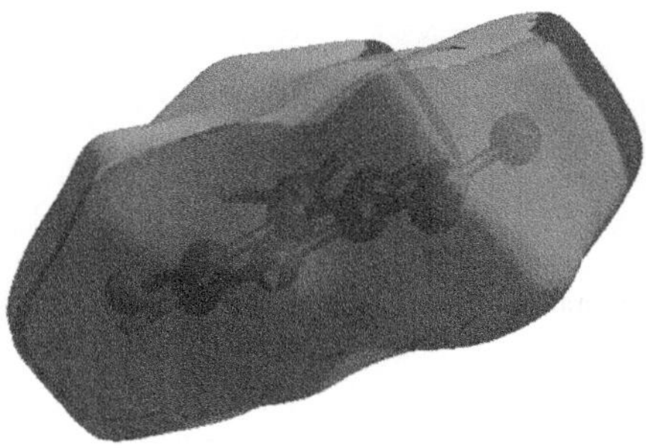

Figure 12.11 2F5NA crystals—fragment patched effect.

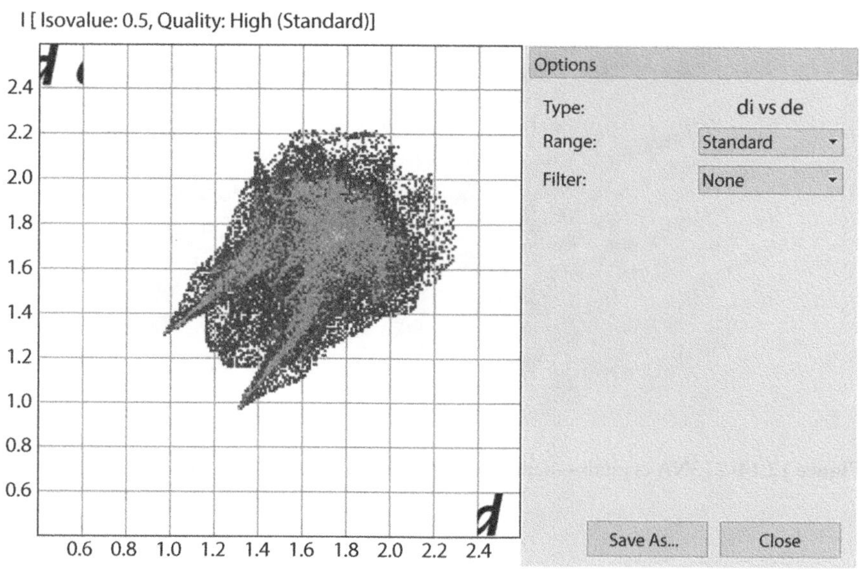

Figure 12.12 2F5NA crystals—fingerprint effect [50–52].

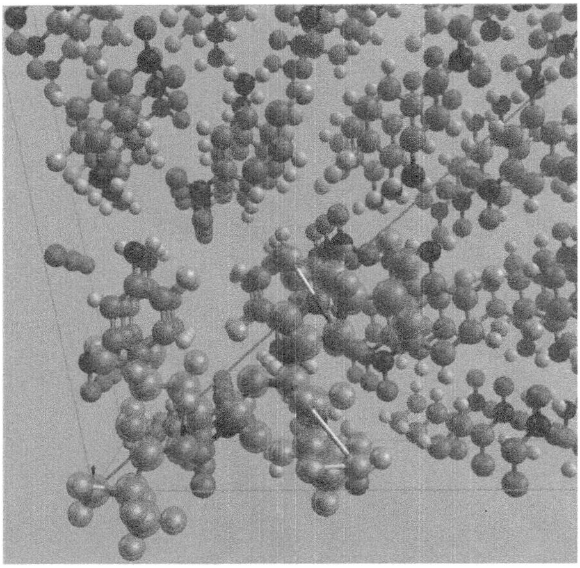

Figure 12.13 2F5NA crystals—peptide link effect [50–52].

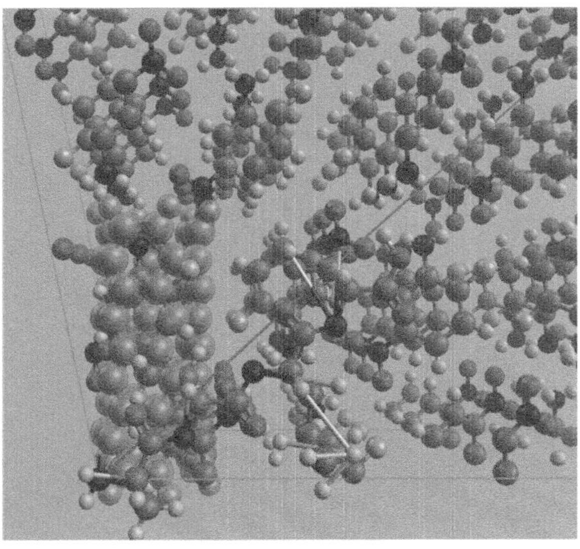

Figure 12.14 2F5NA crystals—nanotube with acidic link effect [50–52].

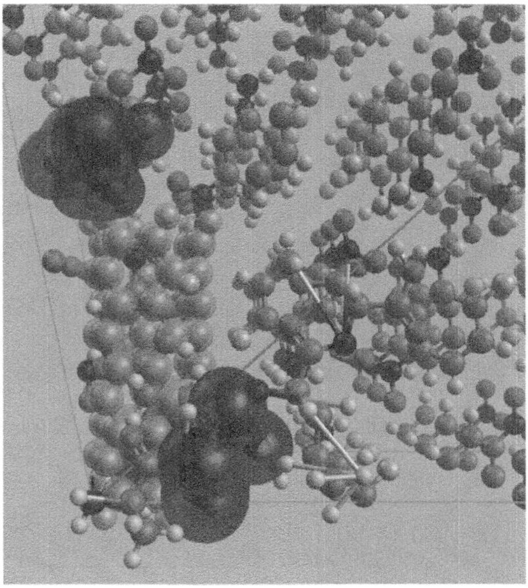

Figure 12.15 2F5NA crystals—weak interactions [50–52].

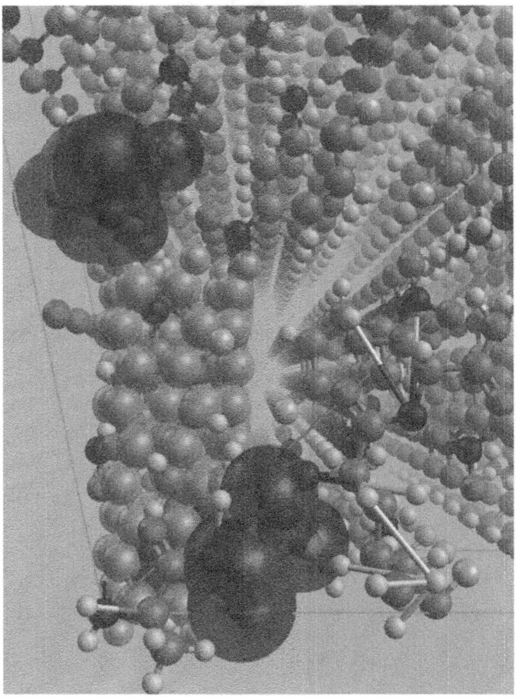

Figure 12.16 2F5NA crystals—5 × 5 × 5 slab [50–52].

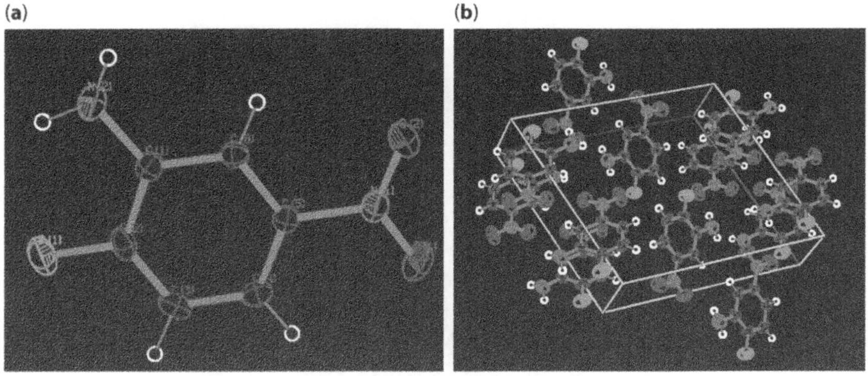

Figure 12.17 (a, b) 2F5NA crystals—Ortep of crystal and unit cell frame work with Ortep [50–52].

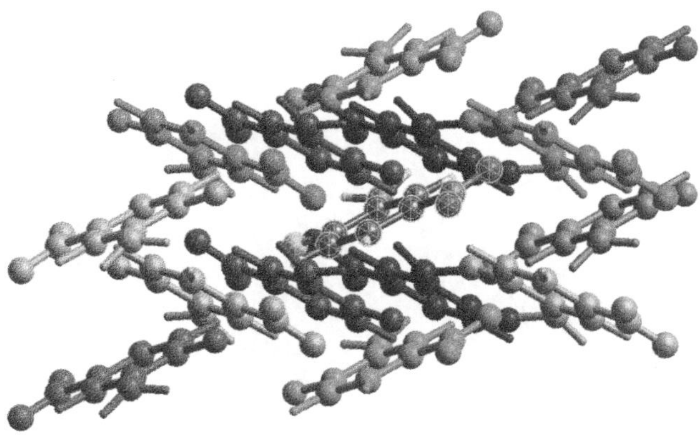

Figure 12.18 2F5NA crystals—interactions mapping with different energies [50–52].

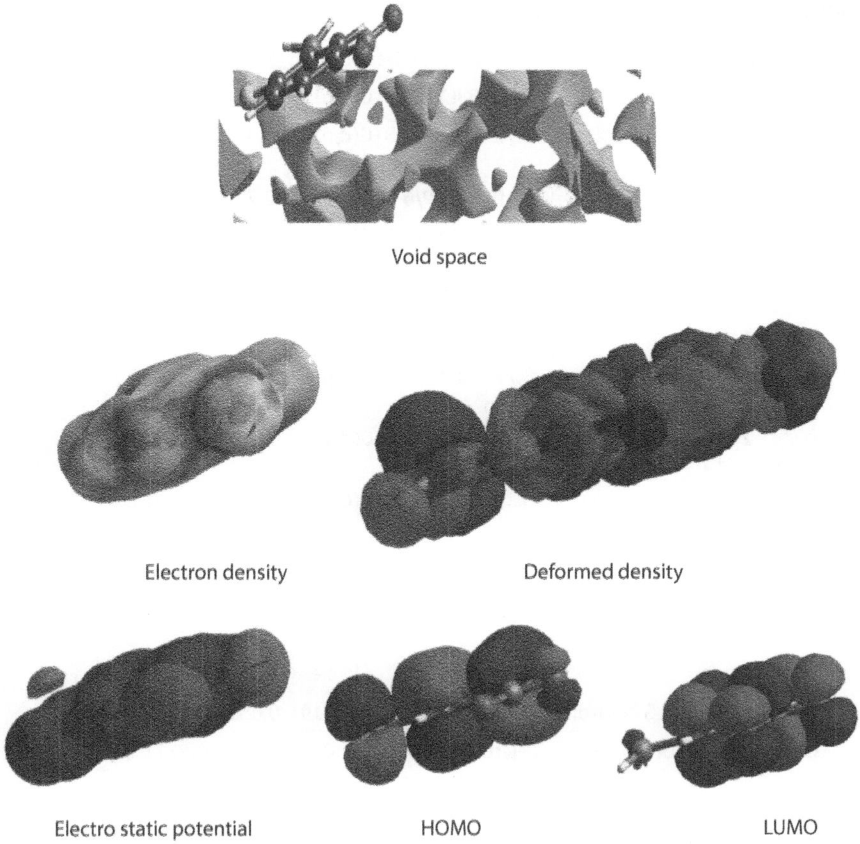

Figure 12.19 Void, electron, deformed densities, potential and frontier orbitals of 2F5NA crystals [50–52].

Table 12.1 Interaction energies and surface info of 2F5NA.

	N	Symop	R	Electron Density	E_ele	E_pol	E_dis	E_rep
	1	-x, -y, -z	8.30	B3LYP/6-31G(d,p)	-1.9	-0.2	-4.7	1.3
	2	x+1/2, -y+1/2, z +1/2	8.72	B3LYP/6-31G(d,p)	1.4	-0.6	-3.5	0.9
	1	-x, -y, -z	7.19	B3LYP/6-31G(d,p)	0.7	-0.2	-10.7	5.3
	2	x+1/2, -y+1/2, z +1/2	8.55	B3LYP/6-31G(d,p)	-14.8	-2.8	-7.4	9.2
	2	x, y, z	3.76	B3LYP/6-31G(d,p)	-2.5	-1.6	-38.7	22.8
	1	-x, -y, -z	5.37	B3LYP/6-31G(d,p)	-0.0	-1.9	-15.6	6.4
	2	-x+1/2, y+1/2, -z +1/2	8.71	B3LYP/6-31G(d,p)	1.4	-1.2	-4.5	2.2
	2	-x+1/2, y+1/2, -z +1/2	6.44	B3LYP/6-31G(d,p)	-6.7	-1.4	-10.2	6.7
	1	-x, -y, -z	6.32	B3LYP/6-31G(d,p)	-34.1	-5.7	-13.4	18.7

Scale factors for benchmarked energy models
See Mackenzie et al. IUCrJ (2017)

Energy Model	k_ele	k_pol	k_disp	k_rep
CE-HF ... HF/3-21G electron densities	1.019	0.651	0.901	0.811
CE-B3LYP ... B3LYP/6-31G(d,p) electron densities	1.057	0.740	0.871	0.618

2F5NA Surface Information

Type Hirshfeld
Resolution High (Standard)
Isovalue 0.5
Volume 157.92 Å^3
Area 168.51 Å^2
Globularity 0.838
2F5NAhericity 0.129

Surface Property Information 7 Properties of 2F5NA
Name Min Mean Max Units

---

d i 0.982 1.658 2.308 Å
d e 0.982 1.675 2.255 Å
d norm -0.230 0.370 1.039

Shape Index -0.992 0.312 0.996
Curvedness -4.307 -0.989 0.153

Fingerprint Breakdown
Filtering fingerprint by element type.
Surface area included (as percentage of the total surface area)
for close contacts between atoms inside and outside the surface.

Inside Outside Atom
Atom C H N O F
C 8.0 6.1 0.4 1.2 1.0 16.7
F 0.7 7.0 0.0 2.1 1.1 10.9
H 3.8 17.5 2.3 13.9 6.1 43.6
N 0.4 3.4 0.0 1.6 0.0 5.5
O 0.8 16.6 1.3 2.2 2.3 23.3
13.8 50.5 4.1 21.0 10.6

12.3 Bioutility

12.3.1 Antibacterial of 2F5NA Crystals

The antibacterial action shown by region of reticence consequences show that the grown-up crystals display the movement (Table 12.2) analogously by way of a typical one. The fallout perceptibly divulged that trials confirmed superior antibacterial commotion when compared with the outstanding compounds in this succession. The bustle of full-grown 2F5NA crystals is admirable in opposition to *E. coli, B. subtilis. K. pneumoniae P. aeruginosa,* and *S. aureus.*

Table 12.2 Biouses of 2F5NA crystals.

Microorganisms used	50μL (2F5NA)	100 μL (2F5NA)	Disc (CAZ 10mcg)	D.H_2O
E. coli	3 mm	4mm	Nil	Nil
B. subtilis	4 mm	3mm	6mm	Nil
K. pneumoniae	3 mm	4mm	10mm	Nil
P. aeruginosa	4 mm	3mm	8mm	Nil
S. aureus	3 mm	4mm	7mm	Nil

12.4 Conclusion

The 2F5NA crystals are well grown and the XRD, tubular generation, super lattice structure, and interactions are portrayed with the proper bioutility. The antibacterial use of full-grown 2F5NA crystals is splendid in resistance to *E. coli, B. subtilis. K. pneumoniae P. aeruginosa*, and *S. aureus* and properly reported. The computational data are well matched with XRD data and provide better scaling and new device formation. The titled organic crystalline specimen is well, effective utility in bio as antifungal, antidiabetic are properly delineated. The interaction energy by HF/B3LYP are given in the tabular representation for energy in kJ/mol; ORTEP of crystal for the molecular way and unit cell by ORTEP are presented for a proper and clear picture of the crystal confirmation. The novelty is mainly for bio medicinal use (antibacterial) and enhanced electronic sectors; the material is having nanotube device use mainly the predominant use of the sample.

References

1. Kalaipoonguzhali, V., Senthilkannan, K., Thirumoorthi, C., Chinnadurai, M., Jayanalina, T., Comparison of adsorption energy, ionization potential and electron affinity of CuS-ACT and CuS-Nit nanostructures monowire for nano device fabrication by computational approach. *Mater. Today: Proc.*, 33, 7, 2759–2760, 2020.
2. Gunasekaran, S. *et al.*, Structural studies on picolinium maleate crystal by density functional methods. *Indian J. Phys.*, 87, 12, 1189–1197, 2013.
3. Senthilkannan, K. *et al.*, Anti diabetic (AD) studies of bis-glycine hydro bromide (45 nm) nano crystals. *Mater. Today: Proc.*, 33, 7, 3201–3202, 2020.
4. Senthilkannan, K. *et al.*, Anti-diabetic activites of ZnO doped with Ce (5 at %) nano particles (NPs). *Mater. Today: Proc.*, 33, 7, 3056–3057, 2020.
5. Senthilkannan, K. *et al.*, Fluorescence, filter,nano tribological studies of 12-(4-Chlorophenyl)-9,9-Dimethyl-9,10-Dihydro-8H-Benzo[A]Xanthen-11(12H)-One-(CPDDHBXH) macro and nano crystals. *Mater. Today: Proc.*, 33, 7, 4163–4166, 2020.
6. Senthilkannan, K., Venkatachalam, K., Jothibas, M., Computational and experimental studies of acetoacetanilide crystals. *AIP Conf. Proc*, vol. 2270, pp. 040014, 1–4, 2020.
7. Senthilkannan, K., Venkatachalam, K., Rajamani, A., Computational analysis of LPNPTH anisotropies for dementia for Alzheimer's syndrome by DFT and molecular harboring. *AIP Conf. Proc*, vol. 2270, pp. 040008, 1–5, 2020.
8. Senthilkannan, K., Sivaramakrishnan, V., Kalaipoonguzhali, V., Chinnadurai, M., Kannan, S., Electronic transport, Homo–Lumo and computational

studies of CuS monowire for nano device fabrication by DFT approach. *Mater. Today: Proc.*, 33, 7, 2746–2749, 2020.
9. Senthilkannan, K. and Gunasekaran, S., Spectroscopic studies and other novel studies of 4 bromo 4' chloro benzylidene aniline (BCBA) crystal - A non linear optical material. *Int. J. Chemtech Res.*, 5, 6, 3051–3058, 2013.
10. Senthilkannan, K., Gayathri Devi, S., Nagarajan, P., Flora, G., Ranadevan, R., Anti diabetic (AD) studies of picolinium maleate nano crystals. *Mater. Today: Proc.*, 33, 3, 3005–3007, 2020.
11. Senthilkannan, K., Ramamurthi, K., Bhakya, K., Sivaramakrishnan, V., Kolanjinathan, M., Ranadevan, R., Hardness, Photoconductivity, Anti-diabetic Studies of L-AlaniniumFumarate (LAF) Crystals. *AIP Conf. Proc*, vol. 2270, pp. 100010, 1–4, 2020.
12. Senthilkannan, K., Baskaran, P., Seenivasan, R., Settu, P., Tribological, filter, FTIR and fluorescence studies of L-Alaninium tartrate (LAT) macro and nano crystals. *Mater. Today: Proc.*, 33, 7, 4148–4150, 2020.
13. Senthilkannan, K., Kaleemullah, K., Abdul, J., Ponnusamy., V.K., Govindan, N.M., Effect of anti microbial and fluorescence on L-Alaninium maleate (LAM) macro and nano crystals. *Mater. Today: Proc.*, 33, 7, 2779–2781, 2020.
14. Senthilkannan, K., Ganesh, G., Abdul Jaffer Ali, H., Krishnaveni Ramamurthi, R., Kaleemullah, K., Anti diabetic (AD) activities of L-valinium picrate (LVP) macro and nano crystals. *Mater. Today: Proc.*, 33, 7, 2738–2740, 2020.
15. Senthilkannan, K., Bhakya, K., Iyanar, M., Growth and influx, AC and DC conductivity studies of L-Alaninium Fumarate (LAF) crystals. *AIP Conf. Proc*, vol. 2270, pp. 100009, 1–4, 2020.
16. Senthilkannan, K., Growth, fluorescence and theoretical studies of B2CPCD crystals – Comparative analysis in macro and nano scaled crystals. *Mater. Today: Proc.*, 33, 7, 4368–4371, 2020.
17. Senthilkannan, K. *et al.*, Anti-diabetic (AD) activities of ZnO doped with Ce (7 at%) nano particles (NP). *Mater. Today: Proc.*, 33, 7, 3053–3055, 2020.
18. Senthilkannan, K. *et al.*, Tribological, filter studies of 3-Bromo-2-Hydroxy benzoic acid (BHBA) macro and nano crystals. *Mater. Today: Proc.*, 33, 7, 4145–4147, 2020.
19. Senthilkannan, K. *et al.*, Electronic transport, Homo-Lumo and computational studies of CuS-ACT monowire for nano device fabrication by software approach. *Mater. Today: Proc.*, 33, 7, 2756–2758, 2020.
20. Senthilkannan, K. *et al.*, Anti microbial and fluorescence activities of L-valinium picrate (LVP) macro and nano crystals. *Mater. Today: Proc.*, 33, 7, 2776–2778, 2020.
21. Senthilkumar, R. *et al.*, Anti-diabetic (AD) and hardness profile of 12-(4-Chlorophenyl)-9,9-Dimethyl-9,10-Dihydro-8H-benzo[a]xanthen-11(12H)-one–(CPDDHBXH) – Comparative analysis of macro and nano crystals. *Mater. Today: Proc.*, 33, 7, 4167–4170, 2020.
22. Sathishkumar, R. *et al.*, Synthesis, Growth and Characterization of 2,5–Dimethyl-N-(3-phenylprop-2-en-1-ylidene) Aniline (2,5–DPPA) single

crystal: A new second order nonlinear optical material for photonic and optoelectronic applications. *Optik*, 226, 2, 1–11, 2020.

23. Patel, R.P. *et al.*, Growth and XRD, elemental, mechanical, dielectric, optical and photoconductivity, and surface morphological characterizations of 2-[4-(Trifluoromethyl) phenyl]-1H-benzimidazole (TFMPHB) crystals for electronic, mechanical applications. *Braz. J. Phys.*, 51, 3, 339–350, 2021.
24. Aarthi, R. *et al.*, Molecular structure-associated pharmacodynamic investigation on benzoyl peroxide using spectroscopic and quantum computational tools. *J. Taibah Univ. Sci.*, 12, 1, 104–122, 2018.
25. Saravanan, P. *et al.*, Biofriendly and competent domestic microwave assisted method for the synthesis of ZnO nanoparticles from the extract of Azadirachta indica leaves. *Mater. Today: Proc.*, 33, 7, 3160–3163, 2020.
26. Saravanan, P. *et al.*, A perspective approach towards appreciable size and cost-effective solar cell fabrication by synthesizing ZnO nanoparticles from Azadirachta indica leaves extract using domestic microwave oven. *J. Mater. Sci. Mater. El.*, 31, 5, 4301–4309, 2020.
27. Saravanan, P. *et al.*, Dielectric and magnetic properties of Allium cepa and Raphanus sativus extracts biogenic ZnO nanoparticles. *J. Mater. Sci. Mater. El.*, 32, 1, 1–14, 2021.
28. Periyathambi, P. *et al.*, Fluorescence and filter characterizations of NaBr-added L-alanine (LANB) – A comparative analysis in macro and nano scaled crystals. *Mater. Today: Proc.*, 33, 3766–3769, 2020.
29. Baskaran, P. *et al.*, Anti-diabetic activities of ZnO doped with Ce (3 at %) nano particles. *Mater. Today: Proc.*, 33, 7, 3051–3052, 2020.
30. Baskaran, P. *et al.*, Anti-diabetic studies of barium paranitro phenolate macro and nano crystals. *Mater. Today: Proc.*, 33, 7, 3058–3060, 2020.
31. Kolanjinathan, M., Senthilkannan, K., Paramasivam, S., Baskaran, P., Iyanar, M., Anti-diabetic studies of 4-(4-chlorophenyl)-7,7-dimethyl-7,8-dihydro-4H-1-benzopyran-2,5(3H,6H)-dione – (CPDMDHHBPHHD) nano crystals. *Mater. Today: Proc.*, 33, 7, 2750–2752, 2020.
32. Kolanjinathan, M. *et al.*, Dielectric, fluorescence, filter, nano tribological and photoconductivity studies of 4-(4-chlorophenyl)-7,7-dimethyl-7,8-dihydro-4H-1-benzopyran-2,5(3H,6H)-dione (CPDMDHHBPHHD) macro and nano crystals. *J. Mater. Sci. Mater. El.*, 27, 4, 16907–16917, 2020.
33. Kolanjinathan, M., Hariharasuthan, R., Sivaramakrishnan, V. *et al.*, XRD, CHNSO, fluorescence, filter-influx, NLO, photoconductivity, hardness and helical spring-fabricated device stress analysis of 2′-chloro-4-methoxy-3-nitrobenzil (CMNB) crystal of different scalings for opto-electronic filter and band gap engineering utilities. *J. Mater Sci. Mater El.*, 32, 10049–10057, 2021.
34. Jothibas, M. *et al.*, Structural, optical and photo catatic activity of Ag doped ZnO nano particles obtained by sol-gel method. *AIP Conf. Proc*, vol. 2162, pp. 020151, 1–7, 2019.

35. Selvaraj, L. *et al.*, AS Anti-diabetic (AD) studies of Bis Glycine Hydro Bromide – BGHB macro crystals milled to nano scale of 219 nm as the preliminary fine particles. *Mater. Today: Proc.*, 33, 7, 3763–3765, 2020.
36. Kishore, N. *et al.*, CO and HCHO adsorption on FeO monowire devices: A DFT study. *Appl. Phys. A*, 123, 11, 706, 1–7, 2017. https://doi.org/10.1007/s00339-017-1330-6.
37. Senthilkannan, K., Gunasekaran, S., Wagish, J.G.R., UV, SEM, powder XRD studies of Acetoacetanilide (AAC) Crystal. *Int. J. Chemtech Res.*, 6, 5, 3187–3190, 2014.
38. Kumar, K. *et al.*, Growth of diethyl 3,3′-[(2,4-dichlorophenyl) methylidene] bis(1H-indole-2-carboxylate)-(D32DMBC) organic NLO single crystal and its optical, thermal, mechanical, dielectric and computational studies. *J. Mater. Sci. Mater. El.*, 31, 23, 1–8, 2020. https://doi.org/10.1007/s10854-020-04594-y.
39. Senthilkannan, K., Venkatachalam, K., Bhakya, K., Sharmidha, B., Kalaivani, M., Gayathri Devi, S., Growth and characterization of Picolinium Maleate (PM) Crystals. *AIP Conf. Proc*, vol. 2270, pp. 10014, 1–4, 2020, https://doi.org/10.1063/5.0019341.
40. Senthilkannan, K., Thamarikannan, P., Kalaipoonguzhali, V., Venkatachalam, K., Kannan, S., Baskar, A., Fluorescence, computational enactments of dimethyl N,N′-[(ethyne-1, 2-di-yl)Bis-(1,4- phenyl-ene carbon-yl)]bis-(l-alaninate) crystals. *AIP Conf. Proc*, vol. 2270, pp. 100008, 1–4, 2020, https://doi.org/10.1063/5.0019334.
41. Senthilkannan, K., Thamaraikannan, P., Kalaipoonguzhali, V., Venkatachalam, K., Kannan, S., Ranadevan, R., Computational IR, Raman studies by DFT program and antidiabetic delineation by harboring of acetoacetanilide crystals. *AIP Conf. Proc*, vol. 2270, pp. 10013, 1–4, 2020, https://doi.org/10.1063/5.0019339.
42. Flora, G. *et al.*, Anti-diabetic (AD) and crystal stiffness characterizations of NaBr-added L-alanine (LANB) – A comparative analysis in macro and nano scale crystals. *Mater. Today: Proc.*, 33, 7, 3937–3941, 2020.
43. Flora, G. *et al.*, Anti diabetic (AD), stiffness and hardness studies of 2-[4-(Trifluoromethyl) phenyl]-1H-benzimidazole crystals - (TFMPHB) macro and nano crystal. *Mater. Today: Proc.*, 33, 4233–4236, 2020.
44. Flora, G. *et al.*, Anti-inflammatory (AI) and crystalline hardness characterisations of 4-(4-chlorophenyl)-7,7-dimethyl-7,8-dihydro-4h-1-benzopyran-2,5(3h,6h)-dione-(CPDMDHHBPHHD) – Comparative analysis of macro and nano scales crystals. *Mater. Today: Proc.*, 33, 3578–3582, 2020.
45. Ganesan, S., Gurunathan, R., Pasupuleti, R.R. *et al.*, Green synthesis of V2O5/ZnO nanocomposite materials for efficient photocatalytic and anti-bacterial applications. *Appl. Nanosci.*, 2021. https://doi.org/10.1007/s13204-021-01923-3.
46. Ganesan, H., Senthilkannan, K., Christy, S. *et al.*, Synthesis, growth, XRD, NLO, CHNSO, computational-structural, dielectric, photoconductivity, hardness and biostudies of diethyl 2-amino-5-{4-[bis (4-methyl phenyl)

amino] benzamido} thiophene-3,4-dicarboxylate (DABMPABTD) macro-, nano crystals for device fabrication, pharma, electronic uses. *J. Mater. Sci. Mater. El.*, 32, 15498–15508, 2021.
47. Maalmarugan, J., Yokeswaran, V., Divya, R. *et al.*, Synthesis, growth, XRD, NLO, CHNSO, structure by theoretical approach, dielectric, absorbance, photoconductivity and bio studies of 4-(4-Acetyl-5-Methyl-1H-1, 2, 3-Triazol-1-yl) Benzonitrile crystals for optical, opto-electronic, and photonics utilities. *J. Mater. Sci. Mater. El.*, 32, 13850–13858, 2021. https://doi.org/10.1007/s10854-021-05960-0.
48. Rajkumar, M., Maalmarugan, J., Flora, G. *et al.*, Growth, characterizations, and the structural elucidation of diethyl-2-(3-oxoiso-1,3-dihydrobenzofuran-1-ylidene)malonate crystalline specimen for dielectric and electronic filters, thermal, optical, mechanical, and biomedical applications using conventional experimental and theoretical practices. *J. Mater. Sci. Mater. El.*, 32, 22822–22839, 2021. https://doi.org/10.1007/s10854-021-06761-1.
49. Senthilkannan, K., Flora, G., Gunasekaran, S., Ali, H.A.J., Vimalan, M., Balasubramanian, S., Extraction of Silver Nanoparticles (Ag-NPs) by green synthesis from aqueous extract of seaweeds and their consequences on HeLa cell line and their utility on soil by spectroscopic tools, in: *Nanotechnology for Advances in Medical Microbiology. Environmental and Microbial Biotechnology*, Springer, Singapore, 2021, https://doi.org/10.1007/978-981-15-9916-3_5.
50. Momma, K. and Izumi, F., VESTA 3 for three-dimensional visualization of crystal, volumetric and morphology data. *J. Appl. Crystallogr.*, 44, 1272–1276, 2011.
51. Spackman, P.R., Turner, M.J., McKinnon, J.J., Wolff, S.K., Grimwood, D.J., Jayatilaka, D., Spackman, M.A., Crystal explorer: A program for Hirshfeld surface analysis, visualization and quantitative analysis of molecular crystals. *J. Appl. Crystallogr.*, 54, 3, 1006–1011, 2021. https://doi.org/10.1107/S1600576721002910.
52. Spek, A.L., Single – crystal structure validation with the program PLATON. *J. Appl. Crystallogr.*, 36, 7–11, 2003.

13

Nano, Peptide Link, Pharma Impact and Electron Density of AMPHB Macro, Nano Crystalline Samples

Senthil Kannan K.[1*], Dayana Lobo F.[2], Gayathri A.[3], Prathebha K.[4], Jacintha Tamil Malar A.[2], Maria Sumathi B.[2], Flora G.[2] and Egbert Selwin Rose A.[5]

[1]*Department of R&D/Physics, Edayathangudy G.S Pillay Arts and Science College (Autonomous – Affiliated to Bharathidasan University – Tiruchirappalli), Nagapattinam, Tamilnadu, India*
[2]*Department of Botany, St. Mary's College – Autonomous, Thoothukudi, Tamilnadu, India*
[3]*Department of CSE, Saveetha School of Engineering, Saveetha Institute of Medical and Technical Sciences, Saveetha University, Chennai, TN, India*
[4]*Department of Physics, Easwari Engineering College, Ramapuram, Chennai, TN, India*
[5]*Department of Botany, St. Joseph's College - Autonomous, Tiruchirappalli, TN, India*

Abstract
The 2-amino-4-methylpyridinium 4-hydroxybenzoate (AMPHB) crystalline macro as well as nano scalings are, respectively, prepared by lucrative evaporation and by the proper milled effect and confirmed the process of synthesis by means of the SXRD methodology and confirmed the monoclinicity of the grown macro specimen, as well as by the effectiveness of the other excel results from theory and practices of the specimen. Nanotube generation is a well-known device fabrication by the theoretical way using software with the crystal structure, thermal ellipsoidal portrayal of the titled crystalline specimen, acidic frame work of the titled specimen, the proper peptide linkage stereo type of rotation specific with groups, optimized force field interactions with/without colored effect of potential impact, Vanderwall's impact for the weak interactions, also in the line of pharmacy/bio the antidiabetic, antifungal, and anti-inflammatory proceedings of both scales and the cloned effect of the proper electron density representation of the AMPHB crystalline sample.

**Corresponding author*: MSCGOLDMEDALIST@YAHOO.IN

Kaushik Pal (ed.) Nanovaccinology as Targeted Therapeutics, (213–226) © 2022 Scrivener Publishing LLC

Keywords: Nano, peptide, Vanderwall's impact, pharma-effect

13.1 Introduction

The organic crystalline materials are subjected to profound uses [1-3], versatile-specific functionalities [4–7], and other major contributions to society [8–13]. The materials have opto electronic and pi-pi* uniqueness than other counterpart materials [14–20]. They are of sound optical usage mainly in SHG/THG NLO [21–25] and in major functionalities in bio/pharma uses, such as bacterial, fungal, diabetic, inflammatory, and so on [26–30]. Here, the present investigation is mainly on SXRD, nanotube generation, peptide linkage, force field, Vanderwall's impact, bioactivity, and cloned effect electron density for the organic titled specimen and specified by both scalings of macro, nano [31–33]. The natural sort of large-scale crystals of AMPHB is the one fully developed by the customary evaporation technique and appropriately changed over to 52 nm by nano level through processing of milled effectiveness. The natural material having clever equipped pharma utilities [34–37]. The natural materials, which are organic, are having very much uncovered uses in electronic-mechano-bio sciences and in innovation, here, in AMPHB, the two scalings are recognized to continue for the nanotube development of AMPHB, upgraded power field adequacy, Vanderwall's effect of the crystal, against bio uses and calming portrayals and announced properly for betterment [38–40]. Subatomic crystals set forward a prosperous layer of discernibly different starting the optical, electronic, and cursory belongings shown by traditionalist resolute, for example, covalent or ionic specimens [41–43]. This happens somewhat because of the regularly weedy intermolecular relations, and somewhat because of the fragile collaboration that might happen among atomic degree of independence. In the advanced occasions, atomic precious stones have ended up being the topic of incredible theoretical and investigational explore. Generally, this has focused roughly mounting an accommodating of the material science of these plans in the request to lash it up for specialized purposes like the run-of-the-mill instance of subatomic gadgets, notwithstanding this, current finishing presentation tries to attempt to grasp the climate of implicate carter in these designs [44–52]. A field of locale of consistently amazing development is that of super subatomic science. The key in at the back this deportment is that the material construction and stuffing laid out by a course of action of particles is set up to an incredible breadth by the intermolecular interfaces, for example, hydrogen bonds and van der Waals dealings.

13.2 Characterizations

13.2.1 XRD and Computational Impactness

The XRD data pose the effectiveness of the lattice parameter and confirm the sample is grown and it also tells the monoclinicity of the sample. The Figures from 13.1 to 13.7 portray the AMPHB crystals with nanotubular fabrication of the nm size with the crystal lattice, thermal ellipsoidal view of molecular representation, acidic frames of the rotations, peptide bonds for left side schema on rotation—L rotator mode; weak interactions mode of the sample, force field interactions and cloned effect with electron density variations are properly shown correspondingly with each figures. The peptide built effect of AMPHB is portrayed by Ala-Val way of amino acidic classification with phi and psi shared the 360° rotation with N and C terminals groups of NH_2 and COOH with A chain mode of L stereo type of rotations.

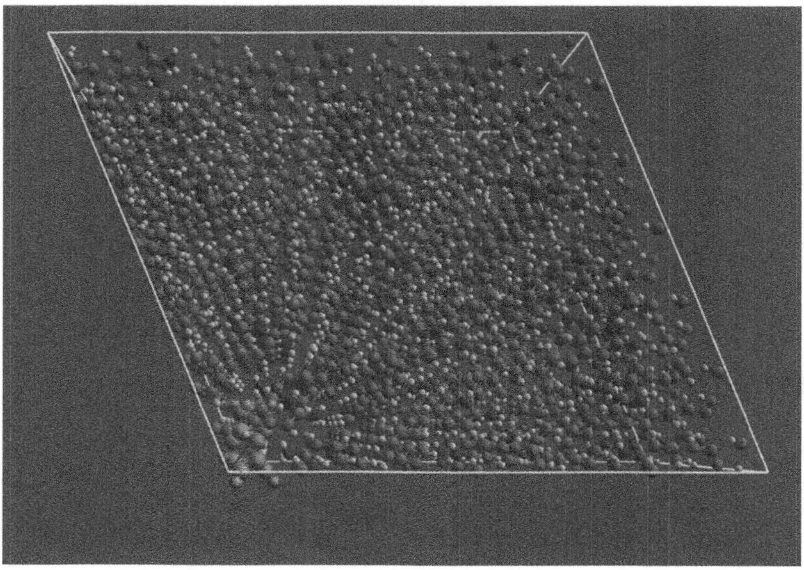

Figure 13.1 Nanotubular fabricated AMPHB crystals with order in 20 nm scaling [50–52].

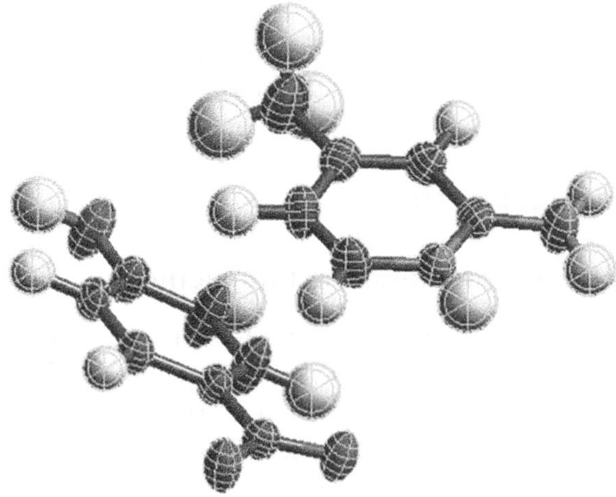

Figure 13.2 Thermal ellipsoidal 50% of AMPHB crystalline molecule [50–52].

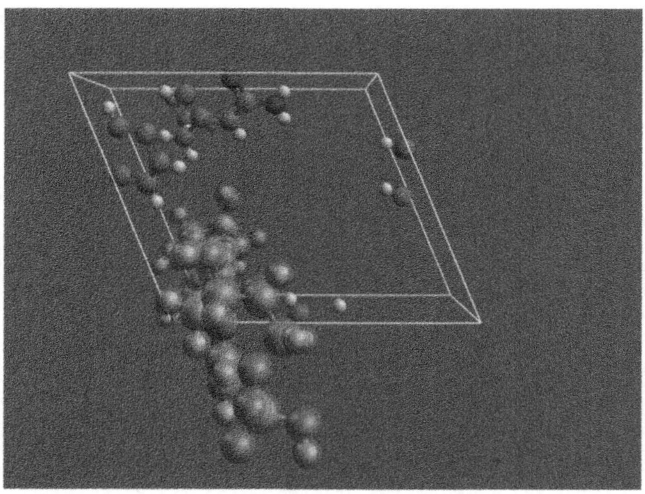

Figure 13.3 Acidic frame built on crystal structure of AMPHB [50–52].

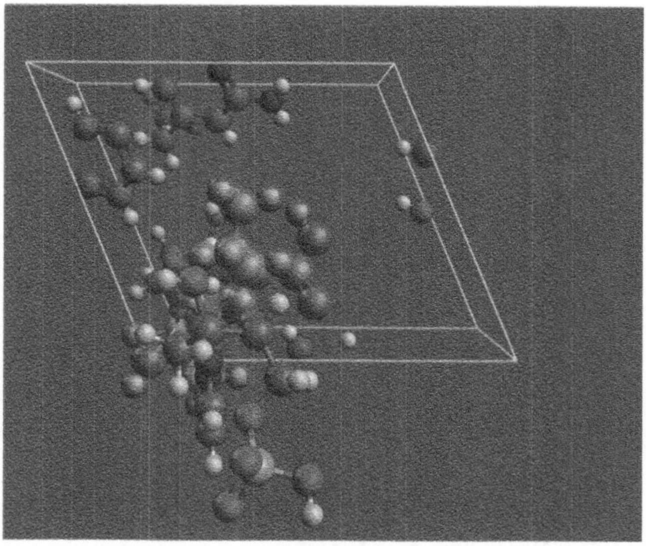

Figure 13.4 Peptide bonds in the G framed network of the crystal proceed for rotations [50–52].

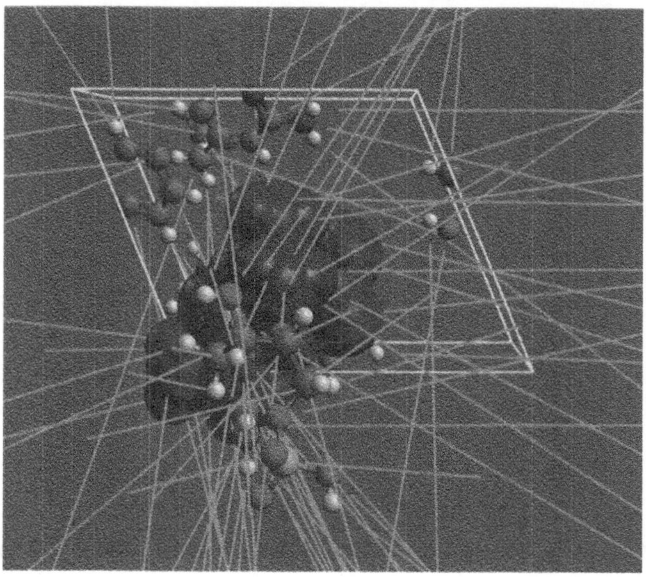

Figure 13.5 Vanderwall's efficiency of AMPHB by software—projection, force field interactions [50–52].

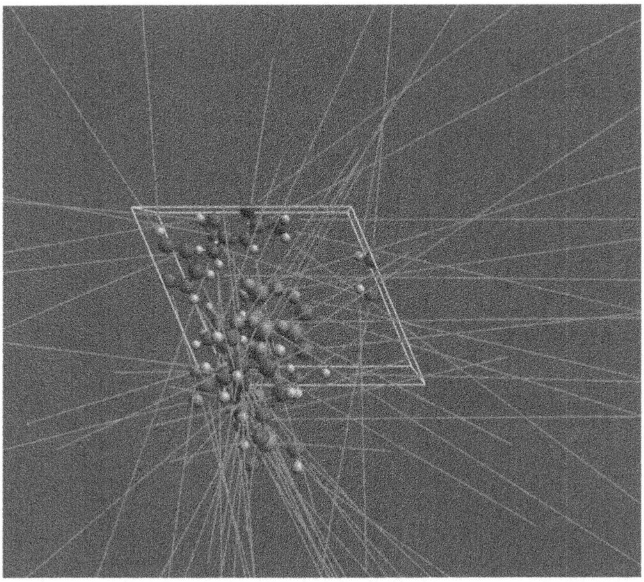

Figure 13.6 AMPHB—optimized force field for the fabricated device with crystal [50–52].

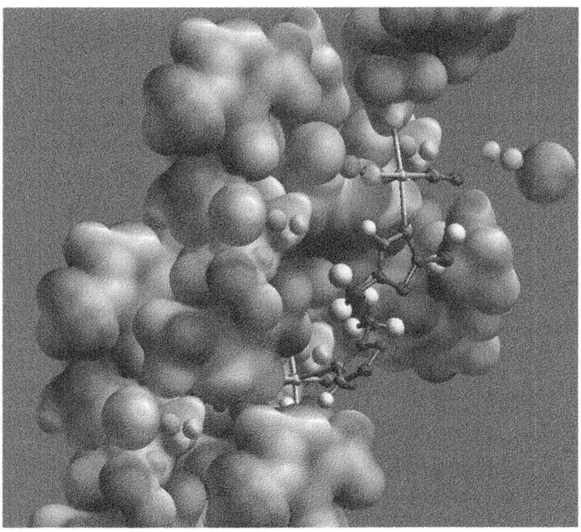

Figure 13.7 Cloned effect with electron density of AMPHB by software [50–52].

13.2.2 Antidiabetic (AD), Anti-Inflammatory (AI), and Anti-Fungal (AF) Effect of AMPHB Macro and Nano Crystals

The antidiabetic character of the AMPHB crystals are considered by means of alpha amylase-AA and Alpha glucosidase-AG and acknowledged as 37.70 and 35.16 for the macro and nano scale for AA and is mainly by the occurrence and presence of pyridine in the crystals and for AG the values are 35.41 and 32.52 nm, the IC_{50} data for the minuscule scale, which is leading than bulk ones for AD efficacy and furnish [25–34]. Also, the AI effect of AMPHB specifies 33.01 and 34.16 for macro and nano for efficiency purpose and better utility for AI effect, the AF effect of *Candida albicans* by the proper control with no effect, standard of 12, 11, and 11 for macro, nano-52 nm and nano-50 nm, the 25, 50, 75, and 100 microliters are measured with AF inhibition as 5:5:NA; 6:6:5; 7:6:5; 7:6:6 for the ascending concentration values and having good impact on AF by the macro, nano-52 and nano-50 scales as mentioned properly in Tables 13.1 to 13.3 for AD, AI, and AF.

Table 13.1 Antidiabetic data for macro and nano AMPHB crystals.

Enzymetic scheme	Macro	Nano
Alpha-amylase	37.70	35.16
Alpha-glucosidase	35.41	32.52

Table 13.2 Anti-inflammatory data for macro and nano AMPHB crystals.

Scheme	Macro	Nano
DPPH	33.01	34.16

Table 13.3 Anti-fungal activity for macro and nano AMPHB crystals.

		Zone of inhibition in mm on *Candida albicans*		
S. no	**Concentration**	**Macro**	**52 nm**	**50 nm**
1	Control	NA	NA	NA
2	Standard	12	11	11
3	25 μL	5	5	NA
4	50 μL	6	6	5
5	75 μL	7	6	5
6	100 μL	7	6	6

NA - not applicable.

13.3 Conclusion

The AMPHB crystalline specimens are respectively prepared by lucrative evaporation and by proper milled effect and confirmed the lattice data by SXRD scheme, as well as by the efficacy of the specimen. Nanotube generation is the device fabrication of the sample by using software with the crystal structure, the structure is 50% thermal ellipsoidal portrayal of the titled crystalline specimen, acidic frame work of the specimen with the proper peptide linkage stereotype of rotation specific with groups are properly enhanced and the optimized force field interactions with Vanderwall's impact for weak interactions, and the antidiabetic character of the AMPHB crystals of alpha amylase-AA and alpha glucosidase-AG and accredited as 37.70 and 35.16 for the macroscale and nanoscale for AA and is mainly by the incidence and existence of mainly the pyridine in the crystals and for AG the values are 35.41 and 32.52, the IC_{50} data for the miniature scale-nm which is foremost than bulk ones for AD efficacy and provide, also the AI effect of AMPHB specifies 33.01 as well as 34.16 for macro and nano for efficiency purpose and better utility for AI effect, the AF effect of *Candida albicans* by the proper control with no effect, standard of 12, 11 and 11 for macro, nano-52 nm and nano-50 nm, the 25, 50, 75, and 100 microliters are measured with AF inhibition as 5:5:NA; 6:6:5; 7:6:5; 7:6:6 for the rising concentration values and having good impact on AF by the macro, nano-52 and nano-50 scales as mentioned properly for AD, AI, and AF.

References

1. Kalaipoonguzhali, V., Senthilkannan, K., Thirumoorthi, C., Chinnadurai, M., Jayanalina, T., Comparison of adsorption energy, ionization potential and electron affinity of CuS-ACT and CuS-Nit nanostructures monowire for nano device fabrication by computational approach. *Mater. Today: Proc.*, 33, 7, 2759–2760, 2020.
2. Gunasekaran, S. *et al.*, Structural studies on picolinium maleate crystal by density functional methods. *Indian J. Phys.*, 87, 12, 1189–1197, 2013.
3. Senthilkannan, K. *et al.*, Anti diabetic (AD) studies of bis-glycine hydro bromide (45 nm) nano crystals. *Mater. Today: Proc.*, 33, 7, 3201–3202, 2020.
4. Senthilkannan, K. *et al.*, Anti-diabetic activites of ZnO doped with Ce (5 at %) nano particles (NPs). *Mater. Today: Proc.*, 33, 7, 3056–3057, 2020.
5. Senthilkannan, K. *et al.*, Fluorescence, filter,nano tribological studies of 12-(4-Chlorophenyl)-9,9-Dimethyl-9,10-Dihydro-8H-Benzo[A]Xanthen-11(12H)-One-(CPDDHBXH) macro and nano crystals. *Mater. Today: Proc.*, 33, 7, 4163–4166, 2020.
6. Senthilkannan, K., Venkatachalam, K., Jothibas, M., Computational and experimental studies of acetoacetanilide crystals. *AIP Conf. Proc.*, vol. 2270, pp. 040014, 1–4, 2020.
7. Senthilkannan, K., Venkatachalam, K., Rajamani, A., Computational analysis of LPNPTH anisotropies for dementia for Alzheimer's syndrome by DFT and molecular harboring. *AIP Conf. Proc.*, vol. 2270, pp. 040008, 1–5, 2020.
8. Senthilkannan, K., Sivaramakrishnan, V., Kalaipoonguzhali, V., Chinnadurai, M., Kannan, S., Electronic transport, HOMO–LUMO and computational studies of CuS monowire for nano device fabrication by DFT approach. *Mater. Today: Proc.*, 33, 7, 2746–2749, 2020.
9. Senthilkannan, K. and Gunasekaran, S., Spectroscopic studies and other novel studies of 4 bromo 4' chloro benzylidene aniline (BCBA) Crystal- A non linear optical material. *Int. J. Chemtech Res.*, 5, 6, 3051–3058, 2013.
10. Senthilkannan, K., Gayathri Devi, S., Nagarajan, P., Flora, G., Ranadevan, R., Anti diabetic (AD) studies of picolinium maleate nano crystals. *Mater. Today: Proc.*, 33, 3, 3005–3007, 2020.
11. Senthilkannan, K., Ramamurthi, K., Bhakya, K., Sivaramakrishnan, V., Kolanjinathan, M., Ranadevan, R., Hardness, Photoconductivity, Anti-diabetic Studies of L -AlaniniumFumarate (LAF) Crystals. *AIP Conf. Proc.*, vol. 2270, pp. 100010, 1–4, 2020.
12. Senthilkannan, K., Baskaran, P., Seenivasan, R., Settu, P., Tribological, Filter, FTIR and fluorescence studies of L-Alaninium tartrate (LAT) Macro and nano crystals. *Mater. Today: Proc.*, 33, 7, 4148–4150, 2020.
13. Senthilkannan, K., Kaleemullah, K., Abdul, J., Ponnusamy., V.K., Govindan, N.M., Effect of anti microbial and fluorescence on L-Alaninium maleate (LAM) macro and nano crystals. *Mater. Today: Proc.*, 33, 7, 2779–2781, 2020.

14. Senthilkannan, K., Ganesh, G., Abdul Jaffer Ali, H., Krishnaveni Ramamurthi, R., Kaleemullah, K., Anti diabetic (AD) activities of L-valinium picrate (LVP) macro and nano crystals. *Mater. Today: Proc.*, 33, 7, 2738–2740, 2020.
15. Senthilkannan, K., Bhakya, K., Iyanar, M., Growth and Influx, AC and DC Conductivity Studies of L-AlaniniumFumarate (LAF) Crystals. *AIP Conf. Proc.*, vol. 2270, pp. 100009, 1–4, 2020.
16. Senthilkannan, K., Growth, fluorescence and theoretical studies of B2CPCD crystals – Comparative analysis in macro and nano scaled crystals. *Mater. Today: Proc.*, 33, 7, 4368–4371, 2020.
17. Senthilkannan, K. *et al.*, Anti-diabetic (AD) activities of ZnO doped with Ce (7 at%) nano particles (NP). *Mater. Today: Proc.*, 33, 7, 3053–3055, 2020.
18. Senthilkannan, K. *et al.*, Tribological, filter studies of 3-Bromo-2-Hydroxy benzoic acid (BHBA) macro and nano crystals. *Mater. Today: Proc.*, 33, 7, 4145–4147, 2020.
19. Senthilkannan, K. *et al.*, Electronic transport, Homo-Lumo and computational studies of CuS-ACT monowire for nano device fabrication by software approach. *Mater. Today: Proc.*, 33, 7, 2756–2758, 2020.
20. Senthilkannan, K. *et al.*, Anti microbial and fluorescence activities of L-valinium picrate (LVP) macro and nano crystals. *Mater. Today: Proc.*, 33, 7, 2776–2778, 2020.
21. Senthilkumar, R. *et al.*, Anti-diabetic (AD) and hardness profile of 12-(4-Chlorophenyl)-9,9-Dimethyl-9,10-Dihydro-8H-benzo[a]xanthen-11(12H)-one –(CPDDHBXH) – Comparative analysis of macro and nano crystals. *Mater. Today: Proc.*, 33, 7, 4167–4170, 2020.
22. Sathishkumar, R. *et al.*, Synthesis, Growth and Characterization of 2,5 – Dimethyl-N-(3-phenylprop-2-en-1-ylidene) Aniline (2,5 DPPA) Single Crystal: A New Second Order Nonlinear Optical Material for Photonic and Optoelectronic Applications. Optik, 226, 2, 1–11, 2020.
23. Patel, R.P. *et al.*, Growth and XRD, Elemental, Mechanical, Dielectric, Optical and Photoconductivity, and Surface Morphological Characterizations of 2-[4-(Trifluoromethyl) phenyl]-1H-benzimidazole (TFMPHB) Crystals for Electronic, Mechanical Applications. *Braz. J. Phys.*, 51, 3, 339–350, 2021.
24. Aarthi, R. *et al.*, Molecular structure- associated pharmacodynamic investigation on benzoyl peroxide using spectroscopic and quantum computational tools. *J. Taibah Univ. Sci.*, 12, 1, 104–122, 2018.
25. Saravanan, P. *et al.*, Biofriendly and competent domestic microwave assisted method for the synthesis of ZnO nanoparticles from the extract of Azadirachta indica leaves. *Mater. Today: Proc.*, 33, 7, 3160–3163, 2020.
26. Saravanan, P. *et al.*, A perspective approach towards appreciable size and cost-effective solar cell fabrication by synthesizing ZnO nanoparticles from Azadirachta indica leaves extract using domestic microwave oven. *J. Mater. Sci. Mater. El.*, 31, 5, 4301–4309, 2020.

27. Saravanan, P. *et al.*, Dielectric and magnetic properties of Allium cepa and Raphanus sativus extracts biogenic ZnO nanoparticles. *J. Mater. Sci. Mater. El.*, 32, 1, 1–14, 2021.
28. Periyathambi, P. *et al.*, Fluorescence and filter characterizations of NaBr-added L-alanine (LANB) – A comparative analysis in macro and nano scaled crystals. *Mater. Today: Proc.*, 33, 3766–3769, 2020.
29. Baskaran, P. *et al.*, Anti-diabetic activities of ZnO doped with Ce (3 at %) nano particles. *Mater. Today: Proc.*, 33, 7, 3051–3052, 2020.
30. Baskaran, P. *et al.*, Anti-diabetic studies of barium paranitro phenolate macro and nano crystals. *Mater. Today: Proc.*, 33, 7, 3058–3060, 2020.
31. Kolanjinathan, M., Senthilkannan, K., Paramasivam, S., Baskaran, P., Iyanar, M., Anti-diabetic studies of 4-(4-chlorophenyl)-7,7-dimethyl-7,8-dihydro-4H-1-benzopyran-2,5(3H,6H)-dione – (CPDMDHHBPHHD) nano crystals. *Mater. Today: Proc.*, 33, 7, 2750–2752, 2020.
32. Kolanjinathan, M. *et al.*, Dielectric, fluorescence, filter, nano tribological and photoconductivity studies of 4-(4-chlorophenyl)-7,7-dimethyl-7,8-dihydro-4H-1-benzopyran-2,5(3H,6H)-dione (CPDMDHHBPHHD) macro and nano crystals. *J. Mater. Sci. Mater. El.*, 27, 4, 16907–16917, 2020.
33. Kolanjinathan, M., Hariharasuthan, R., Sivaramakrishnan, V. *et al.*, XRD, CHNSO, fluorescence, filter-influx, NLO, photoconductivity, hardness and helical spring-fabricated device stress analysis of 2′-chloro-4-methoxy-3-nitrobenzil (CMNB) crystal of different scalings for opto-electronic filter and band gap engineering utilities. *J. Mater Sci. Mater El.*, 32, 10049–10057, 2021.
34. Jothibas, M. *et al.*, Structural, optical and photo catatic activity of Ag doped ZnO nano particles obtained by sol-gel method. *AIP Conf. Proc.*, vol. 2162, pp. 020151, 1–7, 2019.
35. Selvaraj, L. *et al.*, AS Anti-diabetic (AD) studies of Bis Glycine Hydro Bromide – BGHB macro crystals milled to nano scale of 219 nm as the preliminary fine particles. *Mater. Today: Proc.*, 33, 7, 3763–3765, 2020.
36. Kishore, N. *et al.*, CO and HCHO adsorption on FeO monowire devices: a DFT study. *Appl. Phys. A*, 123, 11, 706, 1–7, 2017. https://doi.org/10.1007/s00339-017-1330-6.
37. Senthilkannan, K., Gunasekaran, S., Wagish, J.G.R., UV, SEM, Powder XRD Studies of Acetoacetanilide (AAC) Crystal. *Int. J. Chemtech Res.*, 6, 5, 3187–3190, 2014.
38. Kumar, K. *et al.*, Growth of diethyl 3,3′-[(2,4-dichlorophenyl) methylidene] bis(1H-indole-2-carboxylate)-(D32DMBC) organic NLO single crystal and its optical, thermal, mechanical, dielectric and computational studies. *J. Mater. Sci. Mater. El.*, 31, 23, 1–8, 2020. https://doi.org/10.1007/s10854-020-04594-y.
39. Senthilkannan, K., Venkatachalam, K., Bhakya, K., Sharmidha, B., Kalaivani, M., Gayathri Devi, S., Growth and Characterization of Picolinium Maleate (PM) Crystals. *AIP Conf. Proc.*, vol. 2270, pp. 10014, 1–4, 2020, https://doi.org/10.1063/5.0019341.

40. Senthilkannan, K., Thamarikannan, P., Kalaipoonguzhali, V., Venkatachalam, K., Kannan, S., Baskar, A., Fluorescence, computational enactments of dimethyl N,N′-[(ethyne-1, 2-di-yl)Bis-(1,4- phenyl-ene carbon-yl)]bis-(l-al-aninate) crystals. *AIP Conf. Proc.*, vol. 2270, pp. 100008, 1–4, 2020, https://doi.org/10.1063/5.0019334.
41. Senthilkannan, K., Thamaraikannan, P., Kalaipoonguzhali, V., Venkatachalam, K., Kannan, S., Ranadevan, R., Computational IR, Raman studies by DFT program and antidiabetic delineation by harboring of acetoacetanilide crystals. *AIP Conf. Proc.*, vol. 2270, pp. 10013, 1–4, 2020, https://doi.org/10.1063/5.0019339.
42. Flora, G. *et al.*, Anti-diabetic (AD) and crystal stiffness characterizations of NaBr-added L-alanine (LANB) – A comparative analysis in macro and nano scale crystals. *Mater. Today: Proc.*, 33, 7, 3937–3941, 2020.
43. Flora, G. *et al.*, Anti diabetic (AD), stiffness and hardness studies of 2-[4-(Trifluoromethyl) phenyl]-1H-benzimidazole crystals - (TFMPHB) macro and nano crystal. *Mater. Today: Proc.*, 33, 4233–4236, 2020.
44. Flora, G. *et al.*, Anti-inflammatory (AI) and crystalline hardness characterisations of 4-(4-chlorophenyl)-7,7-dimethyl-7,8-dihydro-4h-1-benzopyran-2,5(3h,6h)-dione-(CPDMDHHBPHHD) – comparative analysis of macro and nano scales crystals. *Mater. Today: Proc.*, 33, 3578–3582, 2020.
45. Ganesan, S., Gurunathan, R., Pasupuleti, R.R. *et al.*, Green synthesis of V2O5/ZnO nanocomposite materials for efficient photocatalytic and anti-bacterial applications. *Appl. Nanosci.*, 2021. https://doi.org/10.1007/s13204-021-01923-3.
46. Ganesan, H., Senthilkannan, K., Christy, S. *et al.*, Synthesis, growth, XRD, NLO, CHNSO, computational-structural, dielectric, photoconductivity, hardness and biostudies of diethyl 2-amino-5-{4-[bis (4-methyl phenyl) amino] benzamido} thiophene-3,4-dicarboxylate (DABMPABTD) macro-, nano crystals for device fabrication, pharma, electronic uses. *J. Mater. Sci. Mater. El.*, 32, 15498–15508, 2021.
47. Maalmarugan, J., Yokeswaran, V., Divya, R. *et al.*, Synthesis, growth, XRD, NLO, CHNSO, structure by theoretical approach, dielectric, absorbance, photoconductivity and bio studies of 4-(4-Acetyl-5-Methyl-1H-1, 2, 3-Triazol-1-yl) Benzonitrile crystals for optical, opto-electronic, and photonics utilities. *J. Mater. Sci. Mater. El.*, 32, 13850–13858, 2021. https://doi.org/10.1007/s10854-021-05960-0.
48. Rajkumar, M., Maalmarugan, J., Flora, G. *et al.*, Growth, characterizations, and the structural elucidation of diethyl-2-(3-oxoiso-1,3-dihydrobenzofuran-1-ylidene)malonate crystalline specimen for dielectric and electronic filters, thermal, optical, mechanical, and biomedical applications using conventional experimental and theoretical practices. *J. Mater. Sci. Mater. El.*, 32, 22822–22839, 2021. https://doi.org/10.1007/s10854-021-06761-1.
49. Senthilkannan, K., Flora, G., Gunasekaran, S., Ali, H.A.J., Vimalan, M., Balasubramanian, S., Extraction of Silver Nanoparticles (Ag-NPs) by Green

Synthesis from Aqueous Extract of Seaweeds and Their Consequences on HeLa Cell Line and Their Utility on Soil by Spectroscopic Tools, in: *Nanotechnology for Advances in Medical Microbiology. Environmental and Microbial Biotechnology*, Springer, Singapore, 2021, https://doi.org/10.1007/978-981-15-9916-3_5.

50. Momma, K. and Izumi, F., VESTA 3 for three-dimensional visualization of crystal, volumetric and morphology data. *J. Appl. Crystallogr.*, 44, 1272–1276, 2011.
51. Spackman, P.R., Turner, M.J., McKinnon, J.J., Wolff, S.K., Grimwood, D.J., Jayatilaka, D., Spackman, M.A., Crystal Explorer: a program for Hirshfeld surface analysis, visualization and quantitative analysis of molecular crystals, *J. Appl. Crystallogr.*, 54, 3,1006–1011, 20212021. https://doi.org/10.1107/S1600576721002910.
52. Spek, A.L., Single – crystal structure validation with the program PLATON. *J. Appl. Crystallogr.*, 36, 7–11, 2003.

14

Super Lattice, Computational Interactions and Bio-Uses of CPDMDP Crystals

Flora G.[1], Christy S.[2], Shobana V.[3], Divya R.[4], Jemma Hermelin Jesy Diaz[5], Pauline Jenifer S.[1], Senthil Kannan K.[6]* and Jacintha Tamil Malar A.[1]

[1]Department of Botany, St. Mary's College – Autonomous, Thoothukudi, Tamil Nadu, India
[2]Department of Information Technology, Saveetha School of Engineering, Saveetha Institute of Medical and Technical Sciences, Saveetha University, Chennai, TN, India
[3]Department of Physics, Mohamed Sathak AJ College of Engineering, Chennai, Tamil Nadu, India
[4]Department of Physics, S.T. Hindu College, Nagercoil, TN, India
[5]Department of Zoology, St. Mary's College – Autonomous, Thoothukudi, Tamil Nadu, India
[6]Department of R&D/Physics, Edayathangudy G.S. Pillay Arts and Science College (Autonomous – Affiliated to Bharathidasan University – Tiruchirappalli), Nagapattinam, Tamil Nadu, India

Abstract
The crystals of macro and nano scales are preferred because of their potential utility in electronic, mechano and bio/pharma utilities; they are preferred because of the impact utility and perfect size and utilities, not by approximation and by accuracy; the CPDMDP (Catena-Poly[[dithiocyanatomanganese(II)]-di-μ-4,4¢-methylenebis(3,5-dimethylpyrazole)]) crystals are successfully grown by solution growth methodology; the formula is $Mn(C_{11}H_{16}N_4)_2(SCN)_2$; base is monoclinic system of bulk crystal and have well intended super cell lattice device construction, nano tubular fabrication, computational interactions and biological utilities, such as anti-diabetic and antioxidant, influx for filter utilities of macro, nano scaled crystals, and long lasting due to pyrazole and presence of manganese and better known by their projected and reported uses. The effectiveness and efficacy is better identified for the CPDMDP based on the chain and by the pyrazole and is having

**Corresponding author*: mscgoldmedalist@yahoo.in

Kaushik Pal (ed.) Nanovaccinology as Targeted Therapeutics, (227–242) © 2022 Scrivener Publishing LLC

nano impact more viable and enabled than the bulk. Alpha-amylase, DPPH, FRAP are for diabetic, oxidant predominant one for data of both scales. The novelty is mainly because of the presence of pyrazole, having projected pharma use; and specifically higher-volume super cell structural interactions and futuristic way in harboring can be proceeded.

***Keywords*:** Super-cell, nano-tubular, interactions, pharma

14.1 Introduction

Crystals are predominant and inevitable in the day-to day-life of an apparatus/components/machines and for human beings by their prolonged and long-lasting uses and have good natural optical materials that are of current interest because they are being used in cutting edge optical information preparing gadgets [1, 2]. Optical properties are significant in the creation of photonic exchanging gadgets, diodes and solar/sunlight-based cells [3–6]. Optical cooperations incorporate distinct recurrence age, the force reliance of the compound, refractive data, dispersing [7–12]. The p-bond framework with suitable electron giver and acceptor gatherings can upgrade the lopsided electronic dispersion prompting an expanded optical nonlinearity [13–20]. The natural materials are better contrasted with inorganic by their serious level of nonlinearity and high harm obstruction. The plan of other organic/natural NLO precious ones of the crystalline type with explicit physical and compound properties is impacted by intermolecular and intramolecular cooperations [31–36]. The intermolecular communications in the translucent construction of the developed CPDMDP crystals were investigated by a Hirshfeld surface and a finger impression plot. Gaussian'09 adaptation E.01 programming bundle utilizing B3LYP technique was utilized to perform DFT computational examinations. To produce Hirshfeld 2D finger impression plots, d_i, d_e and d_{norm} surfaces, curvedness, shape Crystal Explorer program bundle was utilized, for super crystal and nano device fabrication [21–24]. The pyrrazole is an organic matter having discerning proficient pharma uses. The natural crystalline species have all around discovered consumptions in electronic-mechano-bio sciences and in originality, here, the CPDMDP are recognized to continue for the nano tube development, ellipsoidal outline, peptide association of CPDMDP, improved power field—adequacy, Vanderwall's effect of the crystal, hostile to diabetic, antifungal, and mitigating portrayals and revealed [25–28]. Atomic gems set forward a prosperous layer of bodily marvel discernibly different starting the visual, electronic and spur of the moment assets exhibited by conventionalist steadfast like covalent or ionic gems. This happens somewhat because of the typically weedy intermolecular relations, and somewhat because of the sensitive association that might happen among atomic degree of independence [29–34]. In the advanced occasions, subatomic precious stones have ended up being the subject of amazing speculative investigations. Generally, his has focused on roughly mounting a chivalrous of the material science of these plans in the request to tie up for specialized purposes, like the common instance of atomic hardware; notwithstanding this, current fruition presentation attempts to try to fathom the climate of implicate carter in these constructions [35–40]. A field of locale of consistently amazing development is that of super-atomic science [41–43]. This enchanting locale is based ahead the use of individual particles in direct attempt to propose intentional atomic gems that might be utilized for an assortment of specialized purposes. The key in at the back this mentality for construction and stuffing laid out by a game plan of particles is set up to an incredible breadth by the intermolecular interfaces, for example, hydrogen bonds and van der Waals transactions [44–52].

14.2 Computational

The effective calculations and structural changes as well as new structures are properly enunciated, efficiently portrayed using softwares and simulations for the entitled crystalline specimen for the molecule with ball and stick portrayal as seen in Figure 14.1. The 3D effect of the entitled crystals is presented in Figure 14.2, the Halosian effect for crystal projection in Figure 14.3, effective schema of weak interfaces is shown in Figure 14.4, and pixel size and box width elucidation is shown in Figure 14.5. Materials are realized by their utility and projection over a specific domain and here the CPDMDP crystals by their structure adequate for the nano device fabrication as shown in Figure 14.6, the Hirshfeld analysis for CPDMDP is well portrayed for no effect, d_i, d_e, d_{norm}, shape index, curvedness, and fragmented patch with d_i Vs d_e graph as finger printed region in Figure 14.7, weak interaction with color potential effect as in Figure 14.8, the super cell CPDMDP lattice as in Figure 14.9. Voids are very specific in crystals and electron max and min effect are portrayed as electron density and deformation density in the CPDMDP as in Figure 14.10 as given below.

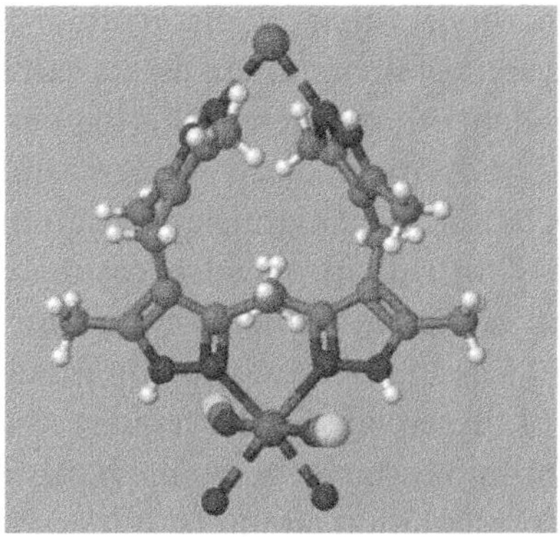

Figure 14.1 Molecule-CPDMDP—Ball and stick depiction.

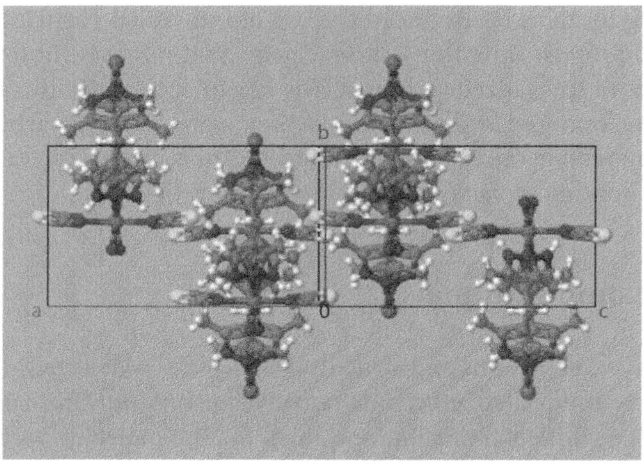

Figure 14.2 CPDMDP—3D effect [50–52].

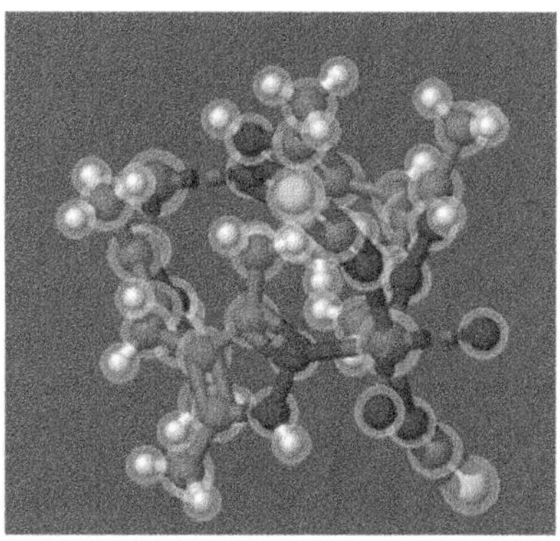

Figure 14.3 CPDMDP—Halosian effect.

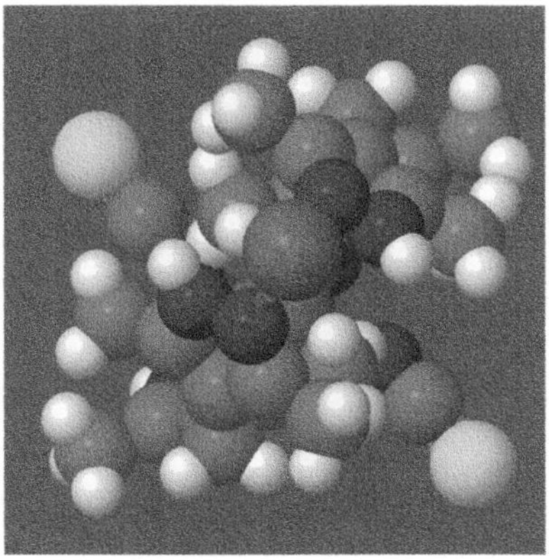

Figure 14.4 Molecule—50% Vanderwall's plan [50–52].

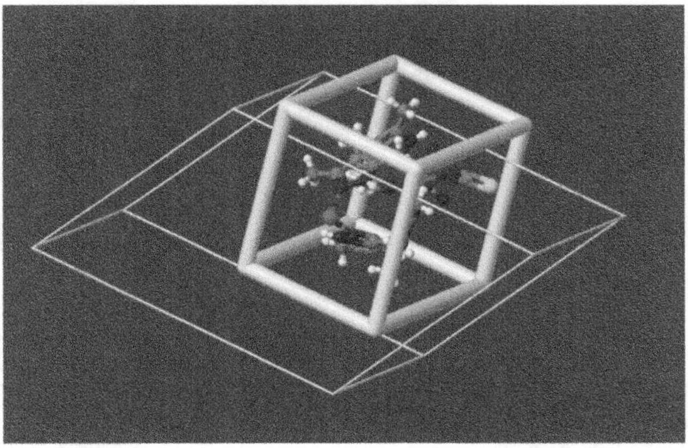

Figure 14.5 CPDMDP—Unit cell of 0.1Å with 1x pixel size and box bounded with 0.5 Å width [50–52].

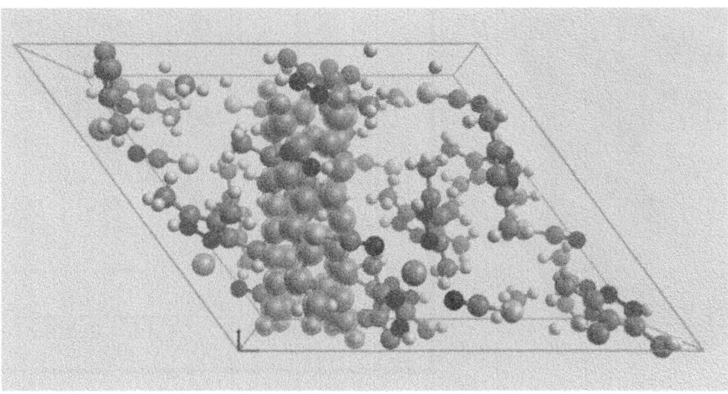

Figure 14.6 CPDMDP—Nano tubular generation built with C-H atoms of 2 × 3 order [50–52].

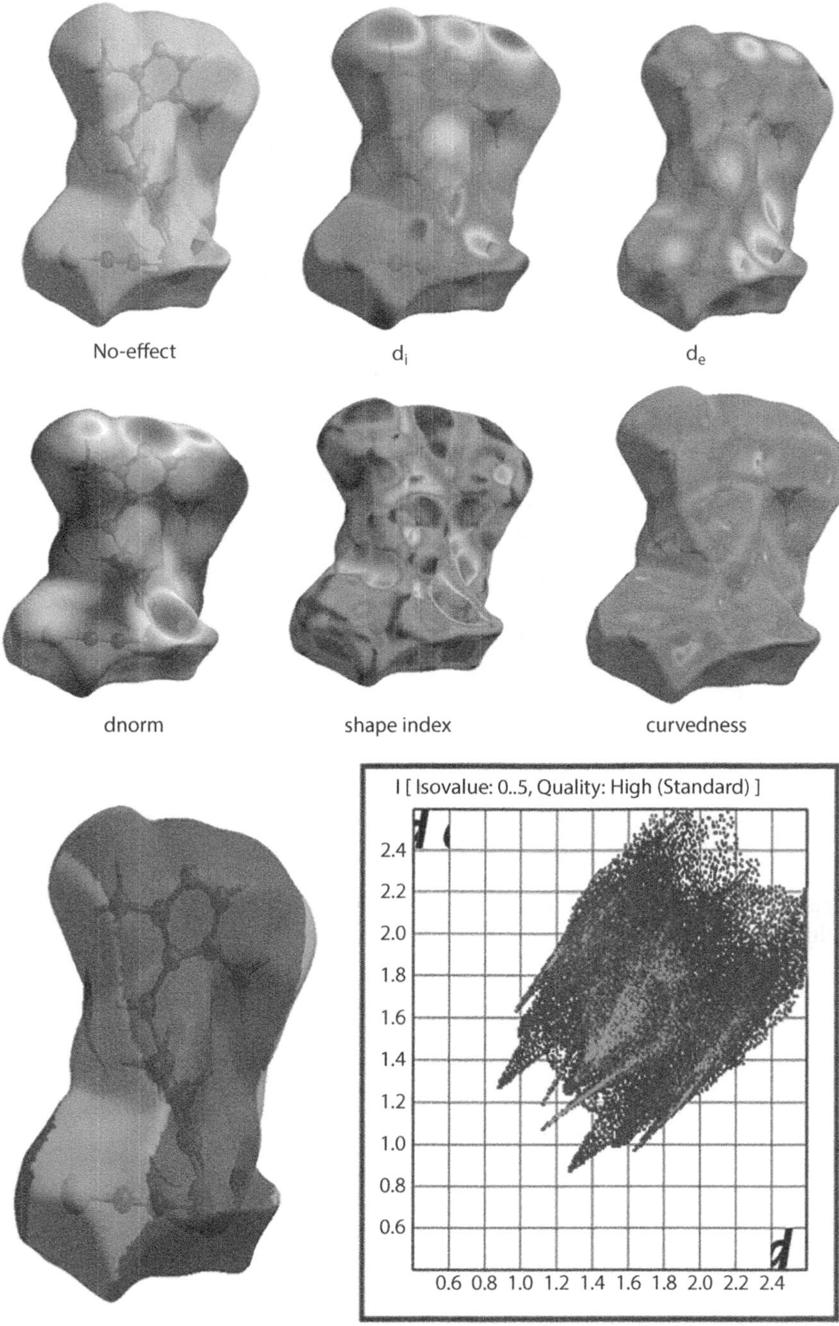

Figure 14.7 CPDMDP—Hirshfeld analysis with finger print effectiveness [50–52].

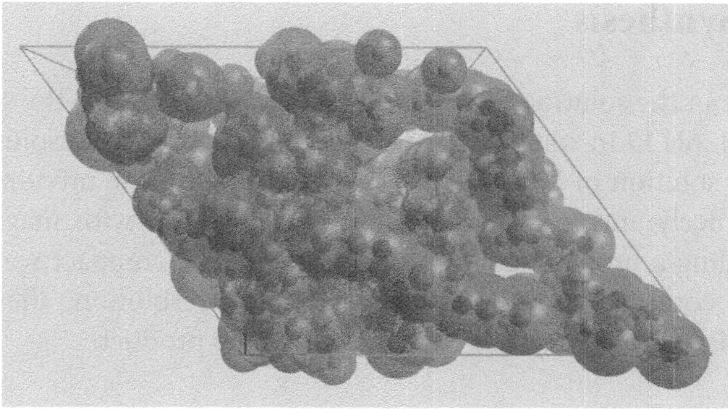

Figure 14.8 CPDMDP—Vanderwall's effect with coloured potential effect [50–52].

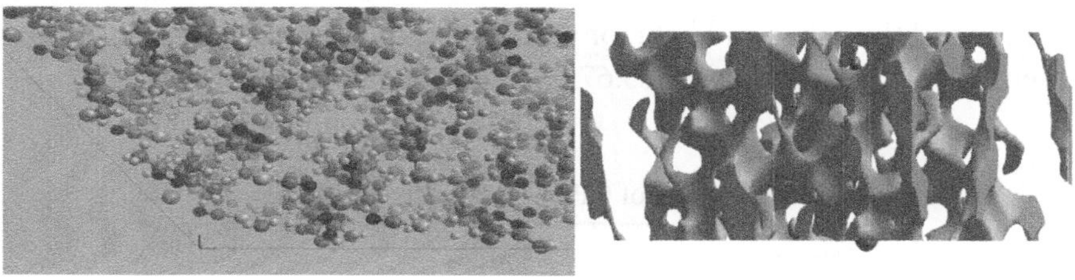

Figure 14.9 CPDMDP—Super crystal lattice with 3 × 3 × 3 scheme (a) Crystalline voids [50–52].

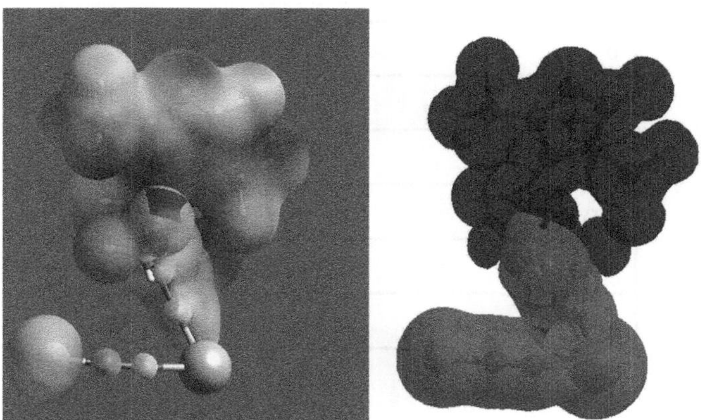

Figure 14.10 CPDMDP - Crystalline voids, electron density and deformation density-software effectiveness [50–52].

14.3 Synthesis

H2mbdpz in the solution of ethanol was properly added to the solution of $Mn(ClO_4)_2.6H_2O$ in water. After the perfect and proper dissolution completion, a solution of NH_4SCN was slowly added to the mixture and was refluxed nicely and in a perfect manner for 2-2.5 h with magnetic stirring, yielding a brown colored precipitate, and the compact was liquified in D.M.F, constructing a precise and complete resolution; after 16 days, pale-reddish colored crystals were yielded as the product.

14.4 XRD

The crystals of CPDMDP are grown by solution growth method; and XRD data reveal the a, b, c and beta for the monoclinic system with space group identity C2/c and volume 3565.67 Å^3 and is mentioned in Table 14.1.

Table 14.1 XRD of CPDMDP macro crystals.

Parameters	**Values**
Empirical formula	$[Mn(C_{11}H_{16}N_4)_2(SCN)_2]$
Crystalline system	Monoclinic
a	21.257Å
b	9.723 Å
c	17.252 Å
Beta	126.610°
Crystal size	6 × 5 × 4 mm^3
Volume	3565.67 Å^3
Space group	C2/c

Table 14.2 Influx of macro, nano CPDMDP crystals.

Influx macro scaling	Influx nano scaling
1.9295 microns	2.4533 microns

14.5 Influx of CPDMDP of Both Scales

Influx value of 1.9295 microns of CPDMDP represents that the macro influx refers that CPDMDP is a high-quality crystal as it is less than 10 microns as the case represents the profile of the system and 2.4533 microns is a nano level influx. So, the CPDMDP macro and nano crystals are used in filter applications especially opto-electronics also as the data are represented in Table 14.2.

14.6 Antidiabetic Activity of Macro, Nano CPDMDP Crystals

Diabetes is a disorder that happens while a person's blood glucose, regularly referred to as blood sugar, rises to dangerously excessive levels. Blood glucose that is derived from meals is our maximum critical supply of energy. Insulin, a hormone produced via way of means of the pancreas, aids glucose absorption into cells for energy production. Sometimes, the human frame no longer produces sufficient or any insulin or insulin will not feature properly. The glucose remains inside the bloodstream and no longer attain the cells. A great deal of glucose inside the bloodstream can cause fitness troubles over time. Diabetes mellitus may be highly controlled primarily with nanotechnology-based techniques, which lessen the hazard of acute and persistent troubles. Nanotechnology's applications in disease diagnosis are fast evolving. These materials are important and indispensable in many areas of human endeavour because of their distinct size-dependent properties. For the treatment of diabetes, many nano formulations with various systems have been created. In particular, the nanoparticles of these samples were more impactful. Nanoparticles have been used *in vitro* and *in vivo* for various applications. Nanoparticles (NPs) and nano crystals are attracting a lot of attention from a therapeutic and diagnostic point of view because of their physicochemical properties that will be more effective, less toxic, and will change medicine with smart outcomes. According to researches, the drug can now be encapsulated into virus-sized nanoparticles. Because nanoparticles can accurately locate damaged cells and deliver medicine to them, they are useful for medication delivery and medicine delivery to the body. The antidiabetic activity of macro and nano CPDMDP crystals is the point of interest of this research. In Table 14.3, the IC50 values for macro and nano crystals of CPDMDP are listed. The maximum normally used and beneficial indicator of a drug's efficacy is half-maximal inhibitory

Table 14.3 AD of macro, nano CPDMDP crystals.

IC 50 values of macro CPDMDP	IC 50 values of nano CPDMDP
39.52	34.45

Table 14.4 AO of macro, nano CPDMDP crystals.

Samples	**% of DPPH for macro scale**	**% of DPPH for nano scale**
CPDMDP	37.34	34.21
Samples	% of FRAP for macro scale	% of FRAP for nano scale
CPDMDP	21.6	19.1

concentration (IC50). It specifies how tons medicinal drugs are needed to barrage an organic technique through half, and consequently serves as a pharmacological efficiency indicator for antagonist drugs. For the antidiabetic activity of CPDMDP crystals, the IC 50 values for macro and nano scales are 39.52 and 34.45, respectively, and the inhibition values growth because the macro scale is transformed to nano size, at the same time as the IC 50 fee decreases, which is suitable for antidiabetic activity work. The presence of pyrazole, as opposed to Magnesium, is in general answerable for CPDMDP's antidiabetic action. When compared to macro particles, nanoparticles are the best source for treating diabetic mellitus. This is also reflected in the outcome.

14.7 Antioxidant Activity

Free radicals are known to have an unpaired electron in the outer orbit, which is responsible to cause various chronic and degenerative diseases like premature aging, cardiac diseases, cancer, organ failure, inflammation, stroke and diabetes. Free radicals are produced in the human body both directly by metabolic processes and indirectly by external factors, like pollution, toxic metals, cigarette smoke, pesticides, industrial emission and poor management of radioactive wastes from various sources, and so on. Every human body system has its own antioxidant defense mechanism to prevent or slow down the damage caused by the free radicals. Some antioxidant substances like lipoic acid and glutothione are naturally produced by the body while other compounds have to be supplemented by food or medication. These compounds are capable to terminate the chain reaction by eliminating the free radical. Potential antioxidants compounds can be identified by *in vitro* experiments, like DPPH and FRAP assays. DPPH is 2,2-diphenyl-1-picrylhydrazyl crystalline powder composed of stable free-radical molecules. In DPPH assay, the radicals are reduced by a hydrogen donor (antioxidant compound). In the present study (Table 14.4), CPDMDP crystal exhibited the highest DPPH scavenging activity (37.34%) in macro scale than nano scale (34.21). FRAP assay deals with the reduction of ferric iron (Fe^{3+}) to ferrous iron (Fe^{2+}) by chemical reaction with the presence of potential antioxidants. Similar to DPPH assay, FRAP assay also reported highest antioxidant activity in macro scale (21.6%) crystals than nano scale (19.1%) of CPDMDP. While comparing the two assays, the values are evident that the radical scavenging capacity of the examined crystal was sensitive to DPPH assay. CPDMDP crystals may act as an efficacious antioxidant by suppressing the free radical activity in the biological system.

14.8 Conclusion

The materials are leading in this universe by means of their prime utility and versatile applications and CPDMDP are of important and best crystal by their diffraction pattern, computational effectiveness by Hirshfeld analysis, void spacing, super cell lattice, nano tubular fabrication and elucidation of structure by software tools and the effectiveness and efficacy is better identified for the CPDMDP based on the chain and by the pyrazole and is having nano impact more viable and enabled than the bulk. Alpha-amylase, DPPH, and FRAP are for diabetic, oxidant predominant one for data of both scales. The novelty is mainly due to presence of pyrazole, having projected pharma use; and specifically higher volume super cell structural interactions and futuristic way in harboring can be proceeded.

References

1. Kalaipoonguzhali, V., Senthilkannan, K., Thirumoorthi, C., Chinnadurai, M., Jayanalina, T., Comparison of adsorption energy, ionization potential and electron affinity of CuS-ACT and CuS-Nit nanostructures monowire for nano device fabrication by computational approach. *Mater. Today: Proc.*, 33, 7, 2759–2760, 2020.
2. Gunasekaran, S. *et al.*, Structural studies on picolinium maleate crystal by density functional methods. *Indian J. Phys.*, 87, 12, 1189–1197, 2013.

3. Senthilkannan, K. *et al.*, Anti diabetic (AD) studies of bis-glycine hydro bromide (45 nm) nano crystals. *Mater. Today: Proc.*, 33, 7, 3201–3202, 2020.
4. Senthilkannan, K. *et al.*, Anti-diabetic activites of ZnO doped with Ce (5 at %) nano particles (NPs). *Mater. Today: Proc.*, 33, 7, 3056–3057, 2020.
5. Senthilkannan, K. *et al.*, Fluorescence, filter, nano tribological studies of 12-(4-Chlorophenyl)-9,9-Dimethyl-9,10-Dihydro-8H-Benzo[A]Xanthen-11(12H)-One-(CPDDHBXH) macro and nano crystals. *Mater. Today: Proc.*, 33, 7, 4163–4166, 2020.
6. Senthilkannan, K., Venkatachalam, K., Jothibas, M., Computational and experimental studies of acetoacetanilide crystals. *AIP Conf. Proc*, vol. 2270, pp. 040014, 1–4, 2020.
7. Senthilkannan, K., Venkatachalam, K., Rajamani, A., Computational analysis of LPNPTH anisotropies for dementia for Alzheimer's syndrome by DFT and molecular harboring. *AIP Conf. Proc*, vol. 2270, pp. 040008, 1–5, 2020.
8. Senthilkannan, K., Sivaramakrishnan, V., Kalaipoonguzhali, V., Chinnadurai, M., Kannan, S., Electronic transport, HOMO–LUMO and computational studies of CuS monowire for nano device fabrication by DFT approach. *Mater. Today: Proc.*, 33, 7, 2746–2749, 2020.
9. Senthilkannan, K. and Gunasekaran, S., Spectroscopic studies and other novel studies of 4 bromo 4' chloro benzylidene aniline (BCBA) Crystal - A non linear optical material. *Int. J. Chemtech Res.*, 5, 6, 3051–3058, 2013.
10. Senthilkannan, K., Gayathri Devi, S., Nagarajan, P., Flora, G., Ranadevan, R., Anti diabetic (AD) studies of picolinium maleate nano crystals. *Mater. Today: Proc.*, 33, 3, 3005–3007, 2020.
11. Senthilkannan, K., Ramamurthi, K., Bhakya, K., Sivaramakrishnan, V., Kolanjinathan, M., Ranadevan, R., Hardness, photoconductivity, anti-diabetic studies of L-AlaniniumFumarate (LAF) crystals. *AIP Conf. Proc*, vol. 2270, pp. 100010, 1–4, 2020.
12. Senthilkannan, K., Baskaran, P., Seenivasan, R., Settu, P., Tribological, filter, FTIR and fluorescence studies of L-Alaninium tartrate (LAT) macro and nano crystals. *Mater. Today: Proc.*, 33, 7, 4148–4150, 2020.
13. Senthilkannan, K., Kaleemullah, K., Abdul, J., Ponnusamy., V.K., Govindan, N.M., Effect of anti microbial and fluorescence on L-Alaninium maleate (LAM) macro and nano crystals. *Mater. Today: Proc.*, 33, 7, 2779–2781, 2020.
14. Senthilkannan, K., Ganesh, G., Abdul Jaffer Ali, H., Krishnaveni Ramamurthi, R., Kaleemullah, K., Anti diabetic (AD) activities of L-valinium picrate (LVP) macro and nano crystals. *Mater. Today: Proc.*, 33, 7, 2738–2740, 2020.
15. Senthilkannan, K., Bhakya, K., Iyanar, M., Growth and influx, AC and DC conductivity studies of L-Alaninium Fumarate (LAF) crystals. *AIP Conf. Proc*, vol. 2270, pp. 100009, 1–4, 2020.
16. Senthilkannan, K., Growth, fluorescence and theoretical studies of B2CPCD crystals – Comparative analysis in macro and nano scaled crystals. *Mater. Today: Proc.*, 33, 7, 4368–4371, 2020.

17. Senthilkannan, K. *et al.*, Anti-diabetic (AD) activities of ZnO doped with Ce (7 at%) nano particles (NP). *Mater. Today: Proc.*, 33, 7, 3053–3055, 2020.
18. Senthilkannan, K. *et al.*, Tribological, filter studies of 3-Bromo-2-Hydroxy benzoic acid (BHBA) macro and nano crystals. *Mater. Today: Proc.*, 33, 7, 4145–4147, 2020.
19. Senthilkannan, K. *et al.*, Electronic transport, Homo-Lumo and computational studies of CuS-ACT monowire for nano device fabrication by software approach. *Mater. Today: Proc.*, 33, 7, 2756–2758, 2020.
20. Senthilkannan, K. *et al.*, Anti microbial and fluorescence activities of L-valinium picrate (LVP) macro and nano crystals. *Mater. Today: Proc.*, 33, 7, 2776–2778, 2020.
21. Senthilkumar, R. *et al.*, Anti-diabetic (AD) and hardness profile of 12-(4-Chlorophenyl)-9,9- Dimethyl-9,10-Dihydro-8H-benzo[a]xanthen-11(12H)-one –(CPDDHBXH) – Comparative analysis of macro and nano crystals. *Mater. Today: Proc.*, 33, 7, 4167–4170, 2020.
22. Sathishkumar, R. *et al.*, Synthesis, Growth and Characterization of 2,5–Dimethyl-N-(3-phenylprop-2-en-1-ylidene) Aniline (2,5 DPPA) single crystal: A new second order nonlinear optical material for photonic and Optoelectronic Applications. *Optik*, 226, 2, 1–11, 2020.
23. Patel, R.P. *et al.*, Growth and XRD, elemental, mechanical, dielectric, optical and photoconductivity, and surface morphological characterizations of 2-[4-(Trifluoromethyl) phenyl]-1H-benzimidazole (TFMPHB) crystals for electronic, mechanical applications. *Braz. J. Phys.*, 51, 3, 339–350, 2021.
24. Aarthi, R. *et al.*, Molecular structure-associated pharmacodynamic investigation on benzoyl peroxide using spectroscopic and quantum computational tools. *J. Taibah Univ. Sci.*, 12, 1, 104–122, 2018.
25. Saravanan, P. *et al.*, Biofriendly and competent domestic microwave assisted method for the synthesis of ZnO nanoparticles from the extract of Azadirachta indica leaves. *Mater. Today: Proc.*, 33, 7, 3160–3163, 2020.
26. Saravanan, P. *et al.*, A perspective approach towards appreciable size and cost-effective solar cell fabrication by synthesizing ZnO nanoparticles from Azadirachta indica leaves extract using domestic microwave oven. *J. Mater. Sci. Mater. El.*, 31, 5, 4301–4309, 2020.
27. Saravanan, P. *et al.*, Dielectric and magnetic properties of Allium cepa and Raphanus sativus extracts biogenic ZnO nanoparticles. *J. Mater. Sci. Mater. El.*, 32, 1, 1–14, 2021.
28. Periyathambi, P. *et al.*, Fluorescence and filter characterizations of NaBr-added L-alanine (LANB) – A comparative analysis in macro and nano scaled crystals. *Mater. Today: Proc.*, 33, 3766–3769, 2020.
29. Baskaran, P. *et al.*, Anti-diabetic activities of ZnO doped with Ce (3 at %) nano particles. *Mater. Today: Proc.*, 33, 7, 3051–3052, 2020.
30. Baskaran, P. *et al.*, Anti-diabetic studies of barium paranitro phenolate macro and nano crystals. *Mater. Today: Proc.*, 33, 7, 3058–3060, 2020.

31. Kolanjinathan, M., Senthilkannan, K., Paramasivam, S., Baskaran, P., Iyanar, M., Anti-diabetic studies of 4-(4-chlorophenyl)-7,7-dimethyl-7,8-dihydro-4H-1-benzopyran-2,5(3H,6H)-dione – (CPDMDHHBPHHD) nano crystals. *Mater. Today: Proc.*, 33, 7, 2750–2752, 2020.
32. Kolanjinathan, M. *et al.*, Dielectric, fluorescence, filter, nano tribological and photoconductivity studies of 4-(4-chlorophenyl)-7,7-dimethyl-7,8-dihydro-4H-1-benzopyran-2,5(3H,6H)-dione (CPDMDHHBPHHD) macro and nano crystals. *J. Mater. Sci. Mater. El.*, 27, 4, 16907–16917, 2020.
33. Kolanjinathan, M., Hariharasuthan, R., Sivaramakrishnan, V. *et al.*, XRD, CHNSO, fluorescence, filter-influx, NLO, photoconductivity, hardness and helical spring-fabricated device stress analysis of 2′-chloro-4-methoxy-3-nitrobenzil (CMNB) crystal of different scalings for opto-electronic filter and band gap engineering utilities. *J. Mater Sci. Mater El.*, 32, 10049–10057, 2021.
34. Jothibas, M. *et al.*, Structural, optical and photo catatic activity of Ag doped ZnO nano particles obtained by sol-gel method. *AIP Conf. Proc*, vol. 2162, pp. 020151, 1–7, 2019.
35. Selvaraj, L. *et al.*, AS Anti-diabetic (AD) studies of Bis Glycine Hydro Bromide – BGHB macro crystals milled to nano scale of 219 nm as the preliminary fine particles. *Mater. Today: Proc.*, 33, 7, 3763–3765, 2020.
36. Kishore, N. *et al.*, CO and HCHO adsorption on FeO monowire devices: A DFT study. *Appl. Phys. A*, 123, 11, 706, 1–7, 2017. https://doi.org/10.1007/s00339-017-1330-6.
37. Senthilkannan, K., Gunasekaran, S., Wagish, J.G.R., UV, SEM, powder XRD studies of Acetoacetanilide (AAC) Crystal. *Int. J. Chemtech Res.*, 6, 5, 3187–3190, 2014.
38. Kumar, K. *et al.*, Growth of diethyl 3,3′-[(2,4-dichlorophenyl) methylidene] bis(1H-indole-2-carboxylate)-(D32DMBC) organic NLO single crystal and its optical, thermal, mechanical, dielectric and computational studies. *J. Mater. Sci. Mater. El.*, 31, 23, 1–8, 2020. https://doi.org/10.1007/s10854-020-04594-y.
39. Senthilkannan, K., Venkatachalam, K., Bhakya, K., Sharmidha, B., Kalaivani, M., Gayathri Devi, S., Growth and characterization of Picolinium Maleate (PM) crystals. *AIP Conf. Proc*, vol. 2270, pp. 10014, 1–4, 2020, https://doi.org/10.1063/5.0019341.
40. Senthilkannan, K., Thamarikannan, P., Kalaipoonguzhali, V., Venkatachalam, K., Kannan, S., Baskar, A., Fluorescence, computational enactments of dimethyl N,N′-[(ethyne-1, 2-di-yl)Bis-(1,4- phenyl-ene carbon-yl)]bis-(l-alaninate) crystals. *AIP Conf. Proc*, vol. 2270, pp. 100008, 1–4, 2020, https://doi.org/10.1063/5.0019334.
41. Senthilkannan, K., Thamaraikannan, P., Kalaipoonguzhali, V., Venkatachalam, K., Kannan, S., Ranadevan, R., Computational IR, Raman studies by DFT program and antidiabetic delineation by harboring of acetoacetanilide crystals. *AIP Conf. Proc*, vol. 2270, pp. 10013, 1–4, 2020, https://doi.org/10.1063/5.0019339.

42. Flora, G. *et al.*, Anti-diabetic (AD) and crystal stiffness characterizations of NaBr-added L-alanine (LANB) – A comparative analysis in macro and nano scale crystals. *Mater. Today: Proc.*, 33, 7, 3937–3941, 2020.
43. Flora, G. *et al.*, Anti diabetic (AD), stiffness and hardness studies of 2-[4-(Trifluoromethyl) phenyl]-1H-benzimidazole crystals - (TFMPHB) macro and nano crystal. *Mater. Today: Proc.*, 33, 4233–4236, 2020.
44. Flora, G. *et al.*, Anti-inflammatory (AI) and crystalline hardness characterisations of 4-(4-chlorophenyl)-7,7-dimethyl-7,8-dihydro-4h-1-benzopyran-2,5(3h,6h)-dione-(CPDMDHHBPHHD) – Comparative analysis of macro and nano scales crystals. *Mater. Today: Proc.*, 33, 3578–3582, 2020.
45. Ganesan, S., Gurunathan, R., Pasupuleti, R.R. *et al.*, Green synthesis of V2O5/ZnO nanocomposite materials for efficient photocatalytic and anti-bacterial applications. *Appl. Nanosci.*, 2021. https://doi.org/10.1007/s13204-021-01923-3.
46. Ganesan, H., Senthilkannan, K., Christy, S. *et al.*, Synthesis, growth, XRD, NLO, CHNSO, computational-structural, dielectric, photoconductivity, hardness and biostudies of diethyl 2-amino-5-{4-[bis (4-methyl phenyl) amino] benzamido} thiophene-3,4-dicarboxylate (DABMPABTD) macro-, nano crystals for device fabrication, pharma, electronic uses. *J. Mater. Sci. Mater. El.*, 32, 15498–15508, 2021.
47. Maalmarugan, J., Yokeswaran, V., Divya, R. *et al.*, Synthesis, growth, XRD, NLO, CHNSO, structure by theoretical approach, dielectric, absorbance, photoconductivity and bio studies of 4-(4-Acetyl-5-Methyl-1H-1, 2, 3-Triazol-1-yl) Benzonitrile crystals for optical, opto-electronic, and photonics utilities. *J. Mater. Sci. Mater. El.*, 32, 13850–13858, 2021. https://doi.org/10.1007/s10854-021-05960-0.
48. Rajkumar, M., Maalmarugan, J., Flora, G. *et al.*, Growth, characterizations, and the structural elucidation of diethyl-2-(3-oxoiso-1,3-dihydrobenzofuran-1-ylidene)malonate crystalline specimen for dielectric and electronic filters, thermal, optical, mechanical, and biomedical applications using conventional experimental and theoretical practices. *J. Mater. Sci. Mater. El.*, 32, 22822–22839, 2021. https://doi.org/10.1007/s10854-021-06761-1.
49. Senthilkannan, K., Flora, G., Gunasekaran, S., Ali, H.A.J., Vimalan, M., Balasubramanian, S., Extraction of Silver Nanoparticles (Ag-NPs) by green synthesis from aqueous extract of seaweeds and their consequences on HeLa cell line and their utility on soil by spectroscopic tools, in: *Nanotechnology for Advances in Medical Microbiology. Environmental and Microbial Biotechnology*, Springer, Singapore, 2021, https://doi.org/10.1007/978-981-15-9916-3_5.
50. Momma, K. and Izumi, F., VESTA 3 for three-dimensional visualization of crystal, volumetric and morphology data. *J. Appl. Crystallogr.*, 44, 1272–1276, 2011.
51. Spackman, P.R., Turner, M.J., McKinnon, J.J., Wolff, S.K., Grimwood, D.J., Jayatilaka, D., Spackman, M.A., Crystal explorer: A program for Hirshfeld

surface analysis, visualization and quantitative analysis of molecular crystals, *J. Appl. Crystallogr.*, 54, 3, 1006–1011, 2021. https://doi.org/10.1107/S1600576721002910.

52. Spek, A.L., Single – Crystal structure validation with the program PLATON. *J. Appl. Crystallogr.*, 36, 7–11, 2003.

15

Biological Effect Nanotubular, Vanderwall's Impact, of 4-Methyl-2-Nitroaniline (4M2NA) Nanocrystals

Senthil Kannan K.[1*], Pauline Jenifer S.[2], Divya R.[3], Raju K.[4], Gayathri A.[5], Jemma Hermelin Jesy Diaz[6], Maria Sumathi B.[2] and Flora G.[2]

[1]*Department of R&D/Physics, Edayathangudy G.S. Pillay Arts and Science College (Autonomous – Affiliated to Bharathidasan University - Tiruchirappalli), Nagapattinam, Tamil Nadu, India*
[2]*Department of Botany, St. Mary's College – Autonomous, Thoothukudi, Tamil Nadu, India*
[3]*Department of Physics, S.T. Hindu College, Nagercoil, TN, India*
[4]*Department of Physics, Easwari Engineering College, Ramapuram, Chennai, TN, India*
[5]*Department of CSE, Saveetha School of Engineering, Saveetha Institute of Medical and Technical Sciences, Saveetha University, Chennai, TN, India*
[6]*Department of Zoology, St. Mary's College – Autonomous, Thoothukudi, Tamil Nadu, India*

Abstract

4M2NA crystalline sample is full-grown by traditional evaporation modus operandi; the present chapter is mainly dealt with the device routed with the effective nano tube production, with the extensive thermal ellipsoidal graph, with proper and finely tuned acidic outlines of network, with the peptide association of 4M2NA, with the optimized force grazing zone-effectiveness, Vanderwall's weak type of interactive impose and impact of the crystal, bio use by the effectiveness of the antidiabetic, antifungal, and anti-inflammatory—the major bio impact analyzes of the titled compound in macro and in nano level scalings to predict the as mentioned major contributions in pharma/bio uses and its functionalities of the both scales with enzymatic facts of the IC_{50} data and is confirmed with nano scalings the prevalence one. The projection of the structural

**Corresponding author*: mscgoldmedalist@yahoo.in

Kaushik Pal (ed.) Nanovaccinology as Targeted Therapeutics, (243–256) © 2022 Scrivener Publishing LLC

impact is counterfitted with the standard theoretical way by the usage of softwares for the impact of atoms or molecules for the structural cases. Because of its novel bio and nanotubular effect, it may have tremendous use and projected pharma utility of other types.

***Keywords*:** Nano tube, weak interaction, 4M2NA, pharma uses, optimization

15.1 Introduction

The organic type of macro crystal 4M2NA is the one full grown by the traditional evaporation method and properly converted to 52 nm by nano level by means of milling [1–7]. The nitro aniline is an organic material having insightful competent pharma uses. The organic crystals are having well-exposed uses in electronic-mechano-bio sciences and in technology. Here, the 4M2NA both scalings are identified to proceed for the nano tube construction [8–15], ellipsoidal illustration, acidic sketches of network, peptide involvement of 4M2NA, optimized force field-effectiveness, Vanderwall's impact of the crystal, antidiabetic, antifungal, and anti-inflammatory characterizations and reported [16–21]. Molecular crystals put forward a prosperous layer of corporeal phenomenon noticeably diverse beginning the ocular, electronic and perfunctory possessions demonstrated by conformist unyielding, such as covalent or ionic crystals [22–27]. This happens partially because of the normally weedy intermolecular relations, and partially because of the delicate interaction that may occur among molecular extent of autonomy. In the modern times, molecular crystals have turned out to be the theme of powerful hypothetical and investigational explore [28–35]. To a large extent, this has centered approximately to the physics of these schemes in the order to strap up it for technical purposes, such as the typical case of molecular electronics, in addition to this finish, at hand recital endeavors to comprehend the environment of incriminate carter in these structures. An arena of region of uniformly powerful movement is that of super-molecular chemistry [36–43]. This enthralling region is based ahead the use of individual molecules in regulating to endeavor to propose purposeful molecular crystals that may be used for a variety of technical purposes. The key in at the rear this attitude is that the crystal structure and stuffing outlined by an arrangement of molecules is established to a great scope by the intermolecular interfaces, such as hydrogen bonds and van der Waals dealings. Molecular crystals of organic molecules are moreover motivating from the genetic and biochemical perception. An indulgent of the hydrogen bond is indispensable to figure out numerous very important biological practices and molecules. Molecular crystals proffer a replica in which to comprehend the environment of the hydrogen bond in biochemical coordination in additional factor [43–52].

15.2 XRD and Computational Data

The 4M2NA crystals are synthesized by proper ratio and analyzed for XRD data and confirmed the monoclinic nature with C2/c space group and a as 13.402 Å b as 9.104 Å and also c as 12.376 Å, $\alpha = 90° = \gamma$ and β is 103.85°, the theoretical confinement molecular arrangement, unit cell, and 3D effect as shown in Figures 15.1a, 15.1b and 15.2 solvent surface and molecular potentials of the entitled compound as in Figure 15.3 and Figure 15.4. Figure 15.5 and Figure 15.6 show the interactions of d_{norms}, internal, external, shape index profile, as well as curvedness and fragmented patch of the 4M2NA. Figure 15.7 shows the standard d_i Vs d_e effect of finger print version of entitled specimen. Figure 15.8 shows the void space details of the 4M2NA; electron-deformation densities and electrostatic potential effect of titled specimen are as shown in Figure 15.9 Figure 15.10 presents the super cell lattice of 4M2NA with specified frame work of acidic, as well as peptide linkage of the entitled specimen, and Figure 15.11 shows the force field portrayal of the specimen.

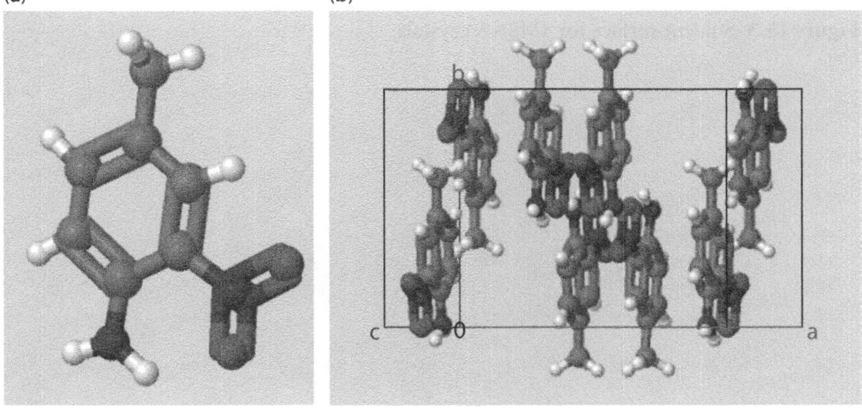

Figure 15.1 (a), (b) Molecular diagram and unit cell by software for 4M2NA crystals [50–52].

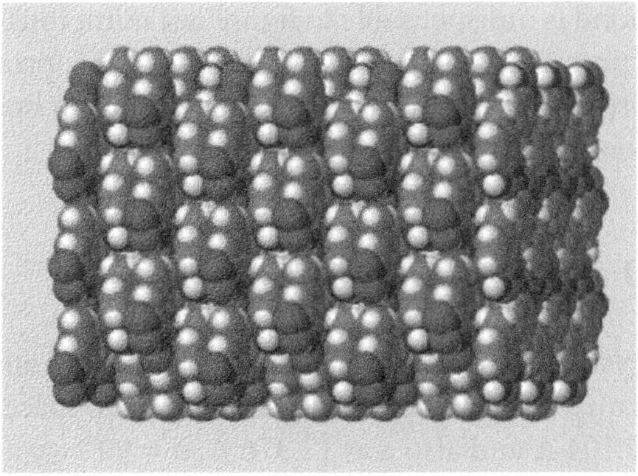

Figure 15.2 3D-pattern for 4M2NA crystals [50–52].

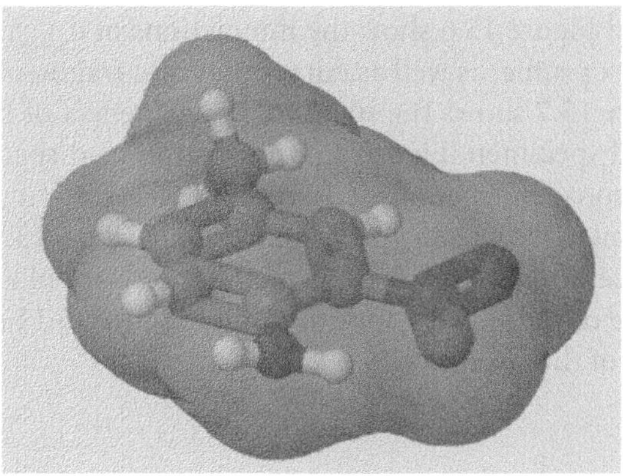

Figure 15.3 Solvent surface for 4M2NA crystals.

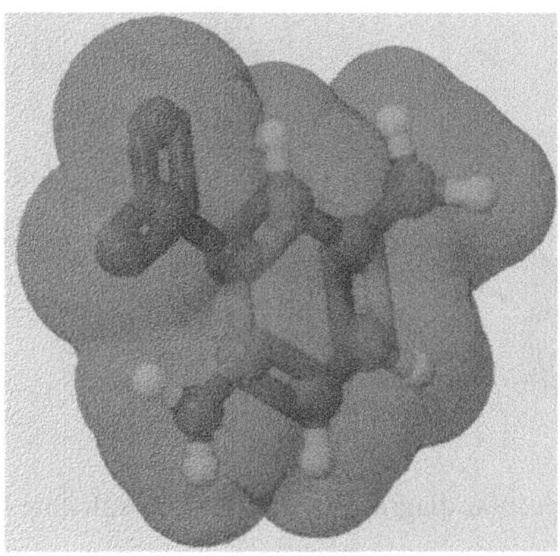

Figure 15.4 Molecular potential for 4M2NA crystals [50–52].

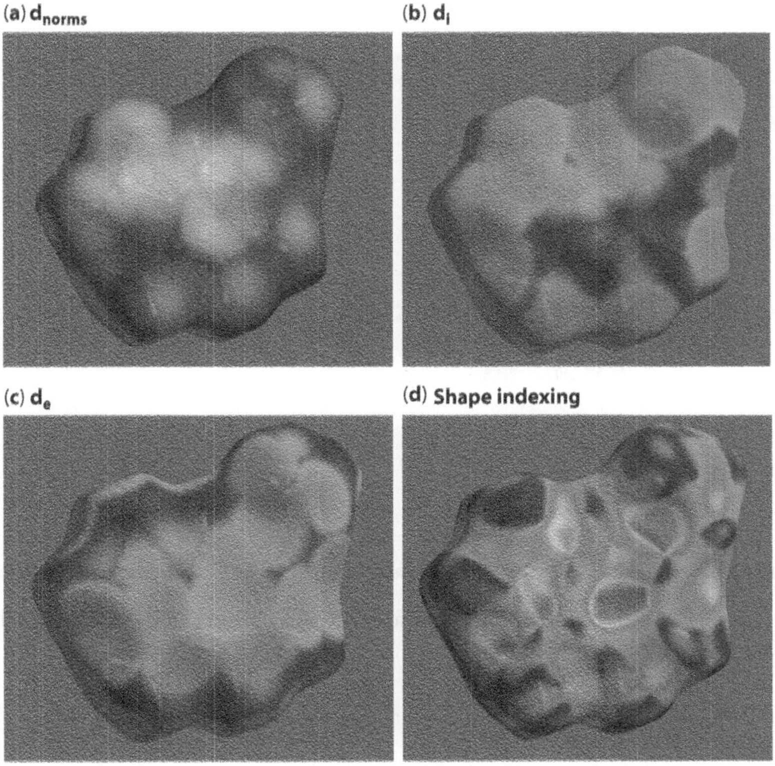

Figure 15.5 (a) Hirshfeld - dnorms for 4M2NA crystals, (b) Hirshfeld - di for 4M2NA crystals, (c) Hirshfeld - de for 4M2NA crystals, (d) Hirshfeld - Shape index for 4M2NA crystals [50–52].

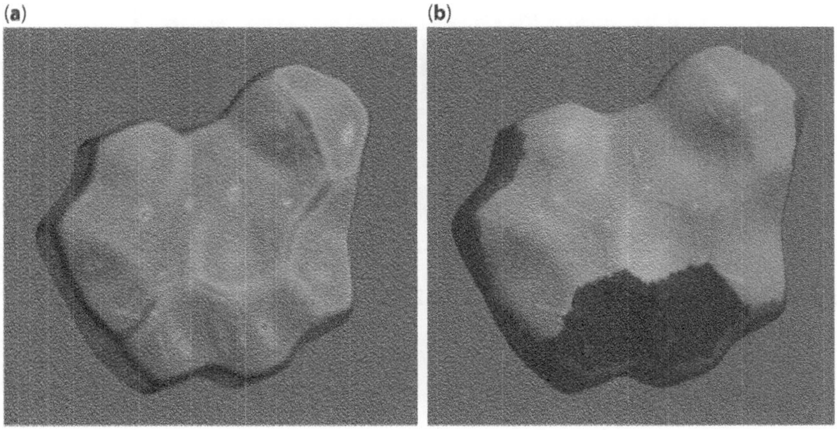

Figure 15.6 (a) Hirshfeld—curvedness for 4M2NA crystals, (b) Hirshfeld—fragmented patch for 4M2NA crystals [50–52].

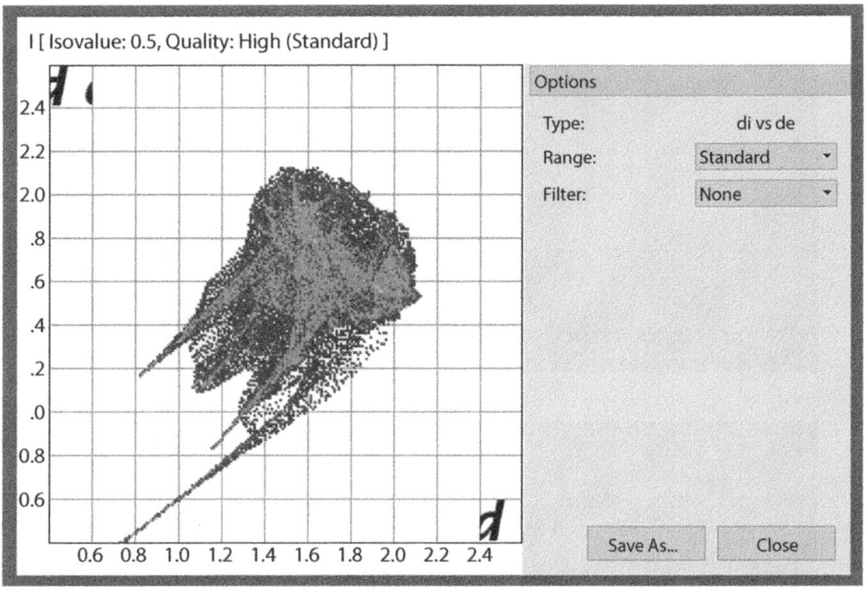

Figure 15.7 Hirshfeld—finger print whole for internal Vs external for 4M2NA crystals [50–52].

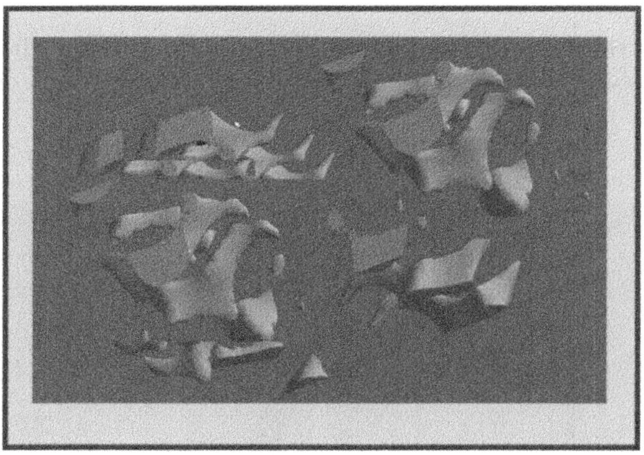

Figure 15.8 Hirshfeld—crystal voids for 4M2NA crystals [50–52].

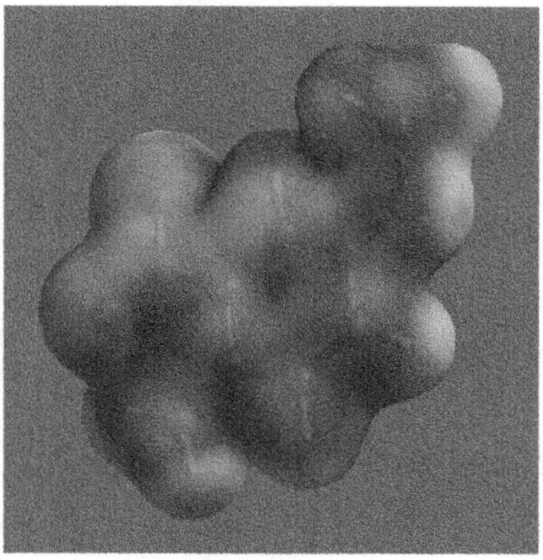

Figure 15.9a Hirshfeld—electron density for 4M2NA crystals [50–52].

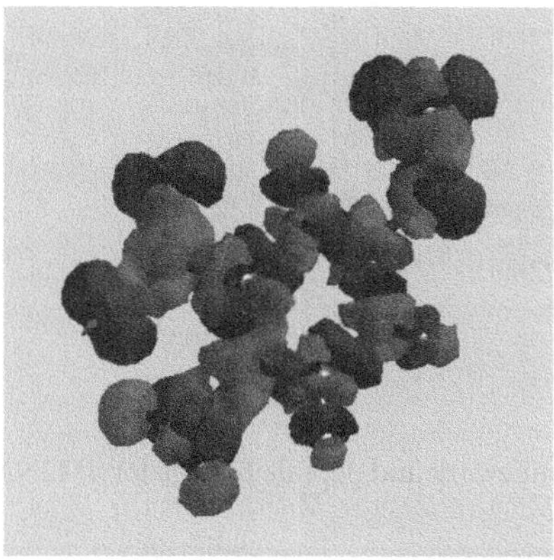

Figure 15.9b Hirshfeld—deformation density for 4M2NA crystals [50–52].

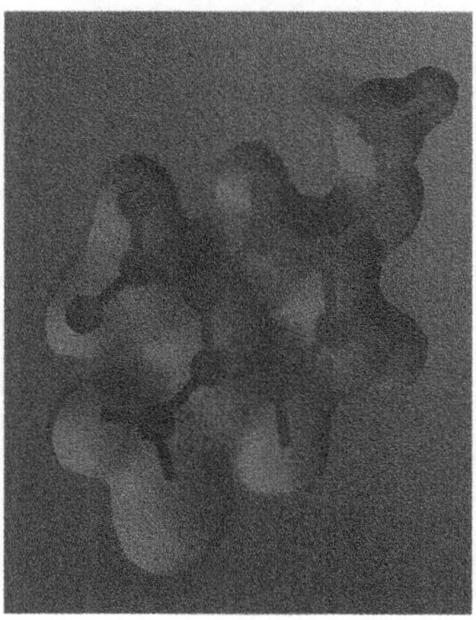

Figure 15.9c Hirshfeld—electrostatic potential for 4M2NA crystals [50–52].

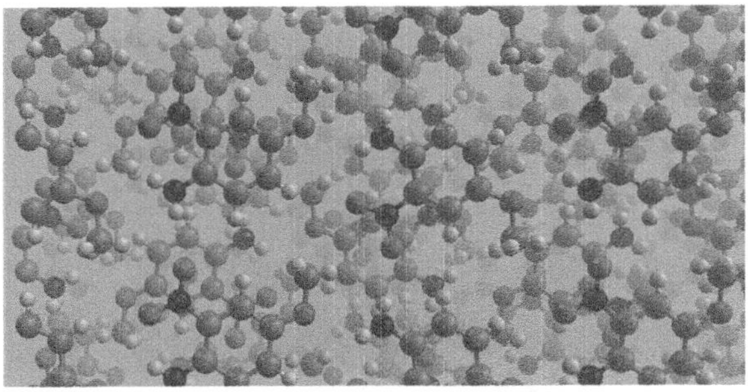

Figure 15.10a Super cell lattice of 4 × 4 × 4 of 3 axes for 4M2NA crystals [50–52].

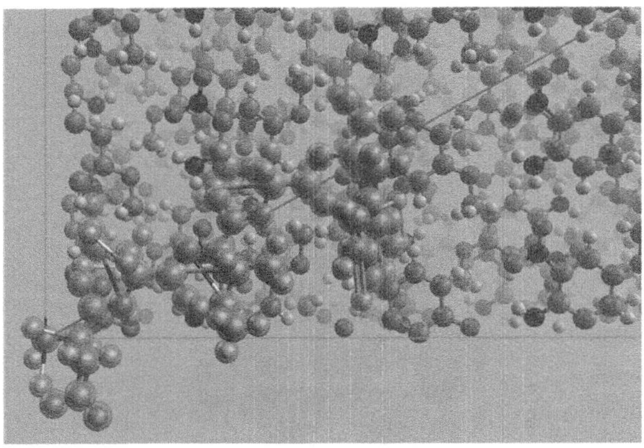

Figure 15.10b Acidic framework and peptide linkage for 4M2NA crystals [50–52].

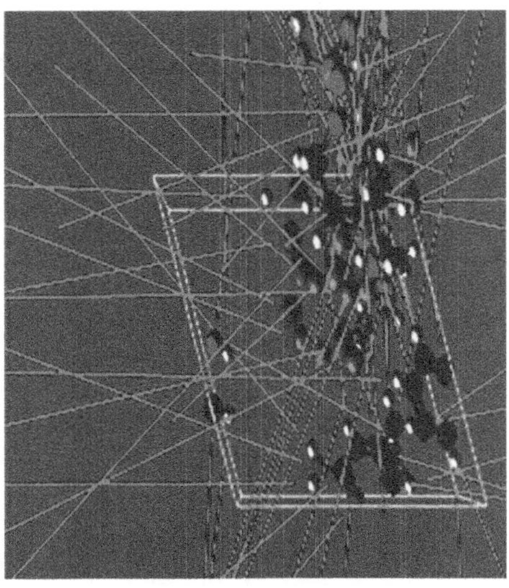

Figure 15.11 Optimized force field for 4M2NA crystals [50–52].

15.3 Biological Activity: Antidiabetic (AD), Anti-Inflammatory (AI), and Antifungal (AF) Effect

The antidiabetic quality of the 4MN2A crystals are measured by way of alpha amylase-AA and alpha glucosidase-AG and accredited as 34.79 and 33.61 for the macro, as well as nano scale for AA and is chiefly by the incident and existence of aniline in the crystalline compound and for AG the values are 34.14 and 33.25, the IC_{50} statistics for the miniature extent-nm which is foremost important than bulkiness ones for AD effectiveness and provide [25–34], also the AI outcome of 4MN2A specifies 35.10, as well as 34.61 for macro and nano for competence intention and enhanced usefulness for AI outcome, the AF consequence of *Candida albicans* by the appropriate control with no outcome, standard of 12, 11 and 11 for macro, nano-52 nm and nano-47 nm, the 25, 50, 75, and 100 microliters are measured with AF inhibition as 6:5:NA; 6:5:5; 9:7:5; 7:6:5 for the ascending concentration values and having good impact on AF by the macro, nano-52, and nano-47 scales.

15.4 Conclusion, Outlook, and Future Aspects

The theoretical outcome of the 4M2NA macro and nanocrystals for the bio activities, as well as the electronic and nano device fabrication with electron density, void space, deformation case as well as molecular potential functions and their relevances by software and Hirshfeld way of analyzing and computed and represented. The nano scale is preferred than the bulk ones in bio cases and in other electronic uses; the crystal super cell lattice has a peptide linkage for other drug utilities. In the near future, the in silico use of the molecular effectiveness with any target can be properly analyzed using software and project for any specific case and identify the *in vivo* and *in vitro* case of drug utility and harboring case study to predict and implement the efficiency. The near future can be proceeded for drug effectiveness.

References

1. Kalaipoonguzhali, V., Senthilkannan, K., Thirumoorthi, C., Chinnadurai, M., Jayanalina, T., Comparison of adsorption energy, ionization potential and electron affinity of CuS-ACT and CuS-Nit nanostructures monowire for

nano device fabrication by computational approach. *Mater. Today: Proc.*, 33, 7, 2759–2760, 2020.

2. Gunasekaran, S. *et al.*, Structural studies on picolinium maleate crystal by density functional methods. *Indian J. Phys.*, 87, 12, 1189–1197, 2013.
3. Senthilkannan, K. *et al.*, Anti diabetic (AD) studies of bis-glycine hydro bromide (45 nm) nanocrystals. *Mater. Today: Proc.*, 33, 7, 3201–3202, 2020.
4. Senthilkannan, K. *et al.*, Anti-diabetic activites of ZnO doped with Ce (5 at %) nano particles (NPs). *Mater. Today: Proc.*, 33, 7, 3056–3057, 2020.
5. Senthilkannan, K. *et al.*, Fluorescence, filter,nano tribological studies of 12-(4-Chlorophenyl)-9,9-Dimethyl-9,10-Dihydro-8H-Benzo[A]Xanthen-11(12H)-One-(CPDDHBXH) macro and nanocrystals. *Mater. Today: Proc.*, 33, 7, 4163–4166, 2020.
6. Senthilkannan, K., Venkatachalam, K., Jothibas, M., Computational and experimental studies of acetoacetanilide crystals. *AIP Conf. Proc*, vol. 2270, pp. 040014, 1–4, 2020.
7. Senthilkannan, K., Venkatachalam, K., Rajamani, A., Computational analysis of LPNPTH anisotropies for dementia for Alzheimer's syndrome by DFT and molecular harboring. *AIP Conf. Proc*, vol. 2270, pp. 040008, 1–5, 2020.
8. Senthilkannan, K., Sivaramakrishnan, V., Kalaipoonguzhali, V., Chinnadurai, M., Kannan, S., Electronic transport, HOMO–LUMO and computational studies of CuS monowire for nano device fabrication by DFT approach. *Mater. Today: Proc.*, 33, 7, 2746–2749, 2020.
9. Senthilkannan, K. and Gunasekaran, S., Spectroscopic studies and other novel studies of 4 bromo 4' chloro benzylidene aniline (BCBA) Crystal- A non linear optical material. *Int. J. Chemtech Res.*, 5, 6, 3051–3058, 2013.
10. Senthilkannan, K., Gayathri Devi, S., Nagarajan, P., Flora, G., Ranadevan, R., Anti diabetic (AD) studies of picolinium maleate nanocrystals. *Mater. Today: Proc.*, 33, 3, 3005–3007, 2020.
11. Senthilkannan, K., Ramamurthi, K., Bhakya, K., Sivaramakrishnan, V., Kolanjinathan, M., Ranadevan, R., Hardness, photoconductivity, anti-diabetic studies of L-Alaninium Fumarate (LAF) crystals. *AIP Conf. Proc*, vol. 2270, pp. 100010, 1–4, 2020.
12. Senthilkannan, K., Baskaran, P., Seenivasan, R., Settu, P., Tribological, filter, FTIR and fluorescence studies of L-Alaninium tartrate (LAT) macro and nanocrystals. *Mater. Today: Proc.*, 33, 7, 4148–4150, 2020.
13. Senthilkannan, K., Kaleemullah, K., Abdul, J., Ponnusamy., V.K., Govindan, N.M., Effect of anti microbial and fluorescence on L-Alaninium maleate (LAM) macro and nanocrystals. *Mater. Today: Proc.*, 33, 7, 2779–2781, 2020.
14. Senthilkannan, K., Ganesh, G., Abdul Jaffer Ali, H., Krishnaveni Ramamurthi, R., Kaleemullah, K., Anti diabetic (AD) activities of L-valinium picrate (LVP) macro and nanocrystals. *Mater. Today: Proc.*, 33, 7, 2738–2740, 2020.
15. Senthilkannan, K., Bhakya, K., Iyanar, M., Growth and influx, AC and DC conductivity studies of L-Alaninium Fumarate (LAF) crystals. *AIP Conf. Proc*, vol. 2270, pp. 100009, 1–4, 2020.

16. Senthilkannan, K., Growth, fluorescence and theoretical studies of B2CPCD crystals – Comparative analysis in macro and nano scaled crystals. *Mater. Today: Proc.*, 33, 7, 4368–4371, 2020.
17. Senthilkannan, K. *et al.*, Anti-diabetic (AD) activities of ZnO doped with Ce (7 at%) nano particles (NP). *Mater. Today: Proc.*, 33, 7, 3053–3055, 2020.
18. Senthilkannan, K. *et al.*, Tribological, filter studies of 3-Bromo-2-Hydroxy benzoic acid (BHBA) macro and nanocrystals. *Mater. Today: Proc.*, 33, 7, 4145–4147, 2020.
19. Senthilkannan, K. *et al.*, Electronic transport, Homo-Lumo and computational studies of CuS-ACT monowire for nano device fabrication by software approach. *Mater. Today: Proc.*, 33, 7, 2756–2758, 2020.
20. Senthilkannan, K. *et al.*, Anti microbial and fluorescence activities of L-valinium picrate (LVP) macro and nanocrystals. *Mater. Today: Proc.*, 33, 7, 2776–2778, 2020.
21. Senthilkumar, R. *et al.*, Anti-diabetic (AD) and hardness profile of 12-(4-Chlorophenyl)-9,9-Dimethyl-9,10-Dihydro-8H-benzo[a]xanthen-11(12H) -one–(CPDDHBXH) – Comparative analysis of macro and nanocrystals. *Mater. Today: Proc.*, 33, 7, 4167–4170, 2020.
22. Sathishkumar, R. *et al.*, Synthesis, growth and characterization of 2,5–Dimethyl-N-(3-phenylprop-2-en-1-ylidene) Aniline (2,5 DPPA) single crystal: A new second order nonlinear optical material for photonic and optoelectronic applications. *Optik*, 226, 2, 1–11, 2020.
23. Patel, R.P. *et al.*, Growth and XRD, elemental, mechanical, dielectric, optical and photoconductivity, and surface morphological characterizations of 2-[4-(Trifluoromethyl) phenyl]-1H-benzimidazole (TFMPHB) crystals for electronic, mechanical applications. *Braz. J. Phys.*, 51, 3, 339–350, 2021.
24. Aarthi, R. *et al.*, Molecular structure- associated pharmacodynamic investigation on benzoyl peroxide using spectroscopic and quantum computational tools. *J. Taibah Univ. Sci.*, 12, 1, 104–122, 2018.
25. Saravanan, P. *et al.*, Biofriendly and competent domestic microwave assisted method for the synthesis of ZnO nanoparticles from the extract of Azadirachta indica leaves. *Mater. Today: Proc.*, 33, 7, 3160–3163, 2020.
26. Saravanan, P. *et al.*, A perspective approach towards appreciable size and cost-effective solar cell fabrication by synthesizing ZnO nanoparticles from Azadirachta indica leaves extract using domestic microwave oven. *J. Mater. Sci. Mater. El.*, 31, 5, 4301–4309, 2020.
27. Saravanan, P. *et al.*, Dielectric and magnetic properties of Allium cepa and Raphanus sativus extracts biogenic ZnO nanoparticles. *J. Mater. Sci. Mater. El.*, 32, 1, 1–14, 2021.
28. Periyathambi, P. *et al.*, Fluorescence and filter characterizations of NaBr-added L-alanine (LANB) – A comparative analysis in macro and nano scaled crystals. *Mater. Today: Proc.*, 33, 3766–3769, 2020.
29. Baskaran, P. *et al.*, Anti-diabetic activities of ZnO doped with Ce (3 at %) nano particles. *Mater. Today: Proc.*, 33, 7, 3051–3052, 2020.

30. Baskaran, P. *et al.*, Anti-diabetic studies of barium paranitro phenolate macro and nanocrystals. *Mater. Today: Proc.*, 33, 7, 3058–3060, 2020.
31. Kolanjinathan, M., Senthilkannan, K., Paramasivam, S., Baskaran, P., Iyanar, M., Anti-diabetic studies of 4-(4-chlorophenyl)-7,7-dimethyl-7,8-dihydro-4H-1-benzopyran-2,5(3H,6H)-dione – (CPDMDHHBPHHD) nanocrystals. *Mater. Today: Proc.*, 33, 7, 2750–2752, 2020.
32. Kolanjinathan, M. *et al.*, Dielectric, fluorescence, filter, nano tribological and photoconductivity studies of 4-(4-chlorophenyl)-7,7-dimethyl-7,8-dihydro-4H-1-benzopyran-2,5(3H,6H)-dione (CPDMDHHBPHHD) macro and nanocrystals. *J. Mater. Sci. Mater. El.*, 27, 4, 16907–16917, 2020.
33. Kolanjinathan, M., Hariharasuthan, R., Sivaramakrishnan, V. *et al.*, XRD, CHNSO, fluorescence, filter-influx, NLO, photoconductivity, hardness and helical spring-fabricated device stress analysis of 2′-chloro-4-methoxy-3-nitrobenzil (CMNB) crystal of different scalings for opto-electronic filter and band gap engineering utilities. *J. Mater Sci. Mater El.*, 32, 10049–10057, 2021.
34. Jothibas, M. *et al.*, Structural, optical and photo catatic activity of Ag doped ZnO nano particles obtained by sol-gel method. *AIP Conf. Proc*, vol. 2162, pp. 020151, 1–7, 2019.
35. Selvaraj, L. *et al.*, AS Anti-diabetic (AD) studies of Bis Glycine Hydro Bromide – BGHB macro crystals milled to nano scale of 219 nm as the preliminary fine particles. *Mater. Today: Proc.*, 33, 7, 3763–3765, 2020.
36. Kishore, N. *et al.*, CO and HCHO adsorption on FeO monowire devices: A DFT study. *Appl. Phys. A*, 123, 11, 706, 1–7, 2017. https://doi.org/10.1007/s00339-017-1330-6.
37. Senthilkannan, K., Gunasekaran, S., Wagish, J.G.R., UV, SEM, Powder XRD Studies of Acetoacetanilide (AAC) Crystal. *Int. J. Chemtech Res.*, 6, 5, 3187–3190, 2014.
38. Kumar, K. *et al.*, Growth of diethyl 3,3′-[(2,4-dichlorophenyl) methylidene] bis(1H-indole-2-carboxylate)-(D32DMBC) organic NLO single crystal and its optical, thermal, mechanical, dielectric and computational studies. *J. Mater. Sci. Mater. El.*, 31, 23, 1–8, 2020. https://doi.org/10.1007/s10854-020-04594-y.
39. Senthilkannan, K., Venkatachalam, K., Bhakya, K., Sharmidha, B., Kalaivani, M., Gayathri Devi, S., Growth and Characterization of Picolinium Maleate (PM) Crystals. *AIP Conf. Proc*, vol. 2270, pp. 10014, 1–4, 2020, https://doi.org/10.1063/5.0019341.
40. Senthilkannan, K., Thamarikannan, P., Kalaipoonguzhali, V., Venkatachalam, K., Kannan, S., Baskar, A., Fluorescence, computational enactments of dimethyl N,N′-[(ethyne-1, 2-di-yl)Bis-(1,4- phenyl-ene carbon-yl)]bis-(l-alaninate) crystals. *AIP Conf. Proc*, vol. 2270, pp. 100008, 1–4, 2020, https://doi.org/10.1063/5.0019334.
41. Senthilkannan, K., Thamaraikannan, P., Kalaipoonguzhali, V., Venkatachalam, K., Kannan, S., Ranadevan, R., Computational IR, Raman studies by DFT pro

gram and antidiabetic delineation by harboring of acetoacetanilide crystals. *AIP Conf. Proc*, vol. 2270, pp. 10013, 1–4, 2020, https://doi.org/10.1063/5.0019339.

42. Flora, G. *et al.*, Anti-diabetic (AD) and crystal stiffness characterizations of NaBr-added L-alanine (LANB) – A comparative analysis in macro and nano scale crystals. *Mater. Today: Proc.*, 33, 7, 3937–3941, 2020.
43. Flora, G. *et al.*, Anti diabetic (AD), stiffness and hardness studies of 2-[4-(Trifluoromethyl) phenyl]-1H-benzimidazole crystals - (TFMPHB) macro and nanocrystal. *Mater. Today: Proc.*, 33, 4233–4236, 2020.
44. Flora, G. *et al.*, Anti-inflammatory (AI) and crystalline hardness characterisations of 4-(4-chlorophenyl)-7,7-dimethyl-7,8-dihydro-4h-1-benzopyran-2,5(3h,6h)-dione-(CPDMDHHBPHHD) – comparative analysis of macro and nano scales crystals. *Mater. Today: Proc.*, 33, 3578–3582, 2020.
45. Ganesan, S., Gurunathan, R., Pasupuleti, R.R. *et al.*, Green synthesis of V2O5/ZnO nanocomposite materials for efficient photocatalytic and anti-bacterial applications. *Appl. Nanosci.*, 2021. https://doi.org/10.1007/s13204-021-01923-3.
46. Ganesan, H., Senthilkannan, K., Christy, S. *et al.*, Synthesis, growth, XRD, NLO, CHNSO, computational-structural, dielectric, photoconductivity, hardness and biostudies of diethyl 2-amino-5-{4-[bis (4-methyl phenyl) amino] benzamido} thiophene-3,4-dicarboxylate (DABMPABTD) macro-, nanocrystals for device fabrication, pharma, electronic uses. *J. Mater. Sci. Mater. El.*, 32, 15498–15508, 2021.
47. Maalmarugan, J., Yokeswaran, V., Divya, R. *et al.*, Synthesis, growth, XRD, NLO, CHNSO, structure by theoretical approach, dielectric, absorbance, photoconductivity and bio studies of 4-(4-Acetyl-5-Methyl-1H-1, 2, 3-Triazol-1-yl) Benzonitrile crystals for optical, opto-electronic, and photonics utilities. *J. Mater. Sci. Mater. El.*, 32, 13850–13858, 2021. https://doi.org/10.1007/s10854-021-05960-0.
48. Rajkumar, M., Maalmarugan, J., Flora, G. *et al.*, Growth, characterizations, and the structural elucidation of diethyl-2-(3-oxoiso-1,3-dihydrobenzofuran-1-ylidene)malonate crystalline specimen for dielectric and electronic filters, thermal, optical, mechanical, and biomedical applications using conventional experimental and theoretical practices. *J. Mater. Sci. Mater. El.*, 32, 22822–22839, 2021. https://doi.org/10.1007/s10854-021-06761-1.
49. Senthilkannan, K., Flora, G., Gunasekaran, S., Ali, H.A.J., Vimalan, M., Balasubramanian, S., Extraction of Silver Nanoparticles (Ag-NPs) by Green Synthesis from aqueous extract of seaweeds and their consequences on HeLa cell line and their utility on soil by spectroscopic tools, in: *Nanotechnology for Advances in Medical Microbiology. Environmental and Microbial Biotechnology*, Springer, Singapore, 2021, https://doi.org/10.1007/978-981-15-9916-3_5.
50. Momma, K. and Izumi, F., VESTA 3 for three-dimensional visualization of crystal, volumetric and morphology data. *J. Appl. Crystallogr.*, 44, 1272–1276, 2011.

51. Spackman, P.R., Turner, M.J., McKinnon, J.J., Wolff, S.K., Grimwood, D.J., Jayatilaka, D., Spackman, M.A., Crystal Explorer: A program for Hirshfeld surface analysis, visualization and quantitative analysis of molecular crystals, *J. Appl. Crystallogr.*, 54, 3, 1006–1011, 20212021. https://doi.org/10.1107/S1600576721002910.
52. Spek, A.L., Single – crystal structure validation with the program PLATON. *J. Appl. Crystallogr.*, 36, 7–11, 2003.

16

Biomedical, Tribological, and Electronic Functionalities of Silver Nanoparticles

Flora G.[1], Ganesan H.[2], Maalmarugan J.[3], Egbert Selwin Rose A.[4], Dayana Lobo F.[1], Divya R.[5], Senthil Kannan K.[6*] and Sheeba M.[7]

[1]*Department of Botany, St. Mary's College (Autonomous), Thoothukudi, TN, India*
[2]*Department of Mechanical Engineering, Sri Ranganathar Institute of Engineering and Technology, Athipalayam, Coimbatore, TN, India*
[3]*Department of EEE, Sri Ranganathar Institute of Engineering and Technology, Athipalayam, Coimbatore, TN, India*
[4]*Department of Botany, St. Joseph's College - Autonomous, Tiruchirappalli, TN, India*
[5]*Department of Physics, S.T. Hindu College, Nagercoil, Tamil Nadu, India*
[6]*Department of R&D/Physics, Edayathangudy G.S. Pillay Arts and Science College (Autonomous - Affiliated to Bharathidasan University - Tiruchirappalli), Nagapattinam, Tamil Nadu, India*
[7]*Department of Zoology, PSGR Krishnammal College for Women, Coimbatore, TN, India*

Abstract
In the current examination, silver nanoparticles were synthesized properly and in a perfect manner with green production procedure using *Mangifera indica* (Mango) leaves and established lucratively customized in all cases. The band gap energy was considered as 393 nm from the spectral conjugated value, which established the manufactured model as the standard Ag nanoparticles. The silver NPs grown by solvothermal method extorted from plant leave and is analyzed for cancer, bacterial, as well as fungi and also for mechano-tribology work as well as electronic filter work. The electronic filter influx for macro is 2.4325 and nano is 2.7692 microns, respectively, as an electronic tool especially for opto-electronics type. The tribological data provided represents the wear and tear and also the mechano use for stress-enhanced value after nano Ag coatings. The HeLa cell lines' effectiveness of the silver sample is well approved and confirmed using the data analysis and

**Corresponding author*: mscgoldmedalist@yahoo.in

Kaushik Pal (ed.) Nanovaccinology as Targeted Therapeutics, (257–266) © 2022 Scrivener Publishing LLC

the assay prepared. In the future, the harboring as well as other bio remediation against such as tumor, malarial using this sample is properly enabled.

Keywords: Mango, Ag-nano, tribology, influx, bio-medication

16.1 Introduction

Nanoparticles are in the range of nanometers in diameter. Being a lot more modest frequencies of apparent light, nanoparticles cannot be perceived with common visual magnifying instruments, necessitating the utilization of electronized magnifying lens, otherwise magnifying lens. For a similar explanation, scatterings in straightforward locale may be clear, though deferrals of superior constituent parts generally disperse a few or all noticeable light episode on them [1–6]. Nanoparticles likewise effectively go through normal channels, for example, normal ceramic candles with the goal that partition from fluids requires extraordinary nanofiltration procedures [7–12]. Numerous disciplines like science, physical science, geography, and other science are related [13–17]. Being at the progress between mass materials and nuclear or atomic designs, they frequently display marvels that are not seen at one or the other scale [18–23]. They are a significant part of environmental contamination, of a kind surface construction, which brings about mechanical properties that are not the same as the mass material [24–27]. Non-round nanonparticles (e.g., crystals, blocks, poles, and so on) display shape-ward and size-subordinate [28–36]. The inorganic materials are subjected to profound uses [37–40], versatile specific functionalities [41–43], and other major contributions to society [44]. The materials have opto electronic uniqueness than the counter parting materials [45]. They are of sound optical usage mainly in electronic [46] and in major functionalities in the bio/pharma uses such as bacterial, fungal, diabetic, inflammatory, and so on [47, 48]. Here, the present investigation is mainly on the PXRD, bio-activity, and nano impactness of tribological as well as influx [43–49].

16.2 Tribological Data

The silver nano coating of 43 nm is coated on the bulk piece of iron and the effectiveness in the stress is 2% increased by this. One can confirm that the sample is so effective in tribological efficiency of wear and tear of the specimen and increase in particle size increases the stress efficiency at proportional rate/pro rata base.

16.3 Influx

The electronic filter influx for macro is 2.4325 and nano is 2.7692 microns, respectively, as an electronic tool especially for optoelectronics type, whereas the thin film influx is 2.6215 microns as the mid value of macro, as well as nano level filter uses.

16.4 HeLa Cell Line, Bacterial and Fungal Utility

The concentration with viability for 50, 100, 150, and 200 μg/ml is properly analyzed as properly reported in Table 16.1 and is having good viability data than earlier silver NPs report on other plants [49]. The bacterial and fungal utility of the Ag NPs are portrayed in Tables 16.2 and 16.3 and describe the activities against the species and their effectiveness are well depicted than the earlier cases as mentioned and practically feasible [49].

Table 16.1 Results of viability test for HeLa cell line after treatment by AgNPs.

S. no.	Concentrations (μg/ml)	Cell viability (%)
1	50	72.58 ± 0.55
2	100	69.94 ± 0.34
3	150	57.28 ± 0.76
4	200	16.64 ± 0.34
5	Control	100 ± 0

Table 16.2 Bactericidal activity of silver nanoparticles synthesized by *Mangifera indica* against garden soil bacterial isolates (Zone of inhibition mm).

Bacteria	Control			A	B	C	D
	W	AgNPs	Strp				
Bacills subtilis	0	7	1 ± 0.07	0	0	0	0
Bacillus spp	0	0	1 ± 0.2	5 ± 0.07	7 ± 0.22	3 ± 0.24	0
Pseudomonas fluorescens	0	0	1 ± 0.02	0	0	0	3 ± 0.76
Pseudomonas spp	0	0	1 ± 0.12	1 ± 0.25	0	0	0

Values are mean of 3 replicate ± SD
A – 1-AgNPs ; B-2-AgNPs ; C- 3-AgNPs ; *D* – 4-AgNPs ; W- Water; AgNPs – Silver NPs; *Strp* - Streptomycin, NIL- Without inhibition.

Table 16.3 Fungicidal activity of silver nanoparticles synthesized by *Mangifera indica* against garden soil fungal isolates (Zone of inhibition (mm)).

Fungi	Control			A	B	C	D
	W	AgNPs	Strp				
Aspergillus flavus	3 ± 0.75	3 ± 0.75	2 ± 0.02	9 ± 0.09	3 ± 0.07	7 ± 0.24	8 ± 0.01
Aspergillus fumigatus	NIL	5 ± 0.06	2 ± 0.005	7 ± 0.35	5 ± 0.01	8 ± 0.77	8 ± 0.15
Alternaria alternata	NIL	NIL	2 ± 0.70	1 ± 0.02	NIL	3 ± 0.75	3 ± 0.017
Cladosporim	NIL	NIL	2 ± 0.034	NIL	NIL	NIL	NIL

Values are mean of 3 replicate ± SD
A – 1-AgNPs ; B-2-AgNPs ; C- 3-AgNPs ; *D* – 4-AgNPs ; W- Water; AgNPs – Silver NPs; *Strp*, Streptomycin; NIL, without inhibition.

16.5 Conclusion

In the present inspection, silver nanoparticles were properly well grown from mango extract and are of 43-nm size; faultless approach prepared by a novel green production practice by means of *Mangifera indica* (mango) folios, ascertained as advantageously employed in all sort of consequences. The silver NPs grown by solvothermal method extorted from plant leave and is analyzed for cancer, bacterial as well as fungi and also for mechanotribology work as well as electronic filter work. The electronic filter influx for macro is 2.4325 and nano is 2.7692 microns respectively as an electronic tool especially for optoelectronics type. The tribological data provided represents the wear and tear and also the mechano use for stress enhanced value after nano Ag coatings. The HeLa cell lines effectiveness of the silver sample is well approved and confirmed using the data analysis and the assay prepared. In the future, the harboring, as well as other bio remediation against, such as tumor, malarial using this sample is properly enabled. Thus, Ag nanoparticles with proper usage in antibacterial, antifungal, and anticancer and are of best mechanotribology property for stress with enhanced value and effective influx value.

References

1. Kalaipoonguzhali, V., Senthilkannan, K., Thirumoorthi, C., Chinnadurai, M., Jayanalina, T., Comparison of adsorption energy, ionization potential and electron affinity of CuS-ACT and CuS-Nit nanostructures monowire for nano device fabrication by computational approach. *Mater. Today: Proc.*, 33, 7, 2759–2760, 2020.
2. Gunasekaran, S. *et al.*, Structural studies on picolinium maleate crystal by density functional methods. *Indian J. Phys.*, 87, 12, 1189–1197, 2013.
3. Senthilkannan, K. *et al.*, Anti diabetic (AD) studies of bis-glycine hydro bromide (45 nm) nano crystals. *Mater. Today: Proc.*, 33, 7, 3201–3202, 2020.
4. Senthilkannan, K. *et al.*, Anti-diabetic activites of ZnO doped with Ce (5 at %) nanoparticles (NPs). *Mater. Today: Proc.*, 33, 7, 3056–3057, 2020.
5. Senthilkannan, K. *et al.*, Fluorescence, filter,nano tribological studies of 12-(4-Chlorophenyl)-9,9-Dimethyl-9,10-Dihydro-8H-Benzo[A]Xanthen-11(12H)-One-(CPDDHBXH) macro and nano crystals. *Mater. Today: Proc.*, 33, 7, 4163–4166, 2020.
6. Senthilkannan, K., Venkatachalam, K., Jothibas, M., Computational and experimental studies of acetoacetanilide crystals. *AIP Conf. Proc.*, vol. 2270, pp. 040014, 1–4, 2020.
7. Senthilkannan, K., Venkatachalam, K., Rajamani, A., Computational analysis of LPNPTH anisotropies for dementia for Alzheimer's syndrome by DFT and molecular harboring. *AIP Conf. Proc.*, vol. 2270, pp. 040008, 1–5, 2020.
8. Senthilkannan, K., Sivaramakrishnan, V., Kalaipoonguzhali, V., Chinnadurai, M., Kannan, S., Electronic transport, HOMO–LUMO and computational

studies of CuS monowire for nano device fabrication by DFT approach. *Mater. Today: Proc.*, 33, 7, 2746–2749, 2020.
9. Senthilkannan, K. and Gunasekaran, S., Spectroscopic studies and other novel studies of 4 bromo 4' chloro benzylidene aniline (BCBA) Crystal- A non linear optical material. *Int. J. Chemtech Res.*, 5, 6, 3051–3058, 2013.
10. Senthilkannan, K., Gayathri Devi, S., Nagarajan, P., Flora, G., Ranadevan, R., Anti diabetic (AD) studies of picolinium maleate nano crystals. *Mater. Today: Proc.*, 33, 3, 3005–3007, 2020.
11. Senthilkannan, K., Ramamurthi, K., Bhakya, K., Sivaramakrishnan, V., Kolanjinathan, M., Ranadevan, R., Hardness, photoconductivity, anti-diabetic studies of L-Alaninium Fumarate (LAF) crystals. *AIP Conf. Proc.*, 2270, 100010, 1–4, 2020.
12. Senthilkannan, K., Baskaran, P., Seenivasan, R., Settu, P., Tribological, filter, FTIR and fluorescence studies of L-Alaninium tartrate (LAT) Macro and nano crystals. *Mater. Today: Proc.*, 33, 7, 4148–4150, 2020.
13. Senthilkannan, K., Kaleemullah, K., Abdul, J., Ponnusamy., V.K., Govindan, N.M., Effect of anti microbial and fluorescence on L-Alaninium maleate (LAM) macro and nano crystals. *Mater. Today: Proc.*, 33, 7, 2779–2781, 2020.
14. Senthilkannan, K., Ganesh, G., Abdul Jaffer Ali, H., Krishnaveni Ramamurthi, R., Kaleemullah, K., Anti diabetic (AD) activities of L-valinium picrate (LVP) macro and nano crystals. *Mater. Today: Proc.*, 33, 7, 2738–2740, 2020.
15. Senthilkannan, K., Bhakya, K., Iyanar, M., Growth and influx, AC and DC conductivity studies of L-Alaninium Fumarate (LAF) crystals. *AIP Conf. Proc.*, 2270, 100009, 1–4, 2020.
16. Senthilkannan, K., Growth, fluorescence and theoretical studies of B2CPCD crystals - Comparative analysis in macro and nano scaled crystals. *Mater. Today: Proc.*, 33, 7, 4368–4371, 2020.
17. Senthilkannan, K. *et al.*, Anti-diabetic (AD) activities of ZnO doped with Ce (7 at%) nanoparticles (NP). *Mater. Today: Proc.*, 33, 7, 3053–3055, 2020.
18. Senthilkannan, K. *et al.*, Tribological, filter studies of 3-Bromo-2-Hydroxy benzoic acid (BHBA) macro and nano crystals. *Mater. Today: Proc.*, 33, 7, 4145–4147, 2020.
19. Senthilkannan, K. *et al.*, Electronic transport, Homo-Lumo and computational studies of CuS-ACT monowire for nano device fabrication by software approach. *Mater. Today: Proc.*, 33, 7, 2756–2758, 2020.
20. Senthilkannan, K. *et al.*, Anti microbial and fluorescence activities of L-valinium picrate (LVP) macro and nano crystals. *Mater. Today: Proc.*, 33, 7, 2776–2778, 2020.
21. Senthilkumar, R. *et al.*, Anti-diabetic (AD) and hardness profile of 12-(4-Chlorophenyl)-9,9-Dimethyl-9,10-Dihydro-8H-benzo[a]xanthen-11 (12H)-one –(CPDDHBXH) - Comparative analysis of macro and nano crystals. *Mater. Today: Proc.*, 33, 7, 4167–4170, 2020.
22. Sathishkumar, R. *et al.*, Synthesis, Growth and characterization of 2,5 - Dimethyl-N-(3-phenylprop-2-en-1-ylidene) Aniline (2,5 DPPA) single

crystal: A new second order nonlinear optical material for photonic and optoelectronic applications. *Optik-International Journal for Light and Electron Optics*, 226, 2, 1–11, 2020.

23. Patel, R.P. *et al.*, Growth and XRD, elemental, mechanical, dielectric, optical and photoconductivity, and surface morphological characterizations of 2-[4-(Trifluoromethyl) phenyl]-1H-benzimidazole (TFMPHB) crystals for electronic, mechanical applications. *Braz. J. Phys.*, 51, 3, 339–350, 2021.
24. Aarthi, R. *et al.*, Molecular structure-associated pharmacodynamic investigation on benzoyl peroxide using spectroscopic and quantum computational tools. *J. Taibah Univ. Sci.*, 12, 1, 104–122, 2018.
25. Saravanan, P. *et al.*, Biofriendly and competent domestic microwave assisted method for the synthesis of ZnO nanoparticles from the extract of Azadirachta indica leaves. *Mater. Today: Proc.*, 33, 7, 3160–3163, 2020.
26. Saravanan, P. *et al.*, A perspective approach towards appreciable size and cost-effective solar cell fabrication by synthesizing ZnO nanoparticles from Azadirachta indica leaves extract using domestic microwave oven. *J. Mater. Sci. Mater. El.*, 31, 5, 4301–4309, 2020.
27. Saravanan, P. *et al.*, Dielectric and magnetic properties of Allium cepa and Raphanus sativus extracts biogenic ZnO nanoparticles. *J. Mater. Sci. Mater. El.*, 32, 1, 1–14, 2021.
28. Periyathambi, P. *et al.*, Fluorescence and filter characterizations of NaBr-added L-alanine (LANB) – A comparative analysis in macro and nano scaled crystals. *Mater. Today: Proc.*, 33, 3766–3769, 2020.
29. Baskaran, P. *et al.*, Anti-diabetic activities of ZnO doped with Ce (3 at %) nanoparticles. *Mater. Today: Proc.*, 33, 7, 3051–3052, 2020.
30. Baskaran, P. *et al.*, Anti-diabetic studies of barium paranitro phenolate macro and nano crystals. *Mater. Today: Proc.*, 33, 7, 3058–3060, 2020.
31. Kolanjinathan, M., Senthilkannan, K., Paramasivam, S., Baskaran, P., Iyanar, M., Anti-diabetic studies of 4-(4-chlorophenyl)-7,7-dimethyl-7,8-dihydro-4H-1-benzopyran-2,5(3H,6H)-dione – (CPDMDHHBPHHD) nano crystals. *Mater. Today: Proc.*, 33, 7, 2750–2752, 2020.
32. Kolanjinathan, M. *et al.*, Dielectric, fluorescence, filter, nano tribological and photoconductivity studies of 4-(4-chlorophenyl)-7,7-dimethyl-7,8-dihydro-4H-1-benzopyran-2,5(3H,6H)-dione (CPDMDHHBPHHD) macro and nano crystals. *J. Mater. Sci. Mater. El.*, 27, 4, 16907–16917, 2020.
33. Kolanjinathan, M., Hariharasuthan, R., Sivaramakrishnan, V. *et al.*, XRD, CHNSO, fluorescence, filter-influx, NLO, photoconductivity, hardness and helical spring-fabricated device stress analysis of 2′-chloro-4-methoxy-3-nitrobenzil (CMNB) crystal of different scalings for opto-electronic filter and band gap engineering utilities. *J. Mater Sci. Mater El.*, 32, 10049–10057, 2021.
34. Jothibas, M. *et al.*, Structural, optical and photo catatic activity of Ag doped ZnO nanoparticles obtained by sol-gel method. *AIP Conf. Proc.*, 2162, 020151, 1–7, 2019.

35. Selvaraj, L. *et al.*, AS Anti-diabetic (AD) studies of Bis Glycine Hydro Bromide – BGHB macro crystals milled to nano scale of 219 nm as the preliminary fine particles. *Mater. Today: Proc.*, 33, 7, 3763–3765, 2020.
36. Kishore, N. *et al.*, CO and HCHO adsorption on FeO monowire devices: A DFT study. *Appl. Phys. A*, 123, 11, 706, 1–7, 2017. https://doi.org/10.1007/s00339-017-1330-6.
37. Senthilkannan, K., Gunasekaran, S., Wagish, J.G.R., UV, SEM, powder XRD studies of Acetoacetanilide (AAC) Crystal. *Int. J. Chemtech Res.*, 6, 5, 3187–3190, 2014.
38. Kumar, K. *et al.*, Growth of diethyl 3,3′-[(2,4-dichlorophenyl) methylidene] bis(1H-indole-2-carboxylate)-(D32DMBC) organic NLO single crystal and its optical, thermal, mechanical, dielectric and computational studies. *J. Mater. Sci. Mater. El.*, 31, 23, 1–8, 2020. https://doi.org/10.1007/s10854-020-04594-y.
39. Senthilkannan, K., Venkatachalam, K., Bhakya, K., Sharmidha, B., Kalaivani, M., Gayathri Devi, S., Growth and Characterization of Picolinium Maleate (PM) Crystals. *AIP Conf. Proc.*, 2270, 10014, 1–4, 2020, https://doi.org/10.1063/5.0019341.
40. Senthilkannan, K., Thamarikannan, P., Kalaipoonguzhali, V., Venkatachalam, K., Kannan, S., Baskar, A., Fluorescence, computational enactments of dimethyl N,N′-[(ethyne-1, 2-di-yl)Bis-(1,4- phenyl-ene carbon-yl)]bis-(l-alaninate) crystals. *AIP Conf. Proc.*, vol. 2270, pp. 100008, 1–4, 2020, https://doi.org/10.1063/5.0019334.
41. Senthilkannan, K., Thamaraikannan, P., Kalaipoonguzhali, V., Venkatachalam, K., Kannan, S., Ranadevan, R., Computational IR, Raman studies by DFT program and antidiabetic delineation by harboring of acetoacetanilide crystals. *AIP Conf. Proc.*, 2270, 10013, 1–4, 2020, https://doi.org/10.1063/5.0019339.
42. Flora, G. *et al.*, Anti-diabetic (AD) and crystal stiffness characterizations of NaBr-added L-alanine (LANB) – A comparative analysis in macro and nano scale crystals. *Mater. Today: Proc.*, 33, 7, 3937–3941, 2020.
43. Flora, G. *et al.*, Anti diabetic (AD), stiffness and hardness studies of 2-[4-(Trifluoromethyl) phenyl]-1H-benzimidazole crystals - (TFMPHB) macro and nano crystal. *Mater. Today: Proc.*, 33, 4233–4236, 2020.
44. Flora, G. *et al.*, Anti-inflammatory (AI) and crystalline hardness characterisations of 4-(4-chlorophenyl)-7,7-dimethyl-7,8-dihydro-4h-1-benzopyran-2,5(3h,6h)-dione-(CPDMDHHBPHHD) – comparative analysis of macro and nano scales crystals. *Mater. Today: Proc.*, 33, 3578–3582, 2020.
45. Ganesan, S., Gurunathan, R., Pasupuleti, R.R. *et al.*, Green synthesis of V2O5/ZnO nanocomposite materials for efficient photocatalytic and anti-bacterial applications. *Appl. Nanosci.*, 2021. https://doi.org/10.1007/s13204-021-01923-3.
46. Ganesan, H., Senthilkannan, K., Christy, S. *et al.*, Synthesis, growth, XRD, NLO, CHNSO, computational-structural, dielectric, photoconductivity, hardness and biostudies of diethyl 2-amino-5-{4-[bis (4-methyl phenyl)

amino] benzamido} thiophene-3,4-dicarboxylate (DABMPABTD) macro-, nano crystals for device fabrication, pharma, electronic uses. *J. Mater. Sci. Mater. El.*, 32, 15498–15508, 2021.

47. Maalmarugan, J., Yokeswaran, V., Divya, R. *et al.*, Synthesis, growth, XRD, NLO, CHNSO, structure by theoretical approach, dielectric, absorbance, photoconductivity and bio studies of 4-(4-Acetyl-5-Methyl-1H-1, 2, 3-Triazol-1-yl) Benzonitrile crystals for optical, opto-electronic, and photonics utilities. *J. Mater. Sci. Mater. El.*, 32, 13850–13858, 2021. https://doi.org/10.1007/s10854-021-05960-0.
48. Rajkumar, M., Maalmarugan, J., Flora, G. *et al.*, Growth, characterizations, and the structural elucidation of diethyl-2-(3-oxoiso-1,3-dihydrobenzofuran-1-ylidene)malonate crystalline specimen for dielectric and electronic filters, thermal, optical, mechanical, and biomedical applications using conventional experimental and theoretical practices. *J. Mater. Sci. Mater. El.*, 32, 22822–22839, 2021. https://doi.org/10.1007/s10854-021-06761-1.
49. Senthilkannan, K., Flora, G., Gunasekaran, S., Ali, H.A.J., Vimalan, M., Balasubramanian, S., Extraction of Silver Nanoparticles (Ag-NPs) by Green Synthesis from aqueous extract of seaweeds and their consequences on HeLa cell line and their utility on soil by spectroscopic tools, in: *Nanotechnology for Advances in Medical Microbiology. Environmental and Microbial Biotechnology*, Springer, Singapore, 2021, https://doi.org/10.1007/978-981-15-9916-3_5.

17

Commercialization of Nanovaccines: Utopia or a Reality?

Amjad Islam Aqib[1]*, Tean Zaheer[2], Muhammad Usman[3], Muhammad Arslan[4] and Khazeena Atta[5]

[1]*Department of Medicine, Cholistan University of Veterinary and Animal Sciences, Bahawalpur, Pakistan*
[2]*Department of Parasitology, University of Agriculture Faisalabad, Pakistan*
[3]*Department of Anatomy and Histology, Cholistan University of Veterinary and Animal Sciences, Bahawalpu, Pakistan*
[4]*Department of Poultry Science, Cholistan University of Veterinary and Animal Sciences, Bahawalpur, Pakistan*
[5]*Institute of Biochemistry and Biotechnology, University of Veterinary and Animal Sciences, Lahore, Pakistan*

Abstract

Nanotechnology recently surfaced to resolve vaccine failures that arise majorly because of the weak immunogenicity of vaccines, *in vivo* instability, need of multiple jabs, and toxicity. This technology equally enhances humoral and cellular immune systems by provoking phagocytic cells, gut and mucosa-associated lymphoid tissues that in turn enhance antigen recognition and presentation. Liposomes, emulsions, polymeric nanoparticles, and graphene oxide nanosheets are some of the examples of nanovaccines. Advanced step is multifunctional nanovaccine that significantly increases immune response being targeted specific, stable delivery system, and efficacious. The technology has created hope for AIDS, malaria, hepatitis B surface antigens, rheumatoid arthritis, and chronic autoimmune. Moreover, multifactorial diseases of animals like foot-and-mouth disease (FMD), brucellosis, Johne's disease, anaplasmosis and bovine respiratory disease complex (BRDC) may be benefited through nanovaccine. Such a useful technology is in its initial phases which is no way spared from constraints, inclusive of which are mainly the process of production of nanoparticles and construction of nanovaccines in sterile condition. Large volumes of solvents and lethargy drying

**Corresponding author*: amjadislamaqib@cuvas.edu.pk

Kaushik Pal (ed.) Nanovaccinology as Targeted Therapeutics, (267–282) © 2022 Scrivener Publishing LLC

process also demand some alternative methods of preparations. In addition to these, intradermal injections leading to dermatological problems, oral administration leading to GIT issues, and nasal administration leading to respiratory problems, and damage to brain and the development of thrombosis are salient constraints associated with applications. Current book chapter summarizes hopes, as well as gaps to achieve the targets for further proposals to work on the gaps.

***Keywords*:** Nanovaccines, development, public health, animal health, constraints, application

17.1 Introduction

Vaccination is the best procedure for lessening high mortality rates, just as decreasing the tremendous social and financial effect related to disorders. Despite the advancement of conventional vaccines, enhancements are needed because of worries about the low immunogenicity of the toxicity, instability, and the requirement for numerous organizations of the vaccines. To defeat the referenced issues, nanotechnology, as of late, has been joined into vaccine improvement. Nanotechnology progressively assumes a significant part in vaccine advancement nanocarrier-based conveyance frameworks that offer a chance to build the cell and humoral immune reactions. The utilization of nanoparticles in vaccine definitions permits upgraded immunogenicity and security of antigen, yet in addition designated enhances targeted delivery and slow delivery.

The nanotechnologies utilized in the ground of vaccines consolidate nanocarriers that have different of courses of action, having characteristics in size and surfaces. A number of nanocarrier vaccine were made and utilized in the delivery of antigens and adjuvants to immune cells with conclusive objective to upgrade a safe immunological reaction. In specific systems, nanocarriers are planned for conveyance of an antigen and an adjuvant. Nanocarriers might work with focusing on just as upheld arrival of antigens to antigen-introducing cells. Effective parts of vaccines dependent on nanotechnology plans keep up with the utilization of nanocarriers in ground of vaccine. Particles under 10 micrometers instantly reached the phagocytic cell, like macrophages. This focus on cell take-up of antigens, as needs be extending the capability of antigen affirmation and demonstration. Solid nanocarriers could shield antigen based on protein vaccine from debasement, work with section into the gut-related lymphoid tissue and mucosa-related lymphoid tissues, conveying them as fit for vaccine movement through oral or mucosal courses. Surface-changed nanocarriers may help the assigned transport of antigens. Immune cells express a collection of surface receptors, including the mannose receptor, scrounger receptor, and Toll-like receptors (TLR). Nanocarriers covered with immune cell focusing on particles, for instance, carbohydrates, antibodies, and peptides, may focus on these overexpressed receptors to work on the capability of antigen and adjuvant transport toward the advancement of explicit and specific immunological reaction in prophylactic vaccinations.

The utilization of nanoparticle that are based on vaccines based on nanotechnology is arising as a unique methodology for inoculation of conventional subunit vaccines. Nanovaccines may actuate quick and durable cell and humoral immunity. Vaccines based on nanoparticles are likewise effortlessly directed via various conveyance courses, including intranasal, intravenous, transdermal, oral, made such that they move through the blood brain boundary. These vaccine developments display expanded heat stability at room temperature, in contrast to customary subunit vaccine. Nanovaccine capacity solidness essentially lessens clinical capacity costs and takes into consideration worldwide conveyance to remote area. Notwithstanding thermal dependability, particles based on nanotechnologycan keep up with antigen protein strength and usefulness for broadened timeframes, which is warranted to get a suitable immune reaction.

Nanotechnology-based vaccines can be intended to imitate the size and shape of microorganisms to advance simple take-up by immune cells. Furthermore, particles are linker and functionalized, for example, alpha-1,2-connected dimannopyranoside, to formulate them as a pathogen for effective take-up. Formerly disguised by immune cells, the nanoparticles corrupt to deliver antigen throughout delayed timeframe. Particles are normally combined from a huge number of regular and engineered biocompatible polymeric materials, considering an "attachment" stage. A variety of nanoparticles is formed considering the control of molecule shape, size, surface charge, and hydrophobicity, and at last self-adjuvating impacts. As a specified benefit, nanovaccines might be valuable for further developing vaccine adequacy in agriculture species. Antigen is utilized as polymeric nanoparticles transporters, additionally, adjuvants might be utilized to further the development of vaccine adequacy and soundness against dairy cattle, leading to resisting sicknesses. The toxicity of nanoparticles is difficult to evaluate, especially when attempting to quickly evaluate various nano formulations for vaccine or different drugs. Large numbers of the unfavorable impacts of nanoparticles on humans are probably going to result from long-term, low-level exposures, which is hard to quantify and requires extremely long trials to be determined.

17.2 Development of Nanovaccines

Vaccine development and vaccination is a phenomenal milestone in the prevention of infectious diseases and eradication of numerous diseases. Several types of vaccines with specific merits and demerits are developed through evolutionary process, including live, attenuated, and killed toxoids [1]. Vaccination is also substantially valuable in minimizing mortality and morbidity. However, vaccine hesitancy demands further considerations for developing more safe vaccines [2, 3]. Successful vaccination entails effective protection against a specific pathogen, memory response generation, and more importantly, the effective antigen delivery system [1]. Whereas the induction of proper immunogenicity and stimulation of vigorous and long-lasting immune response is limited in most of the modern vaccines, use of new advanced delivery system and adjuvants is the valuable solution to compensate these problems [4]. Nanovaccinology or use of nanotechnology in vaccine development is a quite valuable technology for effective vaccine development and induction of long-lasting immune response. This nanoparticle-based synthetic delivery system provide protection to encapsuled antigen from host environment, enhance its presentation and uptake to antigen presenting cells and release antigen in sustainable manner [1, 2]. The antigen delivery to dendritic cells has the key importance for the development of appropriate immune response. This uptake from dedritic cells considerably improved through nanoparticles. Therefore, nanoparticles are the excellent choice for vaccine delivery and adjuvant [5]. Vaccine development through nanotechnology provides nanocarrier-based delivery system that improve the cellular, as well as humoral immune response. The nanoparticles in the vaccine development ensures advanced paybacks, including improved immunogenicity, better antigen stability, and targeted delivery along with sustained antigen release and hence served as antigen depots [6, 7].

17.3 Novel Adjuvants and Delivery System for Nanovaccines

Traditional vaccines had a pivotal role in disease control; however, several limitations, including safety issues for immunocompromised individuals, lack of good protection from some vaccines, wide range of diseases deficient in licensed vaccines, and so on necessitated more advanced solutions. The development of vaccines based on isolated proteins or naked DNA is considered as more safe but poor immunogens and hence less efficacious. Use of adjuvants is the practical solution to improve the efficacy but traditional vaccines used aluminum-based adjuvants that are not always the good choice to generate strong immune response and can induce local immune response [8]. Furthermore, improvements are also required to compensate the instability, bioavailability, surface electric charge, and multiple vaccine administrations. Nanoparticles in nanovaccines is an effective tool not only to overcome the antigen stability and poor immunogenicity but also act as adjuvant [7]. Non-virus DNA vectors are also one of the useful tool for gene therapy with more safety over viral vectors [9]. Vaccine antigens can be encapsulated by nanoparticles or conjugated on the surface. Encapsulated antigens prevent rapid degradation, whereas conjugated antigen present to immune system like pathogen. Some of the nanoparticles has the ability to modulate immune response to antigen by entering in the antigen-presenting cells [10]. The nanoparticles improved the recognition and presentation of antigen by facilitating the uptake by the mucosa and gut-associated lymphoid tissue, as well as phagocytic cell [11]. Nanoparticles possessed good adjuvant properties and hence a good choice for vaccine delivery [12]. Nanotechnology deals with the fabrication and manipulation of matter at a tiny scale of 1 to 100 nm [7]. The smaller size improved the cellular uptake by phagocytic cells including dendritic cells and macrophages and hence improve the antigen presentation and recognition efficiency. Therefore, determination of the particle size for optimum immune response is also an important aspect of nanovaccinology. Nanotechnology-based particles having physical and chemical characteristics that include chemical composition, size of particle, morphology and shape, surface charge and hydrophobicity change the immune response induction [8]. Nanoparticulate vaccine and adjuvants systems predominantly includes viral vectored vaccines, particles, like virus and virosomes, MF59, immunomodulating complexes, polymeric nanoparticles, monophosphoryl lipid A, nondegradable nanoparticles, calcium phosphate nanoparticles, Montanide™, liposomes, proteosomes, and cholesterol-bearing hydrophobized pullulan nanoparticles [7, 11, 13]. Most of the adjuvants improved humoral immune response, whereas some specifically improved cytotoxic T cells response, including viral vectors, Montanide™ ISA 51 and 720, as well as ISCOMs. MPL® and MF59 improved Th1 response while liposomes, virus-like particles and nondegradable nanoparticles produced cellular immunity as well [13]. Viral vector-based vaccines responsible for induction of vigorous cytotoxic T lymphocyte response without any adjuvant and resulted in elimination of virus-infected cells [14]. Virus-like particles (VLPs) are excellent noninfectious nanoparticles and became highly accepted and successful technology in vaccinology [15]. VLPs are safer than live vaccines as they are lacking genetic material of virus and hence not able to replicate [7, 16]. Liposomes are artificially assembled nontoxic molecules, which are composed of phospholipid bilayer shell with aqueous core. These liposomes encapsulating the antigen and improved the uptake of antigen as delivery vehicles [17–19]. Liposomes has enormous potential to induce desired immune response by targeting not only the immune cells but also cell organelles. These also improved the cross-presentation of antibodies and greatly improved the efficacy of vaccines [19]. Several nonbiodegradable materials are also used as adjuvants and for vaccine delivery. These materials include silica [20], carbon [21], polystyrene [22], quantum dots [23] and gold [24]. This material improved the immunogenicity by persisting in the tissues for longer duration [13]. Immunostimulant complexes (ISCOM) are the cage-like nanoparticles that are the combination of phospholipid, protein antigen, cholesterol, and saponin adjuvant Quil A. This spherical structure is utilized for entrapping the antigens that are hydrophobic in nature [25]. Nonviral vectors are the delivery vehicles that carry antigen in the form of RNA or DNA. These vehicles delivered antigen to target cell for induction of immune response [26]. Although nonviral vectors have good potential in vaccinology, they may face the reduced efficiency, which can be improved using some synthetic or natural materials. Nonviral vectors are the safer and more efficacious choice than viral vectors as it not required viral components, more antigen protection and easy production and large scale. Emulsions can be categorized as water-in-oil and oil-in-water and hence having two liquid phases, emulsifier, and excipient [27]. MF59 is the highly famous, safe, potent, and effective adjuvant emulsion for many types of vaccines. MF59 has the potential to take out stronger humoral and cellular immune response than aluminum-based adjuvants [28].

17.4 Success Story

Nanobacteria: Proteosomes, exosomes, liposomes, virosomes, super fluids, nanobeads based on nanoparticles, particle-like virus articles, and bacteriophages are a few examples of nano-sized vehicles that are evaluated here as expected nanocarriers for vaccine delivery to immune system. Nanobacteria are another significant subject for mention here, because of their role in the contamination of vaccines and some complicated disorders. The following are reason for preferring nano technology-based vaccine over conventional vaccines:

- Replacement for conventional adjuvants: nanotechnology-based vaccines exhibited immunogenicity, without occurrence of unusual (Alum) conventional vaccine led to irritation.
- Prolong times of protection and shelf life: Nanotechnology particles-based vaccine deliverance system prevent to utilize poisonous material like thimerosal and formaldehyde and possibly expand strength of vaccine.
- Low frequency of organization for boost: Nanotechnology-based vaccines can be directed for support vaccination less regularly than ordinary vaccine, which are generally multi-injection and dose deliverance systems.

17.5 Nanovaccines in Human Health

Vaccination is the best procedure for lessening high awfulness and mortality rates, just as decreasing the tremendous social and financial effect related with disorders. Vaccines are used to initiate the immune system to stimulate the immune reaction against targets, like malignant growth cells and microbial agents. Different kinds of vaccine might be utilized to treat malignancies, for example, entire tumor cell vaccines, dendritic cell vaccine, antigen or adjuvant vaccine, viral vectors, and DNA vaccine. The immunologic impact is not generally adequate to invert the progression of malignancy, vaccines are, by and large, well tolerated and give helpful anticancer impacts in certain circumstances. Antigen malignant growth vaccines are regularly made up of cancer-related antigen, not typically present on healthy cells, alongside different components (for example adjuvants) used to animate the immune responses against the antigens, bringing about the destruction ofcancerous cells, without destroying other cells, and preventing reformation.

COVID 19: Almost certainly, nanotechnology hold great prospective in the treatment to avoidance of COVID-19. Nanotechnology against COVID-19 use various methodologies, for example, staying away from viral infectivity (a) study of infection-free equipment, such as (PPE) personal protective equipment, to improve security of medical care laborers and formation of antiviral sanitizers and surface protection, which can inactivate the infection and prevent its spread; (b) method of highly specific and sensitive nanotechnology based sensors to rapidly distinguish disease or immune responses; (c) improvement in latest drugs having upgraded action, less toxicity and supported delivery to a target tissue, for instance, toward lungs; and (d) advancement of a nanotechnology-based vaccination to help humoral and cellular immune responses.

Inflexal: Inflexal V, advertised in numerous countries for more than ten years, 4 ordinary product of vaccine dependent on nanoparticle-based technologies. They use virosomes based nanoparticles or particles like virus as adelivery and adjuvant system, and could be stored at 2–8°C.

Inflexal V: Influenza is a critical respiratory issue of human, answerable for passing overall reliably. Inflexal V is made from a blend of 3 monovalent virosome pools, each outlined with explicit glycoproteins HA and NA of one influenzas infection kind strain. The vaccine is biodegradable and contains no thiomersal, formaldehyde, and low degree of ovalbumin. Virosomesantigens to start a solid safe therefore, this item is extraordinarily practical by reflecting natural viral contamination. The resulted material has been supported by number of nations and is equitable adjuvanted influenza immunization authorized for all age gatherings.

Epaxal: Hepatitis An is an extraordinary irresistible problem of liver achieved by the hepatitis A virus, having manifestations of vomit, diarrhea, jaundice, fever, stomach pain and lose bowel movement. This vaccine relies upon formalin inactivated HAV adsorbed to the external surface of virosomes that supplant the adjuvantAluminum hydroxide with phospholipids. A particular injected dose of virosomal HAV vaccine is all around endured and exceptionally immunogenic, with 88% to 97% of seroprotection 14 days after the initial dose.

Gardasil™ and Cervarix™: HPV is a transmit by sexual contact disease that end up with severe sickness that includes genital warts and cervical malignant growths. Cervical cancer is the 2nd general reason for malignant growth passing in women around the world, simply close to breast cancer. HPV leads to numerous cervical cancer cases each year, types 16 and 18 are accountable for about 70%. Gardasil™ and Cervarix™ are subunit vaccines that contain VLPs gathered from majority of capsid proteins. Vaccination with these 2 products has been defended by women in opposition to a high extent of forerunner lesions of cervical cancer brought about by HPV.

17.6 Nanovaccines in Animal Health

Despite their accessibility and widespread use to combat numerous significant pathogens affecting animals, a few of these yield products show different adequacy and protection in the area, need different doses, and not stable under normal circumstances. Nanovaccines have arisen as emerging options in contrast to other customary vaccination stages. Specifically, nanovaccines based on polymer give supported discharge of antigen payloads, balance out such payloads, and persuade upgraded antibody and cell mediated immunological reaction. Nanotechnology based vaccines are constant at room temperature, limiting requirement for cold chain storage. Nanotechnology-based particle stages can be developed for designated the conveyance at the target place through intranasal, aerosol, or oral administration to enhance wanted mucosal immunity.

- Instances of nano emulsion vaccines are recombinant B anthracis spore based and influenza virus. Following the oral course of vaccine stacked on PLGA nanotechnology-based particles, they produce Immunoglobulin type G and Immunoglobulin type A immunological responses explain through are *Helicobacter pylori*, Tetanus pathogen, *Bordetella pertussis* vaccine, and *Bovine para* influenza type III vaccine.
- Recombinant Leishmania SOD is illustration of vaccine that stacked on chitosan nanotechnology-based particles are given through subcutaneous infusion, besides, TB vaccine stacked on chitosan is given by respiratory lot, moreover pneumococcal antigen vaccine and *Streptococci equi* antibody are stacked on chitosan and done through intranasal course.
- Gold particle base nanovaccine is offered against to foot and mouth illness. Skillet *et al.* planned 2 different nanotechnology-based particles stages for mucosal vaccination in opposition to type A FMDV.
- Empty capsid like molecule vaccine which influence horse and known as Africanhorse sickness.
- The utilizations of nanotechnology become the demonstrating ground for untried and more disputable methods from Nano technology vaccine to sex determination in breeding.

Trypanosoma: These days, nanotechnology should show potential part in veterinary medicine.Instance is that the blend of nanocarrier mediated therapy is helpful in dealing of different disorders influencing food produced by animal for human consumed by them. It is prompted that quantum spots (QD) are suggested to be utilized. Likewise, nanovaccine provide for the treatment of trypanosome. This is done by targeted delivery of diminazen (DMZ). The permeable positive nanotechnology-based particles completely focused on trypanosomes. Assessment of clinical boundaries after nanoparticle treatment revealed decrease in allergic conditions. Rhabdovirus and AP-3M2e: The prevention of viral disease especially the rhabdovirus. Spring viremia of carp virus (SVCV) was considered as a model to estimate the probability of targeted nanovaccine in preventing rhabdovirus diseases.3M2e VLP is a potential bivalent nanovaccine, which provides twofold safety against IAV (influenza A virus) and PCV2 (porcine circovirus type 2) both in animals and humans

17.7 Constraints in the Development and Application

Nanoparticle based medicine is the utilization of nanotechnology for the diagnosis, prevention, and treatment of diseases. Nanotechnology-based medicines are few micrometer transporter materials (nanoparticles) considered to work on the biodistribution of typified compounds by conveying them more viably and more specifically to the obsessive (site-explicit medication conveyance), as well as by directing them away from possibly uncommon healthy tissues (site-aversion drug conveyance). The impediments of nanoparticles for the conveyance of vaccines range from concern regards poisonousness of particle, to challenges in creating the materials and introducing antigens in local structure. The formation of appropriate nanoparticles could introduce some specialized difficulties. For instance, although insect cell lines that are generally utilized communicate VLPs, they cannot glycosylate proteins similarly as mammalian cells. For different frameworks, there are worries over the soundness or possible to increase creation. Perhaps, the hindrance with liposome conveyance frameworks is not stable. The manners by which it had defeated is by altering the surface bywater liking polymer, like glycol. This fills in as a boundary to reticuloendothelial framework cells to expand its bloodsystem lifetime.

The production of nanoparticles into biomedical application shows possible toxicity, since certain materials, which should somehow be viewed as protected interpretation of various qualities in a nanoparticulate frame, can here become harmful. For instance, in its natural mineral state titanium dioxide is organically latent, in any case, when directed as a nanoparticle more modest than 20 nm in width it causes an inflammatory response in animals and humans. Essentially, gold is by and large viewed as a protected, inactive material, and is utilized regularly for clinical inserts, notwithstanding, gold nanoparticles with a breadth of 1.4 nm act diversely and had displayed to pervade cells and nuclear membrane and tie irreversibly in theunstable condition of major groove of DNA. This condition is not valid for gold nanoparticles and that of a marginally bigger measurement (15 nm) are considered harmless at up to sixty double rates.

Other poisonousness concern related with nanoparticles is collection inside cells, especially with constantly use for longer time. To be sure, fluorescent quantum dots are seen in the mice after completion of 2 years after giving them injection. As described earlier, the techniques utilized describe that cell dealing of nanoparticles frequently completed utilizing pharmacological inhibitors or altered cell lines. For instance, while Rejman *et al.*, show that treatment of B16 cells with chlorpromazine emphatically inhibit the take-up of negative charge 50 nm polystyrene nanoparticles contrasted with 200 nm particles, dos Santos *et al.*, report an inverse output. By and large, it is maybe better to utilize a blend of different inhibitors and changed cell lines with carefully chose controls. One more issue related with pharmacological inhibitors is their cell line explicit viability, implying that care should be taken when deciphering outcome from investigations and maybe features the requirement for utilizing a few diverse cell lines to reach determinations appropriate to an *in vivo* system.

There are additionally other explicit worries ended parts utilized in nanoparticles. Regardless of quantity of animal vaccines which use ISCOMs, there are vulnerabilities that needs to date forestalled their licensure for the utilization of people. Comparative outcomes have likewise been reported with subcutaneous and intraperitoneal organization of Quil A. where it is accepted so that it led to degradation of the liver. Be that as it may, recorded in rodents, with low poisonousness detailed in bigger earthbound animals, including rhesus monkeys, chickens, canines, or dairy cattle.

17.8 Issues Related to Product Application

Adverse reaction during and after application: Human skin, digestive system and lungs are reliably in direct contact with the climate. However, skin go about as a limit, lungs and digestive system furthermore grant transport (active and passive) of various substances like water, enhancements, or oxygen. Our understanding in this field essentially comes from drug conveyance (drug exploration) and toxicology (xenobiotics) examines. Human skin fills in as a block and no basic parts are taken up through the skin (except for radiation critical to form vitamin D). The lungs exchange oxygen and carbon dioxide with the environment, and some water escapes with warm breathed out air. The digestive system is in close contact with the materials taken up orally; there all supplements (beside gasses) are exchange between the body and the environment. Self-replicating particles that is wild, or "nanorobots," the genuine risks and toxic. The little size of nanomaterials and how their surfaces are acclimated to extend the straightforwardness with which they can connect with biological frameworks—the very characteristics that make them appropriate for applications in drug and industry—makes nanomaterials possibly hurting for individuals and the climate. The following are the three main reasons that can be constraints in vaccine development:

- Nanotechnology-based particles in vaccine may damage the lungs. Environmental pollution also harms the lungs and cause severe disorder. This happens due to their size (that they penetrate lungs) and furthermore that they bring other artificial substances incorporating metals and hydrogen and carbon.
- Nanotechnology-based particles could enter the human body through the skin, lungs, and digestive track. Nanoparticles produce free radicals which cause destruction in the cell and DNA. Once the nanotechnology-based particles enter the body circulatory system and then reach blood brain barrier.
- The body produced resistance to most naturally atom and molecules in which they become in contact. It has no natural immunity and are toxic.

17.9 Characteristics of Nanoparticles Applicable to Public Health

Size: To pass through cell membrane, arrive at the blood and different organs because of their little size. nanotechnology-based particles show high surface to volume ratio (for example the surface area contrasted with the volume) than bigger particles of exact material that was used initially. So, on the surface, a greater number of molecules are present. This might be one reason why nanotechnology-based particles are high in toxicity than bigger particles of a similar composition. The expression of a dose reaction relationship based on molecule size brought about a comparable dose reaction connection between low solubility – less toxicity, particles of various sizes.
Chemical structure and surface attributes: The toxicity of nanoparticles relies on their chemical composition. Nanotechnology-based nanoparticles made less harmful by altering their surface.

Shape: The health impacts of nanoparticles are probably dependent on their shape. A known instance is nanotechnology-based tubes, i.e., nanotubes, which might be of somenanometers in width however length of few micrometers. More toxicity of carbon-based nanotubes is to be formed. Carbon nanotube brought about increased in oxidative pressure and toxicity of cell, which might be deciphered as potential for dermal toxicity.

Despite research in the field of nanomedicine, a couple nano-based drug delivery system has arrived at the market. Some nanoparticles break down easily and their impact on living life are the same with the impacts of the chemicals from which they are produced, other nanoparticles do not degrade frequently. Rather they are assimilated in the body for a longer time, which may cause harmful effect in the body. The toxicity produced by nanotechnology-based particles has been broadly considered, particularly for those nanotechnology materials made for human concern. Safety concern with nanomedicines made it compulsory for focus on the subatomic and molecular level that happen when nanoparticles enter biological system. The hazardous impacts incorporate oxidative pressure, inflammatory reactions, and genotoxicity. There are presently various clinical preliminaries utilizing different nanotechnology-based particle methodologies that exhibit patterns in the rigorousness of undesirable impacts that may be concerned with nanotechnology-basedmedicines. The significant alarm is the affinity for nanotechnology-based particles to initiate the immunological reaction, bringing about slight side effects, as inflammation and more serious side effects that include complement activation-related pseudo allergy to life frightening side effects for example, hypertyrosinemia.

17.10 Conclusion

Nanovaccinology or use of nanotechnology in vaccine development is a quite valuable technology for effective vaccine development and induction of long-lasting immune response. This nanoparticle-based synthetic delivery system provides protection to encapsule antigen from host environment, enhance its presentation and uptake to antigen-presenting cells and release of antigen in a sustainable way. Nanocarrier-based conveyance frameworks offer a chance to upgrade the humoral and cell safe reactions. Vaccine development and vaccination is a phenomenal milestone in the prevention of infectious diseases and eradication of numerous diseases. Several types of vaccines with specific merits and demerits are developed through evolutionary process, including live attenuated, killed and toxoids. Vaccine development through nanotechnology provides nanocarrier-based delivery system that improve the cellular, as well as humoral immune, response. The nanoparticles in the vaccine development ensures advanced paybacks, including improved immunogenicity. Nanovaccines are developed against human and animals. Vaccines are used to initiate the immune system to stimulate the immune reaction against targets, like malignant growth cells and microbial agents. Vaccines developed for human health include Covid 19, Inflexal V, Epaxal and Gardasil™, and Cervarix™. We prefer nanotechnology-based vaccine over conventional vaccine because this avoid the use of toxic material, multi-injection, and multidoses are avoided, traditional adjuvants are substituted. Some of the adverse effects of nanovaccine are that they affect lungs, respiratory system, skin, and immunity. A nanovaccine that shows considerable effect on human effect should be focused on size, shape, and chemical surface and structure of nanoparticles. So nanovaccines play a vital role in securing human and animal health.

References

1. Petkar, K.C., Patil, S.M., Chavhan, S.S. *et al.*, An overview of nanocarrier-based adjuvants for vaccine delivery. *Pharmaceutics*, 13, 4, 455, 2021.
2. Facciolà, A., Visalli, G., Orlando, A., Bertuccio, M. P., Spataro, P., Squeri, R., Picerno, I., & Di Pietro, A. Vaccine hesitancy: An overview on parents' opinions about vaccination and possible reasons of vaccine refusal. *Journal of public health research*, 8, 1, 1436, 2019. https://doi.org/10.4081/jphr.2019.1436
3. Salmon, D.A., Dudley, M.Z., Glanz, J.M. *et al.*, Vaccine hesitancy: Causes, consequences, and a call to action. *Am. J. Prev. Med.*, 49, S391–S398, 2015.
4. Facciola, A., Visalli, G., Lagana, P. *et al.*, The new era of vaccines: The "nanovaccinology. *Eur. Rev. Med. Pharmacol. Sci.*, 23, 7163–7182, 6Fifis T, 2019.
5. Uto, T., Akagi, T., Toyama, M. *et al.*, Comparative activity of biodegradable nanoparticles with aluminum adjuvants: Antigen uptake by dendritic cells and induction of immune response in mice. *Immunol. Lett.*, 140, 36–43, 2011.
6. Demento, S.L., Cui, W., Criscione, J.M. *et al.*, Role of sustained antigen release from nanoparticle vaccines in shaping the T cell memory phenotype. *Biomaterials*, 33, 4957–4964, 2012.
7. Kheirollahpour, M., Mehrabi, M., Dounighi, N.M. *et al.*, Nanoparticles and vaccine development. *Pharm. Nanotechnol.*, 8, 6–21, 2019.

8. Guy, B., The perfect mix: Recent progress in adjuvant research. *Nat. Rev. Microbiol.*, 5, 505–517, 20072007.
9. Hardee, C.L., Arévalo-Soliz, L.M., Hornstein, B.D. *et al.*, Advances in non-viral DNA vectors for gene therapy. *Genes*, 8, 2, 65, 2017.
10. Gregory, A.E., Titball, R., Williamson, D., Vaccine delivery using nanoparticles. *Front. Cell. Infect. Microbiol.*, 4, 3, 13, 2013.
11. Kim, M.G., Park, J.Y., Shon, Y. *et al.*, Nanotechnology and vaccine development. *Asian J. Pharm. Sci.*, 9, 227–235, 2014.
12. Oyewumi, M.O., Kumar, A., Cui, Z., Nano-microparticles as immune adjuvants: Correlating particle sizes and the resultant immune responses. *Expert Rev. Vaccines*, 9, 269, 1095–1107, 2010.
13. Peek, L.J., Middaugh, C.R., Berkland, C., Nanotechnology in vaccine delivery. *Adv. Drug Deliv. Rev.*, 60, 915–928, 2008.
14. Ura, T., Okuda, K., Shimada, M., Developments in viral vector-based vaccines. *Vaccines*, 2, 624–641, 2014.
15. Zeltins, A., Construction and characterization of virus-like particles: A review. *Mol. Biotechnol.*, 53, 92–107, 2013.
16. Pearse, M.J. and Drane, D., ISCOMATRIX® adjuvant for antigen delivery. *Adv. Drug Deliv. Rev.*, 57, 270, 465–474, 2005.
17. Giddam, A.K., Zaman, M., Skwarczynski, M. *et al.*, Liposome-based delivery system for vaccine candidates: Constructing an effective formulation. *Nanomedicine*, 7, 1877–1893, 2012.
18. Li, Z., Ding, S., Li, Y., Study on the immunity protection of 14-3-3–MPLA–liposome vaccine against cystic echinococcosis in mice. *Front. Lab. Med.*, 2, 146–151, 2018.
19. Wang, N., Chen, M., Wang, T., Liposomes used as a vaccine adjuvant-delivery system: From basics to clinical immunization. *J. Control. Release*, 303, 130–150, 2019.
20. Navarro-Tovar, G., Palestino, G., Rosales-Mendoza, S., An overview on the role of silica-based materials in vaccine development. *Expert Rev. Vaccines*, 15, 1449–1462, 2016.
21. Hassan, H.A.F.M., Diebold, S.S., Smyth, L.A. *et al.*, Application of carbon nanotubes in cancer vaccines: Achievements, challenges and chances. *J. Control. Release*, 297, 79–90, 2019.
22. Lambkin, I., Pinilla, C., Hamashin, C. *et al.*, Toward targeted oral vaccine delivery systems: Selection of lectin mimetics from combinatorial libraries, *Pharmaceutical research*, 20, 8, 1258–1266, 2003.
23. Sen, D., Deerinck, T.J., Ellisman, M.H. *et al.*, Quantum dots for tracking dendritic cells and priming an immune response *in vitro* and *in vivo*. *PloS One*, 3, 9, e3290, 2008.
24. Dykman, L.A., Gold nanoparticles for preparation of antibodies and vaccines against infectious diseases. *Expert Rev. Vaccines*, 19, 465–477, 2020.

25. Alexyuk, P.G., Bogoyavlenskiy, A.P., Alexyuk, M.S. *et al.*, Adjuvant activity of multimolecular complexes based on Glycyrrhiza glabra saponins, lipids, and influenza virus glycoproteins. *Arch. Virol.*, 164, 1793–1803, 2019.
26. Ramamoorth, M. and Narvekar, A., Non viral vectors in gene therapy - An overview. *J. Clin. Diagn. Res.*, 9, GE01–GE06, 2015.
27. Shah, P., Bhalodia, D., Shelat, P., Nanoemulsion: A pharmaceutical review. *Syst. Rev. Pharm.*, 1, 24–32, 2010.
28. O'Hagan, D.T., MF59 is a safe and potent vaccine adjuvant that enhances protection against influenza virus infection. *Expert Rev. Vaccines*, 6, 699–710, 2007.

18

Functionalization of Nanobiomaterials in Nanovaccinology

Jyothy G. Vijayan

M. S. Ramaiah University of Applied Sciences, Bengaluru, Karnataka, India

Abstract
Nanovaccines are highly efficient for the treatment of many diseases due to their exact biochemical interactions and active constituents in it. Vaccinations are the best preventive technique used against infectious diseases. To synthesize highly potential vaccines, there is a need to develop new adjuvants and delivery system that improve immunogenicity. Applications of nanotechnology in vaccine synthesis helps to improve the applications based on it. Vaccinations are most efficient preventive measure against infectious diseases. Presently Covid 19 vaccines are on high demand. But still, vaccine hesitance is present in many countries. Vaccine hesitance about COVID-19 virus results from unjustified fear of hypothetical side effects of vaccines and the lack of trust of vaccine safety and efficacy. Nowadays, vaccine development is evolving at a high rate, and the number of candidate vaccine is progressively increasing day by day. This review analyzes the new approach of functionalized bionanomaterial-based nanovaccines and their applications.

Abbreviations

AuNPs	Gold Nanoparticles
BNPs	Bionanoparticles
CNT	Carbon nanotube
HA	Hyluronic acid
MNPs	Magnetic Nanoparticles
NP	Nanoparticles
PCL	Polycaprolactone

Email: jyothyvijayan.res.msruas@gmail.com

Kaushik Pal (ed.) Nanovaccinology as Targeted Therapeutics, (283–300) © 2022 Scrivener Publishing LLC

PEG	Polyethylene Glycol
PEO	Polyethylene Oxide
PNPs	Polymer Nanoparticles
Si NPs	Silica Nanoparticles
TMC	N-Trimethyl Chitosan
VLP	Virus like Particles

Keywords: Nanovaccines, immunogenicity, adjuvants, delivery system and nanotechnology

18.1 Introduction

Nanovaccines are used in different diseases, such as bacterial, viral, cancer, and auto immune disorders. A wide variety of NPs are used as vaccine scaffolds, and efficiency of nanoassembled vaccine depends on different parameters. It includes antigen stability, lack of immunotoxicity, sustained release, flexibility of physical factors, and so on. Vaccines are able to either be kiled or live atteunated antigens. It may not improve desired immune response level. NPs having higher surface properties are able to stimulate the immune system. The hydrophobicity of NPs enhances the release of inflammatory higher adjuvancity compared with conventional vaccine adjuvants making NPs more superior [1].

Nanovaccines are proven to be more efficient than first- and second-generation vaccines because of their low functionalized plasmid DNA, the smart size, and hydrophobicity. Use of bionanomaterials such as chitosan, albumin,peptides, enzyme as nanocarriers for vaccines exhibited long life span and stability to the cancer treatment [2]. Nanovaccines provide efficient cellular pathways and efficient absorption route up to blood vessels. Development in nanotechnology leads to the synthesis of numerous nanostructures, like nanorods, nanoparticles, nanofibers, nanotubes, and nanosheets [3]. Natural or synthetic materials, which are able to incorporate with drugs and self-assemble to form NPS, have been used as drug delivery carriers. Parameters for an effective nanovaccines are as follows: (1) good antigen to develop immunity, (2) an immune adjuvant to costimulate the innate immune system, (3) an effective carrier system. Literature reported that charge, size, and shape of NPs have a major role in antigen uptake. Tunable surface of bionanoparticles give versatile scaffold for different applications, so it can be effectively used in vaccine development [4].

18.2 Characteristics of Functionalized Bionanoparticles

Functionalized BNPs give specific properties that are difficult or impossible to gain using synthetic materials. It gives efficient delivery of BNPs with less cytotoxicity [5]. Functionalization of NPs with oligonucleotide provide fast molecular diagnostics and the identification of nucleic acids. It also detects the intracellular biomolecules like ATP. NPs coated with proteins and antibodies can bond to cell surface receptors which gives targeted delivery [6].

18.3 Functionalization of NPs

NPs possess unique physical attributes that are coupled with biomolecular system. It enables them to use for therapeutic and diagnostic applications. Designed structure of NP monolayer structure can enhance cellular internalization ability, noncytotoxicity, and high bonding capacity. Functionalization of NPs helps them to tune targeted properties, which includes specific recognition needed for biosensing [7]. Generally, NPs are functionalized with different ligands, such as small molecules, surfactants, polymers, dendrimers, and biomolecules.

18.3.1 Functionalization With Different Ligands

Different types of ligands are incorporated in to the surface of NPs making them used in the sensing of biomolecule and cells. It is also applied in intracellular delivery to the diagnosis of different diseases [8]. NPs functionalized with ligand shows affinity toward proteins and cell surface. Molecules have been used for their surface charge in accordance with aromatic stalking and hybridization has a part in sensor synthesis. NPs modified with ligands, which are positively charged, exhibit higher internalization in to the cells [9]. It is comparably less with neutral and negatively charged particles, carboxylated functionalized iron oxide NPs exhibits higher intake in to the cells. In the case of tumor tissue and drug studies, positive NPs were more efficient in delivering drugs to the peripheral cells due to their enhanced uptake. Amine functionalized silica NPs show efficiency in *in vitro* and *in vivo* studies [10].

18.3.2 Polymer Functionalized NPs

Coating NPs with polymers increases the targeting of tumor issues, eg, PEG coating prevents adsorption of blood serum proteins. It enhances the circulation. PEG coated with gold NPs by passive targeting mechanism used for tumor tissue via IR irradiation. Polymer functionalized NPs increase the release of drugs [11].

18.4 Nanomaterials for Vaccine Synthesis

There are many nanomaterials used in the sysnthesis and development of nanovaccines, eg, chitosan, silica, CNT, liposomes, gold, and so on.

18.4.1 Gold NPS

Gold NPs and functionalized Au-NPs are used in the synthesis of sensors, drug delivery, and imaging. Au-NPs are non-toxic in nature. Surface of Au-NPs are developed to attach antigens and adjuvants to synthesize nanovaccines [12].

18.4.2 Silica NPs

Silica NPs are very efficient for different applications. It is highly recommended for vaccine delivery and tumor targeting [13]. Functionalization of SiNPs is synthesized by adding more silanol group on the surfaces. It helps to improve cellular recognition, cellular uptake, and absorption of specific biomolecules. The major limitations for using silica NPs in biomedical field is its toxicity generated from the reducing agents and stabilizers used for the synthesis.

18.4.3 Calcium NPs

For vaccine synthesis calcium phosphate, NPs are mostly used [14]. It is due to their biodegradability and functionalized surface structure. CaPNPs possess good biocompatibility and surface area. Surface functionalized CaPNPs can carry genes in liver also.

18.4.4 Polymeric NPs

Polymers with 10- to 500-nm-sized solid structure are used for different applications, such as in packaging and surface adsorption. Polymers are very efficient for the carrying or releasing of different target-oriented drugs. PNPs are used in drug delivery due to its properties like predictability, chemical stability [15], surface modification, and biocompatibility. PNPs are studied for their progress in mucosal vaccines and used for encapsulated antigen synthesis. PNPs are divided in to natural PNPs and synthetic PNPs. Alginate, hyaluronic acid, and chitosan are the natural PNPs used in the biomedical field.

18.4.5 Inorganic Magnetic NPs

They are also used in vaccine delivery. MNPs are synthesized with the help of magnetic field. Paramagnetic NPs were used in *in vivo* applications also [16].

18.4.6 Chitosan NPs

Many biopolymer is used to make blended adsorbents with chitosan for the removal of pollutants. Biopolymer including gelation, alginate, cellulose are added with chitosan for the contamination process Chitosan has been blended with nanoparticles for water treatment, eg, chitosan/ZnO bionanocomposite. It is used for the removal of acid black from waste water. Chitosan hydrogels are very efficient for the use of the removal of pollutants. It is because of their properties, such as softness and efficiency to store water. Among hydrogels, pH-sensitive hydrogels are good conductors because of the presence of functional groups on it which are ionic in nature and are suitable for the separation. Chitosan beads exhibits excellent properties due to the presence of hydroxyl groups in it. It also exhibits properties, such as acid stability, higher surface area, pore size , chemical stability, and so on [17]. Modification of chitosan is done through physical and chemical methods.

18.4.7 Liposomal NPs

Liposomal NPs are artificially self assembled molecules made up of biodegradabe non-toxic phospholipids bilayer shell with aqueous core. Liposomes can be functionalized to incorporate with hydrophilic/hydrophobic molecules. Liposomal vaccines are used widely because of the addition of different antigens, such as proteins, peptides, and nucleic acids [18] (Table 18.1).

Table 18.1 NPs associated nanovaccines and their applications.

NPs	Nanovaccines	Applications	References
Liposome	DepoDur	Pain relief	[19]
Plasmid	Life Tide	For perinatal morbidity	[20]
Virosomes	Inflexal	Influenza	[21]
DNA vaccine	Apex-IHN	Haematopoietic necrosis	[22]
Dendritic cell	Provenge	Prostate cancer	[23]

18.5 Role of the Surface of NPs on Vaccine Development

Tunable surface of NPs gives a different scaffold for many applications in biomedicines. Different chemical and physical modifications are tried on NP surface and applied in biomedical field. Surface functionalities are fabricated to enhance biomimetic properties which includes noncytotoxicity and specificity for the cells. Sound knowledge about cellular uptake mechanism of functionalized bionanoparticles is essential to apply in the vaccine synthesis development [24]. To gain knowledge in the complex mechanism of NPs in the biosystem helps for the diagnosis of different diseases.

18.6 Nanovaccines: Routes of Administration

Different routes are made with the application of nanovaccines such as oral,by injection, transdermal, ocular, pulmonary and implantation. For that polymers used are PCL, PEG, PLGA, PGA, and so on [25].

18.6.1 Intradermal Routes

Drugs administered by using intradermal routes are applied for the purpose of immunization. Here, drugs are injected in to the epidermal layer of the skin. Drug is slowly released for prolonged effect [26]. Different adjuvants are used here, eg, TMC/HA (N-trimethyl chitosan-hyluronic acid).

18.6.2 Intramuscular Routes

This is used to reach antigen to the langeehans cells. It is used against influenza (H3N1) [27].

18.6.3 Subcutaneous Routes

Here, liposomes are injected subcutaneously to the lymph nodes. PEGylation of liposomes leads to steric stabilization of liposomes and improves the lymphatic uptake at injection site [28].

18.6.4 Oral Routes

DNA vaccines with polymer-based NPs are administered orally through gene therapy [29]. Limitations of oral routs are attributed to the dilution that occurs in gastrointestinal tract as the vaccine travel.

18.6.5 Nasal Routes

Nasal sprays are displayed properties, like small size, easy disposal. It has the ability to reach the mucosal area of the nose [30]. It is encapsulated within NPs and give good adsorption also with the formulation.

18.6.6 Tropical Routes

Here, vaccines are delivered via skin and skin patches to deliver genetic material, eg, plasmid DNA. Here side effects are reduced due to limited toxicity. Here, DNA can be delivered through liposomes and microemulsions. It is used for hepatitis B [31].

18.6.7 Ocular Routes

Here vaccination through ocular mucosa is conducted [32], eg, if eye is exposed to external environment and get infected by antigens, vaccination through ocular is acceptable. The limitation of this approach includes poor drainage, tear turnover, systematic absorption, and corneal permeability.

18.7 Nanovaccines for Different Applications

Nanovaccines are used against pathogens, viruses, bacteria, parasites, and cancer.

18.7.1 Nanovaccines Against Bacteria

Nanovaccines that have been used to treat many diseases have bacterial origin [33–35]. *E. coli* is the most utilized organism in many nanovaccines. Toxins from bacteria also have been used to produce nanovaccines. It is essential to commercialize toxoids against bacteria for human administration.

18.7.2 Nanovaccines Against Pathogens

Many pathogens are arising, such as multidrug-resistant bacteria, mutating viruses, secondary cancer, and so on [36–38]. In this condition. it is very essential to come up with practical solutions to resist the population of pathogens. NPs are found highly effective for wound treatment, prevention of infection, and so on. Nanobiomaterials are proven to be highly efficient in therapeutics, prophylaxis against pathogens, like viruses, bacteria, and parasites.

18.7.3 Nanovaccines Against Viruses

Viral diseases are a great threat to the entire ecosystem. High cost of production is a major challenge to antiviral drug production. Many toxic pathogens like HBV, HIV, are prevented by using nanovaccines, nanoadjuvant, and other medicines [39–41].

18.7.4 Nanovaccines Against Parasites

NPs are used successively against parasitic diseases, such as malaria, toxoplasmosis, anaplasmosis, coccidiosis, and so on. That is, only NPs assembled vaccines are available instead nanovaccines. NPs assembled vaccines are more protectable and higly desirable in nature. Nanovaccines are applicable to parasites, such as ticks, flies, mosquitoes, which causes zoonotic diseases [42–45].

18.7.5 Nanovaccines Against Cancer

Using nanovaccines, cancers of different organs and systems, such as nervous, digestive, reproduction, brain, and endocrine, can be prevented [46, 47]. Bioconjugation with nanoparticles for the formation of nanovaccines helps to improve immune response by providing protection against tumors. The advantage of using nanovaccines includes high precision and high immuno protection.

18.8 Emulsions

Emulsions are used in vaccine synthesis for years and also in vaccine delivery system. Nanoscale emulsions made of two immiscible liquid phases, emulsifiers, and excipients. Liquid of one is dispersed in the other and make a single phase. Here, vaccines are classified into two broad classes: nanosized oil-in-water and nanosized water-in-oil emulsions. Emulsifying agent finally leads to the formation of a film around the globules so that a stable emulsion is produced. Emulsions are thermodynamically unstable and seperate back to oil and water phase. Emulsions can be used in vaccine delivery by carrying antigens inside their core or by mixing with the antigens [48–50]. Nano-emulsions are functionally efficient than larger-sized emulsion. Emulsions are able to permeate the nasal mucosa and carry the antigen to the APCs.

18.9 Nanogels

Nanogel-based vaccines are synthesized by the physical crosslinking with natural polymers. Nanogels are very efficient to synthesize nanovaccines because of its structure. Its structure gives an environment suitable for analytes based on proteins. Radical polymerization is generally used for the synthesis of nanogels. In this process, polymer is produced by adding free radical building blocks. Functionalized nanogels are used for the synthesis of nanovaccines for cancer treatment [51–53].

18.10 Virus-Like Particles (VLP)

VLP resembles structural proteins from viruses. VLP lacks genetic material. VLPs are non-infectious, highly immunogenic and small VLPs are able to load peptides, proteins, nucleic acids and other NPs (Table 18.2).

Table 18.2 Natural andsynthetic sources of nanovaccines.

Exosomes	Proteosomes	Liposomes	Nanobeads	Virosomes
a) Exosome vaccines are used in both humans and animals b) NPs associated are ranged between 30-150n c) NPs originated from endosomal membranes	a) Nanovaccines formulated using proteosomes are safe for humans b) These vesicles are of size between 20-80 nm c) Proteosomes are hydrophilic in nature. So can be uptaken by the immunesystem fastly d) They are used as nanovaccines against influenza, HIV and shigellosis etc.	a) Liposomes are made up of phospholipids which are bilayer and both are hydrophilic and hydrophobic in nature b) Liposomes as drug carrier in nanovaccines helps to improve the therapeutic index and increases the immune reponse. c) Liposomes are able to divide and solubilize the phospholipid cell membranes	a) Most effective immunization techniques b) Here NPs are coated by antigens on their surfaces c) Advantages includes store stability and small dose of administration	a) Virosomes are used for protective immunity b) Vesicular system between virosome and antigen is developed here c) Virosomes helps to transport antigens to the target site

VLPs are noninfectious, small, and immunogenic in nature. VLPs are able to load peptides, proteins, nucleic acids, and other NPs. VLPs can be produced *in vivo* and *in vitro*. VLPs are less expensive and can be used for nanovaccine synthesis. VLPs' self-assembling nanostructures that are used from viral structural proteins.VLPs can be synthesized from capsid proteins, which can be modified to counter pathogenic attacks. VLPs are recommended due to their easy production and the ability to stimulate immune responses [54–57]. Diseases, such as malaria, chikkungunya, influenza, hepatitis, Ebola, corona virus, are fastly studied in clinical stages by using VLP based NPs.

18.11 Applications of Novel Nanovaccines

Nanovaccines are generally provided by topical and oral routes. Topical routs is the most preferred one because it prevents unnecessary invasion to body. It helps antigens to associate with lymphatic system. It prevents unnecessary toxicity. Nanovaccines should be ideal, ie, it should not cause any toxicity, side effects, or pathogenicity. It should be safe. It should not cause any problem to the individual with impaired immune system. Vaccines should not contaminate the environment and are affordable in nature.

18.12 Applications of Functionalized Nanovaccines

High surface area-to-volume ratio of functionalized NPs and their skill development in various formulations, such as nanocrystals, nanoparticles, and nanoclusters, help them to use in different treatment processes against cancer, influenza, and malaria [58–61].

18.12.1 For Cancer Therapy

Functionalized NPs help in the development of nanosized immunotherapy delivery system for cancer. For cancer therapy liposomes, nanosphere and polymeric NP system are used in delivering vaccine antigens. Functionalized NPs work as an adjuvants to antigen-presenting cells and stimulate the immune response with new vaccines. Functionalized NPs act as a vehicle or nanocarrier for targeting tumor in chemotherapies [62–64]. These NPs are nanocarriers with exact size and SA provided by providing selective delivery of antigens to different organs using NPs in cancer treatments helps to reduce toxicity, immunogenicity and biodegradability.

18.12.2 Against Different Infectious Diseases

Use of bionanoparticles in medical field gives the ability to target the disease by crossing the membranes and entering the cells, which may take more time than alternate medicines. But it reduces the side effects and the cost. Adjuvants are added to the vaccines, which help to protect antigen from degradation. In veterinary use, vaccines are generally provided by oral, intramuscular, or intradermal routes. Many nanovaccines in animals are used against cancer recently [65–68].

18.13 Pros and Cons of Using Vaccines

Nanovaccines have various properties and advanced bioavailability, which gives different size, shape, and stability for numerous applications. Nanoemulsion vaccines attained high affinity for the lymphatic system [69]. Novel vaccines are studied for influenza and cancer immunotherapy. New methods, like nanopatch technology, are in high demand because it is pain-free, needle-free, and cost-effective [47]. Development of new vaccines required advanced machines and tools, which makes it more costly. There is a limit in the use of biodegradable polymers, which leads to the loss of immunogenicity in storage [70]. The ability of NPs to overcome the barriers with specific size, shape and charge leads to the increase of the immune response more precisely.

18.13.1 Toxicity of NPs

More than incredible capability and applications of NPs mentioned above, because of unique physicochemical characteristics, unusual and unexpected toxicity of NPs, understanding these properties and how they interact with cells can help develop safer NPs. Composition, size, charge, morphology, hydrophobicity, and route of exposure are significant aspects that affect toxic effects and immune responses elicited by the NPs [71]. Therefore, investigating the toxicity, immune response, and excretion over time of NPs before use is highly necessary. Several studies have identified various cytotoxic properties that make some NPs more toxic than others. Many investigators studied and focused on various aspects of NPs. Several other researchers have focused on improving biocompatibility and limiting the toxicity of NPs.

18.14 Future Aspects

There is a competition developed to find innovative vaccines having low cost, high efficiency, availability of effective antigen delivery. Nanomaterials are a gift for this field and has been used in the structure and design of nanovaccines to regain immunogenicity, lack of toxicity, high stability, and so on. Due to the presence of phagocytic cells, nanovaccines are efficient which leads to an efficient antigen recognition.

Functionalized nanobiobased vaccines have enhanced immunogenicity of nano carrier based vaccines. Multifunctional nanovaccine increases the immune response developed by the target specificity and stable delivery of an antigen. Functionalized nanovaccines need complex purification process and more cost. Scale up procedures needs more time for pharmaceutical applications. Self-assembled bionanovaccines are highly preferred for reducing the obstacles for the improvement of industrial scale up manufacturing regulations.

18.15 Conclusions

NPs are highly used in vaccine delivery due to their incredible capacity and applications. It possesses properties like toxicity, immune response, biocompatibility, size, composition, charge, morphology, and so on. But major threat is related with toxic agents and immune responses. Many reports came up with high cytotoxic effects with NPs than other particles. NPs are very effective adjuvants to stimulate immune responses. Adding antigens to NPs helps to protect them against degradation. It also helps in targeting and controlled release. However, small size and large SA of NPs associated targeted and delivery system cause aggregation and are difficult to handle. Another main issue is related with vaccine safety as it comes to adjuvant approval for human use. Generally, old vaccines strategy involves method used by either killed or live atteunated antigens. Live atteunated vaccines arise clinical disease from mutated/same genotypes. NPs with higher surface properties enables them to strengthen the immune system and immunological response. NPs are hydrophobic in nature releases cytokines. Among new vaccines, the property which helps them to make higher is its superior adjuvancity. This review tries to highlight the progress in the area of functionalized bionanoparticles, modifications, and their uses.

References

1. Fawzy, M., Khairy, G.M., Hesham, A., Rabaan, A.A., El-Shamy, A.G., Nagy, A., Nanoparticles as a novel and promising antiviral platform in veterinary medicine. *Arch. Virol.*, 166, 10, 2673–2682, 2021.
2. Nandedkar, T.D., Nanovaccines: recent developments in vaccination. *J. Biosci.*, *34*, 6, 995–1003, 2009.
3. Simón-Vázquez, R., Peleteiro, M., González-Fernández, Á., Polymeric nanostructure vaccines: Applications and challenges. *Expert Opin. Drug Deliv.*, *17*, 7, 1007–1023, 2020.
4. Singh, L., Kruger, H.G., Maguire, G.E., Govender, T., Parboosing, R., The role of nanotechnology in the treatment of viral infections. *Ther. Adv. Infect. Dis.*, *4*, 4, 105–131, 2017.
5. El-Sayed, N., Korotchenko, E., Scheiblhofer, S., Weiss, R., Schneider, M., Functionalized multifunctional nanovaccine for targeting dendritic cells and modulation of immune response. *Int. J. Pharm.*, *593*, 120123, 2021.
6. Chen, G., Bai, Y., Li, Z., Wang, F., Fan, X., Zhou, X., Bacterial extracellular vesicle-coated multi-antigenic nanovaccines protect against drug-resistant Staphylococcus aureus infection by modulating antigen processing and presentation pathways. *Theranostics*, *10*, 16, 7131, 2020.
7. Zottig, X., Côté-Cyr, M., Arpin, D., Archambault, D., Bourgault, S., Protein supramolecular structures: From self-assembly to nanovaccine design. *Nanomaterials*, *10*, 5, 1008, 2020.
8. Qiu, L., Valente, M., Dolen, Y., Jäger, E., Beest, M.T., Zheng, L., Verdoes, M., Endolysosomal-escape nanovaccines through adjuvant-induced tumor antigen assembly for enhanced effector CD8+ T cell activation. *Small*, *14*, 15, 1703539, 2018.
9. Bros, M., Nuhn, L., Simon, J., Moll, L., Mailänder, V., Landfester, K., Grabbe, S., The protein corona as a confounding variable of nanoparticle-mediated targeted vaccine delivery. *Front. Immunol.*, 9, 1760, 2018.
10. Rosales-Mendoza, S. and González-Ortega, O., Silica-based mucosal nanovaccines, in: *Nanovaccines*, pp. 105–130, Springer, Cham, 2019.
11. Pippa, N., Gazouli, M., Pispas, S., Recent advances and future perspectives in polymer-based nanovaccines. *Vaccines*, *9*, 6, 558, 2021.
12. Zeng, L., Liao, Z., Li, W., Yuan, Q., Wu, P., Gu, Z., Liao, G., Non-covalent glycosylated gold nanoparticles/peptides nanovaccine as potential cancer vaccines. *Chin. Chem. Lett.*, *31*, 5, 1162–1164, 2020.
13. Huang, C., Zhang, L., Guo, Q., Zuo, Y., Wang, N., Wang, H., Zhang, L., Robust nanovaccine based on polydopamine-coated mesoporous silica nanoparticles for effective photothermal-immunotherapy against melanoma. *Adv. Funct. Mater.*, *31*, 18, 2010637, 2021.
14. Mohamed, F.A.N. and Laraba-Djebari, F., Development and characterization of a new carrier for vaccine delivery based on calcium-alginate nanoparticles:

Safe immunoprotective approach against scorpion envenoming. *Vaccine, 34*, 24, 2692–2699, 2016.

15. Nandedkar, T.D., Nanotechnology a path to nanovaccine. *Int. J. Pharma Bio Sci., 3*, 2, 290–292, 2012.
16. Ahmad, M.Z., Ahmad, J., Haque, A., Alasmary, M.Y., Abdel-Wahab, B.A., Akhter, S., Emerging advances in synthetic cancer nano-vaccines: Opportunities and challenges. *Expert Rev. Vaccines, 19*, 11, 1053–1071, 2020.
17. Danesh-Bahreini, M.A., Shokri, J., Samiei, A., Kamali-Sarvestani, E., Barzegar-Jalali, M., Mohammadi-Samani, S., Nanovaccine for leishmaniasis: Preparation of chitosan nanoparticles containing Leishmania superoxide dismutase and evaluation of its immunogenicity in BALB/c mice. *Int. J. Nanomedicine, 6*, 835, 2011.
18. Roopngam, P.E., Liposome and polymer-based nanomaterials for vaccine applications. *Nanomed. J., 6*, 1, 1–10, 2019.
19. Bulbake, U., Doppalapudi, S., Kommineni, N., Khan, W., Liposomal formulations in clinical use: An updated review. *Pharmaceutics, 9*, 2, 12, 2017.
20. Pereira, V.B., Zurita-Turk, M., Saraiva, T.D., Castro, C.P., Souza, B.M., Agresti, P.M., Miyoshi, A., DNA vaccines approach: From concepts to applications, *World Journal of Vaccines*, 4, 50–71, 2014.
21. Bernocchi, B., Carpentier, R., Betbeder, D., Nasal nanovaccines. *Int. J. Pharm., 530*, 1-2, 128–138, 2017.
22. Lamp, I.M.O., DNA vaccine technology–A vaccine breakthrough that could change lives & enable vaccine development programs. *Front. Immunol.* 9:1963.
23. Pereira, V.B., Zurita-Turk, M., Saraiva, T.D., Castro, C.P., Souza, B.M., Agresti, P.M., Miyoshi, A., DNA vaccines approach: From concepts to applications, *World Journal of Vaccines*, 4, 50–71, 2014.
24. Sun, B., Zhao, X., Wu, Y., Cao, P., Movahedi, F., Liu, J., Gu, W., Mannose-functionalized biodegradable nanoparticles efficiently deliver DNA vaccine and promote anti-tumor immunity. *ACS Appl. Mater. Interfaces, 13*, 12, 14015–14027, 2021.
25. Zhao, H., Xu, J., Li, Y., Guan, X., Han, X., Xu, Y., Liu, Z., Nanoscale coordination polymer based nanovaccine for tumor immunotherapy. *ACS Nano, 13*, 11, 13127–13135, 2019.
26. Nandedkar, T.D., Nanovaccines: recent developments in vaccination. *J. Biosci., 34*, 6, 995–1003, 2009.
27. González-Aramundiz, J.V., Peleteiro, M., González-Fernández, Á., Alonso, M.J., Csaba, N.S., Protamine nanocapsules for the development of thermostable adjuvanted nanovaccines. *Mol. Pharm., 15*, 12, 5653–5664, 2018.
28. Sahu, R., Dixit, S., Verma, R., Duncan, S.A., Coats, M.T., Giambartolomei, G.H., Dennis, V.A., A nanovaccine formulation of Chlamydia recombinant MOMP encapsulated in PLGA 85:15 nanoparticles augments CD4+ effector (CD44high CD62Llow) and memory (CD44high CD62Lhigh) T-cells in immunized mice. *Nanomed.: Nanotechnol. Biol. Med., 29*, 102257, 2020.

29. Luo, M., Wang, H., Wang, Z., Cai, H., Lu, Z., Li, Y., Gao, J., A Sting-activating nanovaccine for cancer immunotherapy. *Nat. Nanotechnol.*, *12*, 7, 648–654, 2017.
30. Bernocchi, B., Carpentier, R., Betbeder, D., Nasal nanovaccines. *Int. J. Pharm.*, *530*, 1-2, 128–138, 2017.
31. Renu, S., Wilson, H.L., Tabynov, K., Hiremath, J., Engineered adjuvants and carriers for an animal infectious disease vaccine. *Front. Bioeng. Biotechnol.*, 9, 692634,2021.
32. Lambricht, L., Peres, C., Florindo, H., Préat, V., Vandermeulen, G., Polymer-based nanoparticles as modern vaccine delivery systems, in: *Micro and Nanotechnology in Vaccine Development*, pp. 185–203, 20172017.
33. Chen, G., Bai, Y., Li, Z., Wang, F., Fan, X., Zhou, X., Bacterial extracellular vesicle-coated multi-antigenic nanovaccines protect against drug-resistant Staphylococcus aureus infection by modulating antigen processing and presentation pathways. *Theranostics*, *10*, 16, 7131, 2020.
34. Calderon-Gonzalez, R., Frande-Cabanes, E., Teran-Navarro, H., Marimon, J.M., Freire, J., Salcines-Cuevas, D., Fariñas, M.C., GNP-GAPDH1-22 nanovaccines prevent neonatal listeriosis by blocking microglial apoptosis and bacterial dissemination. *Oncotarget*, *8*, 33, 53916, 2017.
35. Vijayan, V., Mohapatra, A., Uthaman, S., Park, I.K., Recent advances in nanovaccines using biomimetic immunomodulatory materials. *Pharmaceutics*, *11*, 10, 534, 2019.
36. Celis-Giraldo, C.T., López-Abán, J., Muro, A., Patarroyo, M.A., Manzano-Román, R., Nanovaccines against animal pathogens: The latest findings. *Vaccines*, *9*, 9, 988, 2021.
37. Kitiyodom, S., Yata, T., Yostawornkul, J., Kaewmalun, S., Nittayasut, N., Suktham, K., Pirarat, N., Enhanced efficacy of immersion vaccination in tilapia against columnaris disease by chitosan-coated "pathogen-like" mucoadhesive nanovaccines. *Fish Shellfish Immunol.*, *95*, 213–219, 2019.
38. Kingstad-Bakke, B.A., Chandrasekar, S.S., Phanse, Y., Ross, K.A., Hatta, M., Suresh, M., Talaat, A.M., Effective mosaic-based nanovaccines against avian influenza in poultry. *Vaccine*, *37*, 35, 5051–5058, 2019.
39. Ross, K.A., Loyd, H., Wu, W., Huntimer, L., Ahmed, S., Sambol, A., Narasimhan, B., Hemagglutinin-based polyanhydride nanovaccines against H5N1 influenza elicit protective virus neutralizing titers and cell-mediated immunity. *Int. J. Nanomed.*, *10*, 229, 2015.
40. Dhakal, S., Goodman, J., Bondra, K., Lakshmanappa, Y.S., Hiremath, J., Shyu, D.L., Renukaradhya, G.J., Polyanhydride nanovaccine against swine influenza virus in pigs. *Vaccine*, *35*, 8, 1124–1131, 2017.
41. Fusciello, M., Fontana, F., Tähtinen, S., Capasso, C., Feola, S., Martins, B., Cerullo, V., Artificially cloaked viral nanovaccine for cancer immunotherapy. *Nat. Commun.*, *10*, 1, 1–13, 2019.

42. Zaheer, T., Pal, K., Zaheer, I., Topical review on nano-vaccinology: Biochemical promises and key challenges. *Process Biochem., 100*, 237–244, 2021.
43. El Bissati, K., Zhou, Y., Paulillo, S.M., Raman, S.K., Karch, C.P., Roberts, C.W., McLeod, R., Protein nanovaccine confers robust immunity against Toxoplasma. *NPJ Vaccines, 2*, 1, 1–12, 2017.
44. Skwarczynski, M. and Toth, I., Peptide-based subunit nanovaccines. *Curr. Drug Deliv., 8*, 3, 282–289, 2011.
45. Celis-Giraldo, C.T., López-Abán, J., Muro, A., Patarroyo, M.A., Manzano-Román, R., Nanovaccines against animal pathogens: The latest findings. *Vaccines, 9*, 9, 988, 2021.
46. Paulis, L.E., Mandal, S., Kreutz, M., Figdor, C.G., Dendritic cell-based nanovaccines for cancer immunotherapy. *Curr. Opin. Immunol., 25*, 3, 389–395, 2013.
47. Xu, J., Lv, J., Zhuang, Q., Yang, Z., Cao, Z., Xu, L., Liu, Z., A general strategy towards personalized nanovaccines based on fluoropolymers for post-surgical cancer immunotherapy. *Nat. Nanotechnol., 15*, 12, 1043–1052, 2020.
48. Gupta, A., Eral, H.B., Hatton, T.A., Doyle, P.S., Nanoemulsions: formation, properties and applications. *Soft Matter, 12*, 11, 2826–2841, 2016.
49. Fryd, M.M. and Mason, T.G., Advanced nanoemulsions. *Annu. Rev. Phys. Chem., 63*, 493–518, 2012.
50. Solans, C., Izquierdo, P., Nolla, J., Azemar, N., Garcia-Celma, M.J., Nanoemulsions. *Curr. Opin. Colloid Interface Sci.,*10, 3–4, 102–110, 2005.
51. Oh, J.K., Drumright, R., Siegwart, D.J., Matyjaszewski, K., The development of microgels/nanogels for drug delivery applications. *Prog. Polym. Sci., 33*, 4, 448–477, 2008.
52. Chacko, R.T., Ventura, J., Zhuang, J., Thayumanavan, S., Polymer nanogels: A versatile nanoscopic drug delivery platform. *Adv. Drug Deliv. Rev., 64*, 9, 836–851, 2012.
53. Zha, L., Banik, B., Alexis, F., Stimulus responsive nanogels for drug delivery. *Soft Matter, 7*, 13, 5908–5916, 2011.
54. Roldão, A., Mellado, M.C.M., Castilho, L.R., Carrondo, M.J., Alves, P.M., Virus-like particles in vaccine development. *Expert Rev. Vaccines, 9*, 10, 1149–1176, 2010.
55. Zeltins, A., Construction and characterization of virus-like particles: A review. *Mol. Biotechnol., 53*, 1, 92–107, 2013.
56. Dane, D.S., Cameron, C.H., Briggs, M., Virus-like particles in serum of patients with Australia-antigen-associated hepatitis. *Lancet, 295*, 7649, 695–698, 1970.
57. Johnson, J.E. and Chiu, W., Structures of virus and virus-like particles. *Curr. Opin. Struct. Biol., 10*, 2, 229–235, 2000.
58. Ross, K., Adams, J., Loyd, H., Ahmed, S., Sambol, A., Broderick, S., Narasimhan, B., Combination nanovaccine demonstrates synergistic

enhancement in efficacy against influenza. *ACS Biomater. Sci. Eng.*, *2*, 3, 368–374, 2016.
59. Wang, Q., Zhang, Y., Zou, P., Wang, M., Fu, W., She, J., Wu, F., Self-assembly M2e-based peptide nanovaccine confers broad protection against influenza viruses. *Front. Microbiol*, 11, 1961, 2020.
60. Singh, A., Eliciting B cell immunity against infectious diseases using nanovaccines. *Nat. Nanotechnol.*, *16*, 1, 16–24, 2021.
61. Kumar, R., Ray, P.C., Datta, D., Bansal, G.P., Angov, E., Kumar, N., Nanovaccines for malaria using Plasmodium falciparum antigen Pfs25 attached gold nanoparticles. *Vaccine*, *33*, 39, 5064–5071, 2015.
62. Fusciello, M., Fontana, F., Tähtinen, S., Capasso, C., Feola, S., Martins, B., Cerullo, V., Artificially cloaked viral nanovaccine for cancer immunotherapy. *Nat. Commun.*, *10*, 1, 1–13, 2019.
63. Zhu, G., Zhang, F., Ni, Q., Niu, G., Chen, X., Efficient nanovaccine delivery in cancer immunotherapy. *ACS Nano*, *11*, 3, 2387–2392, 2017.
64. Luo, M., Liu, Z., Zhang, X., Han, C., Samandi, L.Z., Dong, C., Gao, J., Synergistic Sting activation by PC7A nanovaccine and ionizing radiation improves cancer immunotherapy. *J. Control. Release*, *300*, 154–160, 2019.
65. Kim, D., Wu, Y., Kim, Y.B., Oh, Y.K., Advances in vaccine delivery systems against viral infectious diseases. *Drug Deliv. Transl. Res.*,12, 1–19, 2021.
66. Gao, A., Liang, H., Shen, Q., Zhou, C., Chen, X.M., Tian, J., Cui, D., Designing a novel nano-vaccine against SARS-CoV-2. *Nano Biomed. Eng.*, *12*, 4, 321–324, 2020.
67. Bhardwaj, P., Bhatia, E., Sharma, S., Ahamad, N., Banerjee, R., Advancements in prophylactic and therapeutic nanovaccines. *Acta Biomater.*, *108*, 1–21, 2020.
68. McGill, J.L., Kelly, S.M., Kumar, P., Speckhart, S., Haughney, S.L., Henningson, J., Sacco, R.E., Efficacy of mucosal polyanhydride nanovaccine against respiratory syncytial virus infection in the neonatal calf. *Sci. Rep.*, *8*, 1, 1–15, 2018.
69. Ge, W., Sui, Y.F., Wu, D.C., Sun, Y.J., Chen, G.S., Li, Z.S., Zhang, X.M., MAGE-1/Heat shock protein 70/MAGE-3 fusion protein vaccine in nanoemulsion enhances cellular and humoral immune responses to MAGE-1 or MAGE-3 *in vivo*. *Cancer Immunol., Immunother.*, *55*, 7, 841–849, 2006.
70. Ni, Q., Zhang, F., Liu, Y., Wang, Z., Yu, G., Liang, B., Chen, X., A bi-adjuvant nanovaccine that potentiates immunogenicity of neoantigen for combination immunotherapy of colorectal cancer. *Sci. Adv.*, *6*, 12, eaaw6071, 2020.
71. Aikins, M.E., Xu, C., Moon, J.J., Engineered nanoparticles for cancer vaccination and immunotherapy. *Acc. Chem. Res.*, *53*, 10, 2094–2105, 2020.

19

Oral Nanovaccines Delivery for Clinical Trials and Commercialization

Dominic Augustine[1], Pushpalatha C.[2*], Sowmya S.V.[1], Chhaya Kumar[2], Elizabeth AbbuVarghese[2] and Gayathri V.S.[2]

[1]*Department of Oral Pathology and Microbiology, Faculty of Dental Sciences, M.S. Ramaiah University of Applied Sciences, MSR Nagar, Bengaluru, Karnataka, India*

[2]*Department of Pedodontics & Preventive Dentistry, Faculty of Dental Sciences, M.S. Ramaiah University of Applied Sciences, MSR Nagar, Bengaluru, Karnataka, India*

Abstract

The field of vaccination has advanced in leaps and bounds; however, effective and novel vaccines are yet to be developed, especially for diseases like acquired immune deficiency syndrome, malaria and tuberculosis. Lack of immune system stimulation, instability, allergenic potential, multiple shots are some of the shortcomings the vaccines in circulation currently carry. Nanotechnology (NT) is a commanding tool that promises to resolve the abovementioned inadequacies. Nanovaccines (NVs) were developed recently where new drugs can be accommodated through nanoparticle (NP) carriers. The similar nanosize between the nano-scaled materials and pathogens ensures optimal trigger response of the immune system resulting in satisfactory cellular and humoral immunity responses. Targeted delivery of NPs result in enhanced antibody response and improved stability coupled with long-time release addresses the many challenges encountered in vaccine development. This chapter aims to comprehensively evaluate the evolution of NVs and their morphology, carriers used, formulation-characterization and NVs' role in immunotherapy with emphasis on recent advances. Although development of NVs is in the infancy stage and few are in the early clinical phases, we firmly believe this new generation of vaccines has great potential for the prevention and treatment of many diseases.

***Keywords*:** Nanotechnology, nanovaccines, nanoparticles, humoral immunity, immunotherapy, targeted delivery

**Corresponding author*: drpushpalatha29@gmail.com

Kaushik Pal (ed.) Nanovaccinology as Targeted Therapeutics, (301–318) © 2022 Scrivener Publishing LLC

19.1 Introduction

Over the past few decades, vaccine development has focused on patient safety and optimum immune system stimulation. However, parenteral vaccine delivery has its own share of shortcomings, like pain during administration, inability to self-administer, anaphylactic reactions, and lack of mucosal immune response. To overcome these disadvantages, researchers have advocated nonparenteral routes, such as oral, nasal, rectal, and vagina. Among these, the oral route seems to be the most preferred as it is easy to administer, possible self-administration, fewer complications, noninvasive, and mass vaccination at a rapid rate is possible [1].

Further, it is a known fact that first pass metabolism, absorption, and bioavailability are few of the significant challenges encountered through the oral route of vaccination. With the advent of nanovaccines, the main focus has shifted to targeted delivery and efficacy. Oral nanovaccines can amplify the effect of conventional oral vaccines that can already cause an appreciable mucosal and systemic response (antigenic-specific systemic antibodies [IgG] in blood and mucosal antigen specific [IgA] antibodies).

In majority of the diseases, the pathogen gains entry through mucosal barriers that are the first site of infection and forms the first line of defence. This makes the concentration of the vaccine in the mucosal regions of paramount importance, further emphasizing the need for specific carriers for target delivery through ONVs. NPs themselves have an inherent immunostimulant property of inducing an antigenic response aided by coencapsulation of multiple antigenic sites.

Stability, storage, and shelf life are some of the important considerations to be made in the mass production of ONVs for commercialization, these factors can be addressed through meticulous formulation and characterization protocols of the ONV [2]. The legal regulations faced with challenges and future scope have also been addressed through his chapter.

19.2 Barriers to Oral Vaccines

Many biological and physiochemical barriers exist; however, the main barrier encountered by oral vaccines is the gastrointestinal system. The influence of the GIT includes the harsh digestive environment, limited absorption, inefficient bioavailability, and the immunotolerant nature of the gut [3]. These barriers could significantly affect the immunological response of the body to the nanovaccine. Researchers have been in the quest for adopting innovative techniques and carrier materials to ensure evasion of barriers to oral vaccine delivery. Failure of vaccines to penetrate the epithelium results in their elimination from the GIT and inability to initiate any type of immune response. Orally delivered vaccines have to depend on active cellular transport. A special cell population called M-fold cells or M cells are located within the Peyer's patches of the intestine. The M cells enable the uptake of antigens however the population of M cells in humans is miniscule impairing efficient vaccine absorption. Generally, M cells could uptake particles ranging from below 1 to 5 μm in size. This makes the M cell a unique target for ONV delivery [4].

The high concentrations of acids, salts, and enzymes create a natural chemical barrier for the uptake of orally delivered vaccines. The key enzyme responsible for proteolytic degradation of the oral vaccine is pepsin, it is active at an acidic environment of pH 2.0. Other enzymes like trypsin, peptidase, and chymotrypsin also facilitate further breakdown of proteins in the small intestine to individual amino acids. Final digestion is executed by few glycoproteins and enzymes, namely glycosidases and protease-peptidases that form the glycocalyx [5]. Immunological epitopes are resistant to digestion, and neutralizing the acidic environment of the intestines can facilitate oral vaccine evasion by enzyme degradation. Research indicates that inactivation of gastric proteases diminishes antigen digestion ensuing increased local-systemic and antibody response [6]. This strategy should be exploited in ONV delivery local-systemic.

Immune tolerance is a well-accepted concept pertaining to substances ingested orally. Certain potentially allergic substances that are consumed on a regular basis though an oral route fail to stimulate an effector response resulting in immune tolerance [7]. From oral vaccine point of view, the mechanism of immune tolerance is an immunological barrier for inciting an immune response to an antigen.

Suppressed immunological response is produced by anti-inflammatory signaling factors produced by the GIT epithelial cells. The gastrointestinal flora, fatty acids, and mucus secreted by goblet cells oppress the anti-inflammatory actions of epithelial and dendritic cells, resulting in tolerance that will favor oral vaccine acceptance [8]. The application of material science to ONVs with detailed physiological properties and immunomodulatory potential will hasten the understanding of bypassing these barriers, thereby enhancing maximum bioavailability of the vaccine.

19.3 Evolution of Oral Nanovaccines

A nanovaccine is an amalgamation of an antigen incorporated with a carrier that is made up of either polymeric, lipid, metallic, proteinic, or graphene type material [9]. Researchers have attempted to formulate a multitude of organic and inorganic nanoparticles for vaccine development. Preparing nanoparticles for vaccine development with appropriate bio-properties and other with unique physicochemical and morphological properties have been described [10]. The evolution of conventional vaccines and nanovaccines is exhibited in Figure 19.1.

The advent of ONV is a relatively new concept in the domain of vaccine development. Recently, researchers have explored the use of ONV to tackle diseases in fish. Chitosan, polylactic-co-glycolic acid, nanopoliplexes, and virus-like particles (VLPs) have been used for oral nanovaccine development. Researchers concluded that ONV have showed remarkable possibilities for application in fish aquaculture, which surely will be adopted by the industry in the following years. Researchers have also demonstrated the use of Salmonella subunit chitosan nanoparticles (NPs)-based vaccine in chicken, they successfully demonstrated targeting of surface F-protein

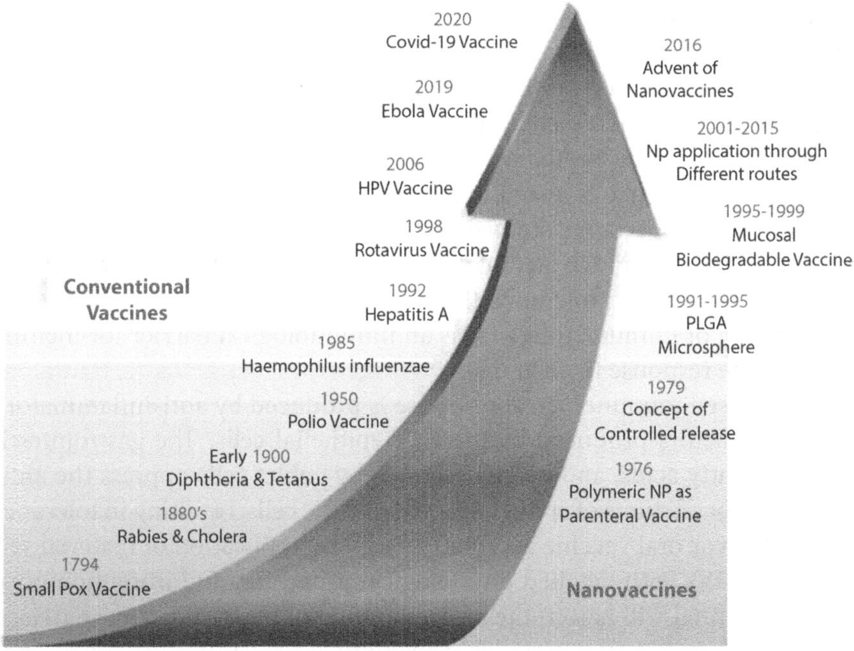

Figure 19.1 The evolution of conventional vaccines and nanovaccines.

coated chitosan NPs to immune cells when delivered orally to layer chickens, the particles were localized in ileal Peyer's patches [11].

19.4 Oral Delivery of Nanovaccines

Nanotechnology aims to deliver a vaccine in an innovative way with minimal side effects. An ideal ONV should be delivered with a sound knowledge of gastrointestinal molecular physiology. ONV may require multiple doses compared with those administered parenterally for an optimum and sustained effect. The drawback of repeated administration could be oral tolerance where a vaccine fails to induce an immunogenic response. Another hurdle faced during oral delivery of vaccines is the nonavailability of effective stimulants required to initiate an immune response.

Each antigen type may act differently, hence all ONVs cannot be delivered in the same manner. Degradation of the antigen or proposed drug to be used as a vaccine can be prevented by using a NP coat or carrier material that is resistant to the physiological barriers. NPs also carry the inherent ability to cause a certain degree of immunostimulant property themselves [1].

The delivery of ONV should be performed with an ideal carrier that will ensure targeted delivery and cause a satisfactory systemic and mucosal immune response. Targeted delivery of ONV can be achieved by specific deposition and enhanced absorption through the Peyer's patches that are dome shaped areas consisting of lymphoid follicles and M cells. The DCs and antigen-presenting cells (APCs) are scattered throughout the lamina propria and intestinal epithelium, which are crucial sites for ONV delivery. Successful delivery of ONV is dictated by its active transport across the intestinal epithelium by M cells and enterocytes succeeded by DC and APCs processing of the ONV, resulting in an immunogenic response [12].

The enterocytes partake in antigen uptake by two mechanisms. The ONV can be transported between the cells through a mechanism of paracellular leak, molecules with a size above 1 μm are transported this way between cellular spaces. At the surface of the intestinal lining epithelium another process called transcellular transport can occur where the antigen in internalized by the enterocyte at its apical end and expelled at its basolateral surface [13]. An ideal ONV delivery should enable sufficient protection from the barriers and degradative enzymes, optimum delivery to the target site, and should be able to stimulate an antigenic immune response. Few oral nanovaccines developed until now have been displayed in Table 19.1.

Table 19.1 Commercially available oral vaccines with details.

Sl no.	Disease	Brand	Formulation	Composition
1	Cholera	Dukoral	Suspension	Whole killed Vibrio cholerae
2	Cholera	Orochol	Lyophilized	Live recombinant lacking CTA
3	Cholera	PXVX0200	Solution	Live-attenuated oral cholera vaccine strain
4	Gastroenteritis	RotaTeq	Solution	Attenuated pentavalent live rotavirus
5	Gastroenteritis	Rotarix	Suspension	Live attenuated monovalent rotavirus
6	Polio	Vario	Liquid	Trivalent, bivalent, and monovalent
7	Acute Respiratory Disease	Ardovax	Enteric coated tablets	Live Adenovirus Vaccine
8	Typhoid	Vivotif	Enteric coated tablets	Live-attenuated strain of Salmonella typhi
9	Bird flu	PXVX0103	Capsule	Live adenoviral-based vaccine
10	HIV	N/A	Intraepithelial needle delivery	HIV-1 Envelope SOSIP trimer

19.5 Immune Response to Oral Nanovaccines

The success of an ONV depends on the immune response its capable of producing that can be quantified by humoral antibodies released in the body. The cellular signalling interplay begins with the processing of the ONV by the DCs and APCs. The DCs process the antigen by fragmenting them into smaller components. The antigen enriched DCs migrate to the Peyer's patches, gut-associated lymphoid tissue (GALT) and intestinal lymph nodes where they trigger the $CD4^{+}$ helper T lymphocytes. The $CD4^{+}$ T cells stimulate the B lymphocytes causing their differentiation into specific IgA$^+$ B cells. Differentiation and maturation in the GALT results in production of plasma cells that can specifically secrete high affinity secretory IgA (sIgA). The sIgA is responsible for mucosal immunity against pathogens [1].

Optimum immune response is also governed by the size of the ONV particles. A study by Wang *et al.* analyzed the influence of various-sized particles (130 nm, 430 nm, and 1–2 mm) loaded with antigen bovine serum albumin for the purpose of generating mucosal and systemic antibodies following oral administration [14]. It was noted that higher immune responses (IgA and IgG) were obtained for the smaller particles (130 and 430 nm) compared with larger particles (1–2 mm). The researchers concluded that particles below 500 nm are better absorbed by M-cells and enterocytes than larger particles. In a contrasting study, Gutierro *et al.* reported a higher IgG titre with 1-mm-sized particles compared to 200 and 500 nm particles [15].

Awaad *et al.* measured PPs' uptake efficiency using single-sized (95, 130, 200, 340, 695, and 1050 nm) particles and suggested that a particle size ranging from 95 to 200 nm was an optimal size for efficient vaccine effect rather than a larger particle size (>300 nm) [16]. A large-scale study with multiple-sized particles using different platforms is the need of the hour to comprehensively determine the effect of ONV size and its correlation with antigen uptake.

19.6 Oral Nanovaccines Carriers

In recent years, researchers have bioengineered several NP platforms with broad applications pertaining to new therapies. The NP design has a significant impact on function of the vaccine embedded in it [10]. The immunogenicity of the NP can be regulated by controlling their morphological properties, namely size, surface area, overall surface charge, loading capability, and penetration ability. Further discussion on nanocarriers is divided into man-made or natural carriers and synthetic carriers [17].

19.6.1 Natural Nanovaccine Carriers

Virus-like particles (VLPs) are well known to be successfully employed as nanovaccines. As new technology unveils better understanding of the VLPs, it is believed that these carriers will revolutionize nanovaccine development. They have a productive surface and are capable of carrying an array of biological molecules. VLPs of various viruses have been confirmed as very immunogenic and are already in use as nanovaccines in humans or animals.

The linking of VLPs to antigenic molecules is also known to improve the immunogenic response induced by the nanobioparticles. Bacterial spores are biological structures capable of encasing an ONV as they have protective coats. They are promising structures for ONV development. Bacterial spores are a shell by nature that is dormant and highly resistant as they contain multiple coats of protein. The antigenic sequence can be made to fuse with the spore coat protein, also the antigen can be integrated with the bacillus gene through fusion. When orally delivered, these modified genes can act on the gastrointestinal system [18].

Exosomes are small endogenous (50–100 nm), spherical vesicles produced and released by the defence cells of the body, mast cells few epithelial cells and APCs. They have a well-defined chemical composition chiefly made up of proteins and are released to regulate intercellular communication. Exosomes are formed by fusion of the endosomal membrane with the plasma membrane of the cell, following this fusion they are released as extracellular exosomes. Few exosomes can induce apoptosis by suppressing T-cell signaling. Research indicates that exosomes from APCs and DCs can stimulate T-cell clones resulting in their recruitment producing immunity [19].

Bacteriophages are viruses, which parasitize a bacterium by infecting it and reproducing inside it. Few well-analyzed phage strains have shown that antigenic genes can be delivered successfully. It has also been demonstrated that phage vaccines are capable of carrying foreign proteins fused to their regular coat protein. When antigenic proteins are fused on bacteriophages with nanotechnology, it results in efficient recognition by APCs [20].

19.6.2 Synthetic Nanovaccine Carriers

SuperFluids can be employed for delivering antigens in a sustained release manner following encapsulation or coating as nanospheres, they are often used with polar solvents. Superfluidity is the characteristic property of a fluid with zero viscosity, which is capable of flowing without loss of any kinetic energy. The use of SuperFluids reduce the exposure of the ONV to harsh external gastric environment, thereby increasing its bioavailability. Overall, SuperFluids amplify the action of the encapsulated vaccine in producing an antigenic response. The polymer encapsulation is cost-effective and several nanotechnology-based manufacturing steps can be skipped in its bio fabrication. This controlled release system has the capacity to deliver different types of antiviral vaccines in either plasmid form, DNA fragment, or as an inactivated virus particle. SuperFluid nanoencapsulation technology can be efficiently utilized for oral delivery of controlled-release vaccine antigens to treat diseases [21].

Proteosomes are ideal vaccine delivery carriers as they are NP in nature, they are comparable to the electron microscopic size of viruses, they are hydrophobic and relatively safe for *in vivo* use. Proteosomes are currently being researched to develop nanovaccines for viral infections like influenza, respiratory syncytial virus and AIDS [22].

Nanobeads serve as effective immunization tools when conjugated with adjuvants. Alum is a routinely used material in humans, it produces impressive antibody responses; however, the cell-mediated responses are often compromised. The size of nanobeads employed is crucial, at a size of 40 nm, it mimics many viruses and results in inducing a moderate T-cell response [23]. The immune responses of nanobeads have been evaluated in an animal study where antigen bound to nanobeads were used in sheep model. The researchers reported a satisfactory cell-mediated and humoral immune response and no adverse reactions were witnessed. This makes the use of nanobeads in animals an ideal candidate to induce immunogenic response.

Liposomes are vesicles made of a spherical lipid bilayer and an inner aqueous compartment fabricated *in vitro.* Since then, liposomes have been employed as carriers in the field of vaccinology. Literature review highlight liposomes are endocytosed transferring their contents to the immune cells promoting the development of T cell-independent immune responses and resulting in development of long-term immunity. The abovementioned statements confirm that liposomes are ideal candidates for the induction of cell mediated immunity. The mechanism through which they modulate their action is still largely unknown and hence they are still not approved for immunization processes.

Virosomes are manufactured from liposomes by combination with fusogenic viral proteins. Virosomes are incapable of replication as they are pure fusion-active vesicles. Their surface property of viral proteins can be exploited for active targeting and specific delivery of antigen [24]. Synthetic viral envelopes are ideal to be made into nanovaccine formulation to deliver adjuvants to APCs [25]. Virosomal nanovaccines have been clinically approved by the World Health Organization (WHO) as superior agents for immune response induction [26].

19.7 Formulation Strategies and Characterization of Oral Nanovaccines

For formulation and characterization of nanovaccines, nanoscale carriers are already in use and are currently approved or under clinical trials. The nanoscale vaccine systems are generally formulated to contain 3 essential elements: an antigen, against which immune responses need to be induced; an adjuvant, to facilitate the interaction between antigen and immune cells and a delivery system to ensure that the components are delivered to the right target area [27]. The means of formulation strategies & characterization in few noted studies are discussed here. The mode of delivery of the ONV can be made through the following formulations:

A. Lipid-Based Vehicles

A study by Liu employed cationic liposomes for oral delivery of an influenza vaccine encoding a gene. The *in vivo* study was performed on mice at an immunization rate of 3 times a week. It was noted that not humoral and cell-mediated immunity were stimulated against the influenza virus. The authors concluded that the cationic liposome formulation is effective through an oral delivery route against viruses [28].

An interesting study by Yu modified the Newcastle disease (ND) vaccine (LaSota strain) by combining it with gypenosides (GPS)/liposome and delivered the same through an oral immunization of chickens. The authors reported an enhanced lymphocyte proliferation with increased specific antibody titer and cytokine secretion [29].

A recent study by Dewangan formulated and charatcterized HBsAg loaded PLGA nanoparticles, HBsAg loaded solid lipid nanoparticles and HBsAg loaded liposomes. On performing in vitro analysis, it was reported that the HBsAg loaded PLGA nanoparticle formulation showed greater entrapment, nano sized, and good release pattern. The authors concluded that the prepared formulation can be used to produce cellular and humoral immune response clinically [30].

An interesting formulation called bilosomes have been extensively used for oral vaccine delivery, these are non-ionic lipid-based vesicles containing biodegradable and biocompatible bile salts (sodium deoxycholate). Shukla *et al.* used bilosomes containing the recombinant hepatitis B surface antigen through oral delivery in mice. GALT showed ready uptake of bilosomes demonstrating both systemic as mucosal responses [31]. Bilosomes can also enhance the bioavailability of drugs, increase their efficacy, and enable toentrap proteins and antigens [32].

B. Immune Stimulating Complexes

ISCOMs are cage-like structures of 30 to 40 nm in diameter composed of glycosides that are present in cholesterol, Quil A, antigens, and phospholipids. An innovative study used the technique of oral vaccination of mice with ISCOMs incorporating herpes simplex virus type 2 (HSV-2) antigens (HSV-specific glycoproteins, gB2, gD1, gE1, and gG2). The authors reported a substantial production of systemic and local immune responses. Another study involving oral immunization of mice with two doses of influenza A/Sichuan/87 ISCOM vaccine demonstrated significant upregulation of humoral IgG2a subclass antibody and ensured protection thereof. It is certain that ISCOM should be considered as a potential oral delivery system [33].

C. Metal-Based NPS

Metallic NPs are relatively non-biodegradable, have rigid structures, and are simple to synthesize. Gold has been used in the field of nanomedicine due to its therapeutic effect and its inert nature [34]. It has been demonstrated that chitosan functionalized gold NPs (CsAuNPs) can be used as a carrier fortetanus toxoid (TT). Oral immunization of mice with CsAuNPs induced up to 28-fold immune response. The use of adjuvant can amplify this effect and provide stability of mucosal vaccines [35]. Silver NPS are nontoxic and have been widely used due to their low cost and ease of production. They find common application as antimicrobials and larvicidals. A note worthy study used silver nanoparticles and delivered a single oral dose to 1-day-old chicks with encapsulated H5 DNA vaccine. An immediate cellular immune response with cytokine production was noticed. The H5 plasmid from the intestine of the chick was even demonstrated within 1 hour of post-immunization delivery through polymerase chain reaction [36].

D. Polymeric-Based NPs

Due to their biocompatibility, stability in harsh environment, ease of mass production, sustained drug release, and adjuvant properties, the polymeric-based NPs are favored for their role in nanovaccine development [37]. The commonly used polymer-based NP is Poly lactic-co-glycolic acid (PLGA). PLGA has been approved for human and veterinary drug delivery by the American Food and Drug Administration (FDA).

A study by Ashhurst and coworkers employed PLGA to carry *M. tuberculosis* lipoprotein MPT83 with trehalose-dibehenate (TDB) adjuvant, the formulation was delivered to mice through a mucosal route. The authors reported a strong anti-MPT83 antibody response [38]. *Bacillus subtilis* produces a biopolymer called poly (γ-glutamic acid) (PGA). γ-PGA NPs have shown to induce cellular and humoral immune responses and have been used extensively for vaccine development. Researchers have noted the deposition of γ-PGA in Peyer's patches of mice after oral administration with enhanced levels of chemokines and T cells [39].

Chitosan is a linear biocompatible polymer used to encapsulate a wide range of biologicals, such as vaccines and peptides. It acts by stimulating the dendritic cells (DC) and lymphocytes. High levels of interleukin 10 were noticed following vaccination of mice accompanied by booster doses at 2-week interval.

Alginate is a hydrophilic polysaccharide obtained from the brown seaweed. It was approved by the U.S. Food and Drug Administration to be delivered orally due to its low toxicity and biocompatibility. In an interesting study by Seong and co-workers' oral immunization of mice with polysaccharide antigen of *Streptococcus pneumonia* coated with alginate showed effective protection against the same pathogen [40].

E. Carbon-Based NPS

Carbon-based NPS are synthesized by utilizing silica as a template and sucrose as a carbon source. Carbon NPs contain large mesopores and macropores, this could encapsulate a considerable amount of antigen and could be an attractive antigen delivery system. Bovine serum albumin (BSA) is frequently used as an antigen and loaded into carbon NPs. Oral immunization of mice with BSA/ carbon NPs induced IgG in serum and mucosal IgA aided by T-helper cell immune responses [41].

19.8 Regulations and Challenges for Oral Nanovaccines Delivery

For commercialization of any vaccine its imperative to obtain a regulatory approval from the governing agency of the concerned country. It is mandatory to assure safety and quality not only during the manufacturing process but also after delivery of the vaccine, this requires comprehensive testing of the ONV ensuring its safety prior to administration.

To ensure the ONV is environmentally safe and healthy a sound knowledge of the ONV fate in air, water and most importantly the human body is required. There are several ethical, legal, and social issues associated with nanocarrier-based systems in developed and underdeveloped countries. Clarity in intellectual property rights is another gray area that needs to be addressed. Nanoparticulate systems face several hurdles due to policy guidelines and possible societal risks. The devices required to detect human and environmental nanocarrier system hazards are not well developed. Regulatory challenges associated with vaccine systems must be emphasized while developing vaccine delivery systems. With the constant advance in the vaccine delivery system, the manufacturer and researchers must overcome problems related to regulatory compliance during *in vitro*, preclinical, and clinical trial phases. Regulatory agencies have provided generalized guidelines for vaccines, adjuvants and nanocarriers for their clinical evaluation. Adjuvanted vaccine usually will require independent molecular characterization. Therefore, its obligatory for the manufacturer to justify the clinical benefits of the vaccine and the adjuvant. Data of *in vitro* and/or *in vivo* studies are needed to justify the rationale for including the specific adjuvant in the vaccine formulation and for determining the dosage. The proof-of-concept studies should have a clear methodology for formulation and reproducible results. Toxicity studies are essential to indicate the formulation as nontoxic and well tolerated by the body prior to administration.

In the Unites States, "The Centre for Biologics Evaluation and Research (CBER) of the US Food and Drug Administration (FDA)" regulates vaccines development and approval. The European pharmaceutical legislation governs Europe and, in general, the WHO Collaborating Centres and WHO Expert Committee on Biological Standardization (ECBS) works in close collaboration with national regulatory authorities of individual countries for regulation of vaccines [1].

The WHO has cleared India's vaccine regulatory system for maintaining international standards, paving the way for easy export of vaccines produced in the country. The National Regulatory Authority of India (NRA) and its affiliated institutions now meet WHO efficacy indicators for a functional vaccine regulatory system. India's Rs 19,000-crore vaccine industry accounts for exports worth 13 billion US dollars to 150 countries. India is a major vaccine producer that has 12 major vaccine manufacturing facilities. Hence, it is necessary that all ONVs be cleared by authentic licenses by government regulatory agencies to ensure not only patient safety and efficacy but also safeguard the best interests of the manufacturer or team of researchers.

19.9 Future Perspectives

Targeted ONV delivery should aim to deliver the formulation at the desired location and ensure uptake by the cells resulting in an optimum immunological response. Insight into these immunological mechanisms can inform the design of next-generation oral vaccines to harness critical functions to elicit immunity. Even though ONVs are delivered through the oral route with minimal systemic toxicity, the individual patient variability is an important challenge affecting its performance. The host factors include gastric pH and microbial flora [42].

The preclinical *in vitro* results should be validated multiple times and results of toxicity studies should be verified on appropriate models for each formulation and its concentration. Suitable animal model experiments need to be conducted to conclude the efficacious potential and safety index of a formulation.

Advent of artificial intelligence and machine learning can be adopted for *in silico* analysis. Through high-throughput screening (HTS), molecular docking, and binding energy calculations, we can now estimate the potential binding of a target antigen to its receptors [43]. This innovative concept is now being employed to study the interaction of several drug molecules and its target areas. HTS was revolutionary in the initial steps in the successful delivery of noncoding RNAs. For the treatment of hereditary transthyretin amyloidosis, a lipid NP composed of siRNA was found through HTS of more than 300 ionizable lipids [44].

Recently, the information collected from HTS studies have been used for the critical development of COVID-19 mRNA vaccines. It is expectable that in the coming years, the combination of HTS of NP formulations with biological organic compounds and RNA sequencing machine learning tools to determine the biological impact of the released drugs will have a significant impact in the design of more efficient drug delivery systems [44, 45].

19.10 Conclusion

Although the development of ONV for humans is at its infancy and past trials have been largely unsuccessful, the development of NPs and innovative biomaterials offer promising new vistas for ONV development. These materials are capable of providing a synergistic effect by acting as both carrier and adjuvant.

Nanotechnology may provide us a new choice for safe and effective vaccines. However, frequency of boost, refrigeration of vaccines, and routes of administration are still challenges for vaccines distribution in small areas or villages of some countries. Nanovaccines are expected to be more effective, convenient, and economic than conventional vaccines. The advancement in material delivery systems bridge the gap between vaccine delivery and immunological challenges. With the ever-changing vaccine technology in force coupled with advances in genetic engineering fabrication of biomolecules and synthetic particles has scaled new heights. The biomaterial field should work hand in glove with biomolecules to design the delivery of ONVs. These technologies may open the fore front for effective ONV development.

References

1. Karandikar, S., Mirani, A., Waybhase, V., Patravale, V.B., Patankar, S., Nanovaccines for oral delivery-formulation strategies and challenges, in: *Nanostructures for Oral Medicine*, pp. 263–293, Elsevier, Amsterdam, Netherlands, 2017 Jan 1.
2. Thakur, N., Thakur, S., Chatterjee, S., Das, J., Sil, P.C., Nanoparticles as smart carriers for enhanced cancer immunotherapy. *Front. Chem.*, 8, 597806, 2020.
3. Frizzell, H. and Woodrow, K.A., Biomaterial approaches for understanding and overcoming immunological barriers to effective oral vaccinations. *Adv. Funct. Mater.*, 30, 37, 1907170, 2020 Sep.
4. des Rieux, A., Fievez, V., Garinot, M., Schneider, Y.J., Préat, V., Nanoparticles as potential oral delivery systems of proteins and vaccines: A mechanistic approach. *J. Control. Release.*, 10116, 1, 1–27, 2006 Nov.
5. Pali-Schöll, I. and Jensen-Jarolim, E., Anti-acid medication as a risk factor for food allergy. *Allergy.*, 66, 4, 469–77, 2011 Apr.
6. Ibañez, A.E., Coria, L.M., Carabajal, M.V., Delpino, M.V., Risso, G.S., Cobiello, P.G., Rinaldi, J., Barrionuevo, P., Bruno, L., Frank, F., Klinke, S., A bacterial protease inhibitor protects antigens delivered in oral vaccines from digestion while triggering specific mucosal immune responses. *J. Control. Release.*, 28220, 18–28, 2015 Dec.
7. Allaire, J.M., Crowley, S.M., Law, H.T., Chang, S.Y., Ko, H.J., Vallance, B.A., The intestinal epithelium: Central coordinator of mucosal immunity. *Trends Immunol.*, 139, 9, 677–96, 2018 Sep.
8. Sun, C.M., Hall, J.A., Blank, R.B., Bouladoux, N., Oukka, M., Mora, J.R., Belkaid, Y., Small intestine lamina propria dendritic cells promote de novo generation of Foxp3 T reg cells via retinoic acid. *J. Exp. Med.*, 204, 8, 1775–85, 2007 Aug 6.

9. Das, A. and Ali, N., Nanovaccine: An emerging strategy. *Expert Rev. Vaccines.*, 20, 10, 1273–90, 2021 Oct 3.
10. Karthikeyan, S., Bhatlu, M.L., Sukanya, K., Jayan, N., Nanovaccination: Evolution and review. *J. Crit. Rev.*, 7, 7, 971–5, 2020.
11. Szeto, G.L. and Lavik, E.B., Materials design at the interface of nanoparticles and innate immunity. *J. Mater. Chem. B*, 4, 9, 1610–8, 2016.
12. Renu, S., Markazi, A.D., Dhakal, S., Lakshmanappa, Y.S., Shanmugasundaram, R., Selvaraj, R.K., Renukaradhya, G.J., Oral deliverable mucoadhesive chitosan-salmonella subunit nanovaccine for layer chickens. *Int. J. Nanomed.*, 15, 761, 2020.
13. Mabbott, N.A., Donaldson, D.S., Ohno, H., Williams, I.R., Mahajan, A., Microfold (M) cells: Important immunosurveillance posts in the intestinal epithelium. *Mucosal Immunol.*, 6, 4, 666–77, 2013 Jul.
14. Tennant S.M., Muhsen K., Pasetti M.F. Gut Immunology and Oral Vaccination. In: Giese M. (eds.) *Molecular Vaccines,* Springer, Vienna, 2013 Jan 18.
15. Wang, T., Jiang, H., Zhao, Q., Wang, S., Zou, M., Cheng, G., Enhanced mucosal and systemic immune responses obtained by porous silica nanoparticles used as an oral vaccine adjuvant: Effect of silica architecture on immunological properties. *Int. J. Pharm.*, 436, 1-2, 351–8, 2012 Oct 15.
16. Gutierro, I., Hernandez, R.M., Igartua, M., Gascon, A.R., Pedraz, J.L., Size dependent immune response after subcutaneous, oral and intranasal administration of BSA loaded nanospheres. *Vaccine,* 21, 1-2, 67–77, 2002 Nov 22.
17. Awaad, A., Nakamura, M., Ishimura, K., Imaging of size-dependent uptake and identification of novel pathways in mouse Peyer's patches using fluorescent organosilica particles. *Nanomed.: Nanotechnol., Biol. Med.*, 8, 5, 627–36, 2012 Jul 1.
18. Gill, P., Nanocarriers, nanovaccines, and nanobacteria as nanobiotechnological concerns in modern vaccines. *Sci. Iranica.*, 20, 3, 1003–13, 2013 Jun 1.
19. Plummer, E.M. and Manchester, M., Viral nanoparticles and virus-like particles: Platforms for contemporary vaccine design. *Wiley Interdiscip. Rev.: Nanomed. Nanobi.*, 3, 2, 174–96, 2011 Mar.
20. Le Pecq, J.B., Dexosomes as a therapeutic cancer vaccine: From bench to bedside. *Blood Cells Mol. Dis.*, 35, 2, 129–35, 2005.
21. Ghaemi, A., Soleimanjahi, H., Gill, P., Hassan, Z., Jahromi, S.R., Roohvand, F., Recombinant λ-phage nanobioparticles for tumor therapy in mice models. *Genet. vaccines Ther.*, 8, 1, 1–7, 2010 Dec.
22. Castor, T.P. and Castor Trevor, P., *Polymer microspheres/nanospheres and encapsulating therapeutic proteins therein*, Patent 7,708,915, 2010.
23. Lesinski, G.B. and Westerink, M.J., Novel vaccine strategies to T-independent antigens. *J. Microbiol. Methods,* 47, 2, 135–49, 2001 Nov 1.
24. Schijns, V.E. and Lavelle, E.C., Trends in vaccine adjuvants. *Exp. Rev. Vaccines.*, 10, 4, 539–50, 2011 Apr 1.

25. Sharma, R. and Yasir, M., Virosomes: A novel carrier for drug delivery. *Int. J. Pharm. Tech Res.*, 2, 4, 2327–39, 2010.
26. Almeida, J., Edwards, D.C., Brand, C., Heath, T., Formation of virosomes from influenza subunits and liposomes. *Lancet*, 306, 7941, 899–901, 1975 Nov 8.
27. Marchisio, P., Esposito, S., Bianchini, S., Dusi, E., Fusi, M., Nazzari, E., Picchi, R., Galeone, C., Principi, N., Efficacy of injectable trivalent virosomal-adjuvanted inactivated influenza vaccine in preventing acute otitis media in children with recurrent complicated or noncomplicated acute otitis media. *J. Pediatr. Infect. Dis.*, 28, 10, 855–9, 2009 Oct 1.
28. Peres, C., Matos, A.I., Conniot, J., Sainz, V., Zupančič, E., Silva, J.M., Graca, L., Gaspar, R.S., Preat, V., Florindo, H.F., Poly (lactic acid)-based particulate systems are promising tools for immune modulation. *Acta Biomater.*, 48, 41–57, 2017 Jan 15.
29. Liu, J., Wu, J., Wang, B., Zeng, S., Qi, F., Lu, C., Kimura, Y., Liu, B., Oral vaccination with a liposome-encapsulated influenza DNA vaccine protects mice against respiratory challenge infection. *J. Med. Virol.*, 86, 5, 886–94, 2014 May.
30. Yu, Y., Wang, D., Abula, S., Hu, Y., Zhao, X., Huang, Y., Liu, J., Wu, Y., Wang, D., Tao, Y., Pan, H., The immunological adjuvant activity of gypenosides liposome against Newcastle disease vaccine. *Int. J. Biol. Macromol.*, 60, 116–21, 2013 Sep 1.
31. Dewangan, H.K., Different Approaches for Nanovaccine Formulation and Characterization, in: *IOP Conference Series: Materials Science and Engineering*, vol. 1116, IOP Publishing, p. 012042, 2021 Apr 1.
32. Shukla, A., Khatri, K., Gupta, P.N., Goyal, A.K., Mehta, A., Vyas, S.P., Oral immunization against hepatitis B using bile salt stabilized vesicles (bilosomes). *J. Pharm. Pharm. Sci.*, 11, 1, 59–66, 2008 Mar 3.
33. Palekar-Shanbhag, P., Lande, S., Chandra, R., Rane, D., Bilosomes: Superior Vesicular Carriers. *Curr. Drug Ther.*, 15, 4, 312–20, 2020 Aug 1.
34. Mohamedi, S.A., Heath, A.W., Jennings, R., A comparison of oral and parenteral routes for therapeutic vaccination with HSV-2 ISCOMs in mice; cytokine profiles, antibody responses and protection. *Antivir. Res.*, 49, 2, 83–99, 2001 Feb 1.
35. Carabineiro, S.A., Applications of gold nanoparticles in nanomedicine: Recent advances in vaccines. *Molecules.*, 22, 5, 857, 2017 May.
36. Barhate, G., Gautam, M., Gairola, S., Jadhav, S., Pokharkar, V., Enhanced mucosal immune responses against tetanus toxoid using novel delivery system comprised of chitosan-functionalized gold nanoparticles and botanical adjuvant: Characterization, immunogenicity, and stability assessment. *J. Pharm. Sci.*, 103, 11, 3448–56, 2014 Nov 1.
37. Jazayeri, S.D., Lim, H.X., Shameli, K., Yeap, S.K., Poh, C.L., Nano and Microparticles as Potential Oral Vaccine Carriers and Adjuvants Against Infectious Diseases. *Front. Pharm.*, 12, 1399, 2021 Jun 2.

38. Calzoni, E., Cesaretti, A., Polchi, A., Di Michele, A., Tancini, B., Emiliani, C., Biocompatible polymer nanoparticles for drug delivery applications in cancer and neurodegenerative disorder therapies. *J. Funct. Biomater.*, 10, 1, 4, 2019 Mar.
39. Ashhurst, A.S., Parumasivam, T., Chan, J.G., Lin, L.C., Flórido, M., West, N.P., Chan, H.K., Britton, W.J., PLGA particulate subunit tuberculosis vaccines promote humoral and Th17 responses but do not enhance control of Mycobacterium tuberculosis infection. *PloS One*, 13, 3, e0194620, 2018 Mar 19.
40. Kim, E., Yang, J., Sung, M.H., Poo, H., Oral Administration of poly-gamma-glutamic acid significantly enhances the antitumor effect of HPV16 E7-expressing Lactobacillus casei in a TC-1 mouse model. *J. Microbiol. Biotechnol.* 29, 9, 1444–1452, 2019.
41. Oliveira, C.R., Rezende, C.M., Silva, M.R., Borges, O.M., Pêgo, A.P., Goes, A.M., Oral vaccination based on DNA-chitosan nanoparticles against Schistosoma mansoni infection. *J. Sci. World*, 2012, 01-11, 2012 Oct.
42. Wang, J.J., Zeng, Z.W., Xiao, R.Z., Xie, T., Zhou, G.L., Zhan, X.R., Wang, S.L., Recent advances of chitosan nanoparticles as drug carriers. *Int. J. Nanomed.*, 6, 765, 2011.
43. Tyagi, P., Pechenov, S., Subramony, J.A., Oral peptide delivery: Translational challenges due to physiological effects. *J. Control. Release.*, 287, 167–76, 2018 Oct 10.
44. Tomé, I., Francisco, V., Fernandes, H., Ferreira, L., High-throughput screening of nanoparticles in drug delivery. *APL Bioeng.*, 5, 3, 031511, 2021 Sep 1.
45. Adams, D., Gonzalez-Duarte, A., O'Riordan, W.D., Yang, C.C., Ueda, M., Kristen, A.V., Tournev, I., Schmidt, H.H., Coelho, T., Berk, J.L., Lin, K.P., Patisiran, an RNAi therapeutic, for hereditary transthyretin amyloidosis. *New Engl. J. Med., 379*, 1, 11–21, 2018.

Index

Printed and bound by CPI Group (UK) Ltd, Croydon, CR0 4YY
17/09/2026
14964274-0005